MEDICAL TERMINOLOGY

A Self-Learning Text

"They certainly give strange and new-fangled names to diseases."

PLATO (427–347 B.C.)
The Republic, Book III

MEDICAL TERMINOLOGY

A Self-Learning Text

Jacqueline Joseph Birmingham, R.N., B.S.N., M.S.
Hartford Hospital, Hartford, Connecticut

SECOND EDITION

with 29 color illustrations by Don Wittig

THE C.V. MOSBY COMPANY

St. Louis • Baltimore • Philadelphia • Toronto • 1990

Mosby

Editor: Richard A. Weimer
Assistant editor: Rina A. Steinhauer
Project manager: Suzanne Seeley
Production editor: Shauna Burnett Sticht
Book designer: Susan E. Lane
Cover designer: Brad Cowan

SECOND EDITION

Previous edition copyrighted 1981

Printed in the United States of America

The C.V. Mosby Company
11830 Westline Industrial Drive, St. Louis, Missouri 63146

Birmingham, Jacqueline Joseph.
Medical terminology : a self-learning text / Jacqueline Joseph Birmingham : with 29 color illustrations by Don Wittig.—2nd ed.
p. cm.
Includes bibliographic references.
ISBN 0-8016-0259-9
ISBN 10259 (Instructor's Guide)
1. Medicine—Terminology. I. Title.
[DNLM: 1. Nomenclature. W 15 B618m]
R 123.B5 1990
610'.14—dc20
DNLM/DLC
for Library of Congress 89-13078
CIP

M/D/D 9 8 7 6 5 4 3 2

To

Sarah Ellen

our second to fly

CONTENTS

INTRODUCTION

The purpose of *Medical Terminology: A Self-Learning Text* is to give the reader the opportunity to acquire knowledge necessary for beginning to understand medical terminology. A self-learning text is designed to allow the learner to master specific information without an instructor.

The body of information in this book is presented in small, easily learned portions developed for the adult learner. Objectives are stated, content related to those objectives is given, and immediate feedback is provided in the form of tests.

Unlike most programmed texts, the feedback follows the discussion of a complete set of objectives. The flow of learning is not constantly interrupted by questions and blank spaces. Ideas, concepts, and sets of information are fully developed, and then the level of understanding is tested.

Self-directed, independent study and self-paced learning are factors that will aid the learner.

This text is designed to be used by those persons who are beginning a career that requires the understanding of medical terms. It is intended to give learners an opportunity to gain first the fundamentals of medical terminology and to build from there in whatever design their needs call for.

The content is limited to *basic* facts needed to learn medical terminology. Because most of the language of medicine is based on Latin and Greek, the rules of construction of the terms are well established. You *can* learn the fundamentals of terminology with a self-learning text.

This text can be used by the following groups:

1 Persons entering health professions.
2 Professional persons who need to understand medical terminology. Lawyers, counselors, and insurance people are among the professionals who could benefit from this book.
3 Persons enrolled in a course on medical terminology or those being self-taught.
4 Teachers who are preparing lectures on body systems. The derivation of medical terms given in this book will help teachers and learners make word associations. For example, the term *glomerulus* means "small ball of yarn," and this association will help recall the anatomy of this structure.

This book is organized by systems. The human body is the focal point of medicine. In most cases when you study the human body, you study it by systems, such as the endocrine or nervous system, and in most cases, when you treat illness, you treat it by system.

The organization of this book is modeled after the actual practice of medicine. Each chapter is designed to give a flow of information somewhat like the flow of the practice of medicine; each of the chapters on systems opens with information relative to the descriptive anatomy and general physiology of that system. The chapter then moves to selected terms related to diagnosis of pathological conditions, and it concludes with terms related to the treatment of disorders related to that system.

Terms are introduced and analyzed. The basic assumption is that new knowledge is learned and retained if it is based on old knowledge. Thus, the analyses given of terms, definitions, and meanings of terms are associated with known English words, and are somewhat general. The translations are informal because at times an exact translation may be as confusing as the term itself.

In addition, terms are grouped in lists to build knowledge. For example, if learners come across the term *glaucoma,* they may not remember its definition, but they may remember that it is associated with the eye. They may also associate it with a list of terms on the fluids of the eye. By making an association between a term and a specific area of the body, the reader has more opportunity for learning.

The medical terminology in this book is limited to the practice of clinical medicine. Clinical medicine deals with the diagnosis and treatment of diseases.

Terminology dealing with genetics, internal cell structure, embryology, and research are not included. Proper names have not been included except in a very few instances.

Terms selected came from the following categories: general terms, commonly used terms, terms used by more than one specialized field of the allied health professions, terms a lay person should know, terms other professionals such as lawyers and insurance personnel would find helpful to know.

The terms presented in this book are a selected group, and the book is not intended to replace a medical dictionary. It may be used as a reference work in addition to other selected references.

Terms introduced may be prefixes, suffixes, root words, combining forms of root words, or complex combinations. The analysis of complex terms is done not only to give their meaning, but to also aid in learning to spell medical words.

USE OF THIS BOOK IN A COURSE IN MEDICAL TERMINOLOGY

Although this book is designed as a self-learning text, some direction may be needed by those persons in a specific allied health field who are using it as a text in a terminology course.

All persons should complete Part I, Chapters 1 to 5. Part II, chapters 6 to 22 contain terms on systems. For coordination with other required classes the instructor must select chapters to be studied first. For example, a radiology student will need the chapters on the skeletal system before the chapters on the eye or the reproductive system.

Because the first five chapters are required reading before any other chapters are begun, by the time students are ready for a chapter assignment on systems, they should have completed the study of that system in anatomy and physiology. This enhances their learning.

For those specialties that spend more time on some systems than on others, this book can act as a reference for terms that will not be used frequently by that specialty. For example, respiratory therapy students undoubtedly remember the names of the parts of the respiratory system, but they may not remember the names of all the parts of the integumentary system. This book can then act as a quick reference for them.

Following is a selection of allied health specialties along with a suggested sequential list of chapters for that specialty. The best sequence is one that correlates with other subjects, especially anatomy and physiology.

SUGGESTED STUDY SEQUENCE

Radiologic Technology

Chapters
1 to 5 required
6 Skeletal System
8 Articular System
7 Muscular System
14 Digestive System
13 Respiratory System
10 Cardiovascular System
11 Hematologic System (optional)
12 Lymphatic System
9 Nervous System
15 Urinary System
16 Endocrine System
17 Male Reproductive System
18 Female Reproductive System
19 Integumentary System
20 The Eye
21 The Ear
22 Thinking and Feeling

Physical Therapy

Chapters
1 to 5 required
9 Nervous System
6 Skeletal System
7 Muscular System
8 Articular System
10 Cardiovascular System
11 Hematologic System
12 Lymphatic System
13 Respiratory System
14 Digestive System
19 Integumentary System
22 Thinking and Feeling
15 Urinary System
16 Endocrine System
17 Male Reproductive System
18 Female Reproductive System
20 The Eye
21 The Ear

Pharmacy Technology*

Chapters
1 to 5 required
19 Integumentary System
6 Skeletal System
8 Articular System
7 Muscular System
9 Nervous System
22 Thinking and Feeling
14 Digestive System
20 The Eye
21 The Ear
10 Cardiovascular System
11 Hematologic System
13 Respiratory System
12 Lymphatic System
16 Endocrine System
18 Female Reproductive System
17 Male Reproductive System
15 Urinary System

* The sequence for pharmacy technology students can vary greatly depending on other courses.

Respiratory Therapy

Chapters
1 to 5 required
13 Respiratory System
10 Cardiovascular System
12 Lymphatic System
11 Hematologic System
9 Nervous System
6 Skeletal System
7 Muscular System
8 Articular System
14 to 22 in sequence

Surgical Technology

Chapters
1 to 5 required
19 Integumentary System
14 Digestive System
15 Urinary System
18 Female Reproductive System
17 Male Reproductive System
13 Respiratory System
21 The Ear
20 The Eye
10 Cardiovascular System
6 Skeletal System
7 Muscular System
8 Articular System
9 Nervous System
11 Hematologic System
12 Lymphatic System
16 Endocrine System
22 Thinking and Feeling

Emergency Medical Technology

Chapters
1 to 5 required
13 Respiratory System
10 Cardiovascular System
11 Hematologic System
6 Skeletal System
14 Digestive System
9 Nervous System
18 Female Reproductive System
20 The Eye
22 Thinking and Feeling
15 Urinary System
12 Lymphatic System
16 Endocrine System
17 Male Reproductive System
19 Integumentary System
21 The Ear

Medical Records Personnel

Study chapters in the order presented.

Medical Technology (Medical Laboratory Technicians)

Chapters
1 to 5 required
11 Hematologic System
10 Cardiovascular System
12 Lymphatic System
15 Urinary System
16 Endocrine System
6 Skeletal System
7 Muscular System
8 Articular System
9 Nervous System
13 Respiratory System
14 Digestive System
17 Male Reproductive System
18 Female Reproductive System
19 Integumentary System
20 The Eye
21 The Ear
22 Thinking and Feeling

DIRECTIONS FOR USE OF THIS SELF-LEARNING TEXT

A self-learning text is exactly what it says it is: a book for you to use by yourself.

Each chapter in this text contains a set of clearly stated objectives, content specific to those objectives, a pretest/posttest, and answers to the test.

To progress through the book follow these directions:

If you feel that you already have the knowledge outlined in the objectives for the chapter, take the pretest/posttest found at the end of the first chapter. Correct your test with the answers on the pages that follow. If you answered all the questions correctly, go on to the next chapter. If you did not answer all the questions correctly, go back to the beginning of the chapter and read the objectives and the content. Then take the pretest/posttest again, and once again correct your test.

If you *know* you do not have the information, start by reading the objectives and content of the chapter. After you have done so, take the pretest/posttest and correct it with the answers found on the following page.

The first five chapters of this book contain basic information necessary for understanding terminology. They should be completed before going on to any of the chapters containing terms on systems.

The terms introduced in each chapter are defined by analyzing the parts of the term. For example, the term *osteochondroma* can be broken down into *osteo, chondr,* and *oma.* It is a tumor (*oma*) made up of bone (*osteo*) and cartilage (*chondr*). Throughout the book the word part is in parentheses following the meaning of the term or part of the term.

Terms are introduced through each chapter. The new terms are listed in two ways: in anatomical or alphabetical order.

The terms may be listed in anatomical order, that is, in the sequence in which the structure being described can be divided. For example, terms on the digestive system are introduced in order from the mouth to the anus.

If the anatomical listing would not enhance learning, an alphabetic sequence is used. Terms related to diseases and treatment of diseases are all listed alphabetically.

The terms introduced are in the singular form. The reader is encouraged to carefully review the list of suffixes that form plurals. You may even wish to copy the plural-forming suffixes on an index card for ready reference.

The tests are designed to determine basic knowledge. In the tests in Chapters 6 to 22 there are several sets of questions in which the learner is directed to match terms in column A with definitions in column B. This method tests the learner's ability to associate the term with a brief definition. To make the test more challenging the learner should cover the list of terms in column A with a piece of paper and write the correct term to the right of column B. This will allow the student the opportunity to recall the term and also to have practice writing out the term. This extra step will reinforce learning.

Also, when lists of terms are given to be used to complete statements that follow, the learner is encouraged to cover the list and attempt to recall the terms.

You are encouraged to read through the entire chapter before concentrating on learning terms. This will give you background on the system you are studying, which will enhance learning.

AUTHOR'S NOTE

Since the printing of the first edition, much has occurred in the field of medicine. The AIDS epidemic and the expansion of transplantation have occurred. Because both affect multiple systems, new information has been integrated into the text and special glossaries have been developed.

The formation of terms in medicine has not changed, thus the strength of this book based on basic word parts still has a strong foundation in the language of medicine.

PUBLISHER'S NOTE

An Instructor's Guide is available to be used with this text.

ACKNOWLEDGMENTS

It is with sincere appreciation that I acknowledge the following people who directly and indirectly assisted in preparation of the second edition of this book. The work done by Lawrence S. Carlton, M.D., and Virginia H. Corcoran, M.L.S., in the preparation of the first edition has endured the years and remains vital for the second edition. The work done by my daughters Wendy and Sarah, and my husband Ron deserves special acknowledgment. Thank you all.

Jackie Birmingham

PART ONE

1 BASIC WORD PARTS

OBJECTIVES

At the end of this chapter you will be able to do the following:

1 Identify the parts of a word.
2 Define the following terms:
  word root
  compound word
  combining form
  prefix
  suffix

ELEMENTS OF MEDICAL TERMS

Medical terms are made up of many different elements. The parts of a word are as follows:

word root
combining form of a word root
prefix
suffix

Words are made up of one or more of these word parts.

Word Root

A word root or root word is the main part of a word. It may be a complete word but is not necessarily a complete word. In the following list of words the word root is in italics:

*tendon*itis
*coll*oid
spasm
*mast*ectomy

In *tendon*itis and *spasm,* the main part of the word is a complete word, whereas in *coll*oid and *mast*ectomy the main part of the word is a word root.

Medical root words come from many sources. The most frequent sources are Latin and Greek, although many other languages contribute words or parts of words.

Compound Words

Compound words are made of two or more words. Some examples of compound words are:

newborn
foot-drop
headache

A root word may be a noun, pronoun, or verb.

Combining Forms

The purpose of combining forms of root words is very direct. The combining form makes the word easier to pronounce.

A combining form of a word root may be made by adding a vowel to the word root. The vowel *o* is most frequently used. The other vowels, *a, e, i,* and *u,* are used less frequently.

Examples of the combining form of a word root are shown in the following list. The word root is in *italic* letters and the combining vowel is in parentheses.

orth(o)pedic
bacteri(o)genic
quadr(i)plegic

If a word root ends in a vowel, in most cases another vowel is not added. Vowels are dropped in some words in which two vowels would be in sequence. Example: osteo + otomy = osteotomy.

It must be noted that some vowels have a specific meaning and thus cannot be dropped without changing the meaning of the word. In this case the vowel is not a combining form but a word part. Example: hemi + opia = hemiopia.

Adjoining word parts that end and begin with the *same* consonant do not need a combining vowel because the word is easily pronounced. In some instances a prefix that is added to the beginning of a word may end in one of several different consonants depending on the consonants in the word parts that follow it. An example of this is the prefix *in-*, which means "without." The consonant *n* changes to the same consonant in the root word.

*in*operative
*im*measurable
*il*logical

This makes the word easier to pronounce.

Combining forms are merely convenience forms and do not influence the meaning of a root word.

When you study, learn the *meaning* of the word parts. It is important to know the difference between a vowel that is a combining vowel and a vowel that is a part of a root word. Example: *hem, hemo* means "blood," while *hemi* means "half."

Root words from different languages, especially Latin and Greek, normally are not mixed. Example: ad + renal = adrenal are Latin word parts meaning "above the kidney." Epi + nephr = epinephr(ine) are Greek word parts meaning "above the kidney." There are many exceptions to this rule, however.

The origin of root words and word parts is not included in this work. It is not as important to know the origin of a word part as it is to know its meaning.

Prefix

A prefix is a word part that is placed (*fix*) at the *beginning* or front (*pre*) of another word or word part. A prefix may be a syllable, a group of syllables, or a word. It is joined to the beginning of a word to alter its meaning or to create a new word. Example: peri (around) + ocular (the eye) = periocular, which means "around the eye."

Suffix

A suffix is a word part that is added *(fix)* to the *end* of a word or word part. The term *suffix* is a derivation of the word meaning "to fasten." Example: neuro (nerve) + tripsy (crushing) = neurotripsy, "crushing of the nerve."

Medical terms are terms which deal with the diagnosis and treatment of disease, and with the maintenance of health. Each term has a limited and definite meaning. Terms used in medicine may be simply root words, or they may be various combinations of root words and word parts.

Pronunciation of medical terms is not especially difficult once you have become familiar with them. Vowels and consonants in medical terms sound the same as in any other English term; therefore they are easy to pronounce. Frequent use of medical terms in your specialty will greatly enhance your ability to pronounce medical terms. Pronunciation keys are not included in this book. Consult your dictionary for correct pronunciation.

PRETEST/ POSTTEST FOR CHAPTER 1

Fill in the blanks:

1. A word root, or root word, is the ________ part of a word.
2. A word root may be a ________, ________, or a ________.
3. A combining form of a root word is made by adding ________________ to the root. The most common one is ____.
4. The purpose of combining forms is ____________________________.
5. If a root word ends in a vowel, in most cases another vowel ________ added.
6. It is important to know the difference between a vowel that denotes a ________ and a vowel that is part of a ________________.
7. When joining word parts that end and begin with the same consonant, a combining vowel ________ used.
8. Some prefixes will end in several different ________ to make them easier to pronounce.
9. A prefix is a word part added to the ________ of a word.
10. A suffix is a word part added to the ________ of a word.
11. Medical terms are terms which deal with ________ and ________ of disease and ________ of health.

PRETEST/ POSTTEST **ANSWERS** FOR CHAPTER 1

1. main
2. noun, pronoun, verb
3. a vowel, o
4. to make the compound word easier to pronounce

5. is not
6. combining form, root word
7. is not
8. consonants
9. beginning
10. end
11. diagnosis, treatment, maintenance

2 PREFIXES

OBJECTIVES

At the end of this chapter you will be able to do the following:

1 Define *prefix.*
2 Describe functions of prefixes.
3 List and define prefixes for each function.

PREFIX

A prefix is a word part that is placed at the beginning of a word. The word *prefix* is made up of a prefix and a word.

Pre means "before," and *fix* means "attach"; therefore *prefix* means "attach before."

Prefixes come from Latin and Greek; therefore there may be two different prefixes with the same meaning, or a prefix may have more than one meaning or use. In most cases a Latin prefix is used with a Latin root word and a Greek prefix with a Greek word.

Prefixes are commonly prepositions. Prepositions are words used to show relationships of a word to other words. Prefixes are added to root words to show the relationship of the word to other words.

A prefix may also be an adverb, which is used to modify a word.

A prefix may be a syllable or a group of syllables. In some instances it is a complete word also.

It is helpful for learning purposes to distinguish between a prefix and a combining form of a root word. Most of the prefixes in this chapter do not include combining forms of root words.

Root words will be learned in the chapters devoted to their proper body systems; in this way it will be easier to associate them with their meaning.

Sets of Prefixes

For the purpose of study the prefixes have been divided into sets according to the various functions.

1 prefixes related to position regarding time and place
2 prefixes describing position in relation to other parts

3 prefixes related to type
4 prefixes describing direction
5 prefixes describing number
6 prefixes related to size and amount
7 prefixes denoting color

Tables 2-1 to 2-7 show the seven sets of prefixes. Use one set at a time; study the prefix and its meaning. Examples are listed to help you learn the prefix. Some prefixes have more than one meaning and may be found in more than one set. It is difficult to determine the placement of some prefixes because of the generality of their meaning. The prefixes have been put in sets for the convenience of study and also to help you make associations. For example, the prefix *ter(t)-* meaning "third" is in the set of prefixes relating to position regarding time and place. The prefix *tri-* is in the set of prefixes describing number. Making the association will help you learn differences in prefixes. The term *tertiary* means "third in order," and the word *triplets* means "three offspring at one birth."

Although this listing of prefixes is broadly comprehensive, you may come across prefixes that have not been included. In this case, add the prefix to the list so that you will have a complete list to meet your needs.

TABLE 2-1
Set 1: Prefixes Related to Position Regarding Time and Place

Prefix	Meaning	Example	Definition
ana-	up, back again	anabolism	building up
ante-	before	antepartum	before delivery
cata-, kata-	down, through	catabolism	breaking down
gen-	beginning, origin	genesis	origin of anything
meta-	beyond, over, between, change, or next to	metacarpal	next to the wrist (refers to a bone of the hand)
noct(i)-	night	nocturnal	occurring in the night
nyct(o)-	night	nyctalgia	pain during the night
post-	after	postpartum	after delivery
pre-	before	prenatal	before birth
prim-	first	primary	first in order
prot(o)-	first	prototype	original form
sym-, syn-	together, union	synergetic	working together
telo-	end	telophase	final phase of mitosis
ter(t)-	third	tertiary	third in order

TABLE 2-2
Set 2: Prefixes Describing Position in Relation to Other Parts

Prefix	Meaning	Example	Definition
acro-	extremity, tip	acrocyanosis	bluish color of hands and feet
anti-	against	antidote	action against a poison
apo-	separation or derivation from	aponia	separation of the mind, confusion
circum-	around	circumoral	around the mouth
contra-	opposite, against	contralateral	opposite side
dorso-, dorsi-	back	dorsiflexion	bending to the back of hand, foot, or spine
ecto-	outside, misplaced	ectopic	not in the intended place
endo-	within	endocardial	within the heart
epi-	on, over, upon	epigastric	over the stomach
eso-	within	esoteric	hidden within
extra-	outside of, in addition to, beyond	extracorporeal	outside the body
fore-	before, in front	forebrain	front part of brain
hyper-	above, excessive, beyond	hyperactive	excessive activity
hypo-	below, under	hypodermic	under the skin
infra-	below	infracostal	below the ribs
inter-	between parts	intercellular	between the cells
intra-	within a part	intracellular	within a cell
juxta-	near	juxtaspinal	near the spinal column
medi-	middle	medial	near the midline of the body
meso-	middle	mesoderm	middle layer of skin
ob-	against	obstruction	blocking of a structure
para-	beside, beyond	paraspinal	beside the spine
peri-	around	perinatal	around the time of birth
pro-	for, in front of, before	prophylaxis	guard against, prevent
schisto-	split, divide	schistothorax	splitting of thorax
schizo-	split, divided	schizonychia	splitting nails
sub-	beneath	subcostal	beneath the ribs
super-	excessive, above	superciliary	hairs above the eyes
supra-	above, over	suprapubic	above the pubic bone
tele-	distant, far	telangiectasia	dilation of capillaries and terminal arteries

TABLE 2-2
Set 2: Prefixes Describing Position in Relation to Other Parts *(continued)*

Prefix	Meaning	Example	Definition
trans-	across, through, over, beyond	transabdominal	through the abdominal wall
ultra-	excessive, extreme	ultrasonic	sound waves beyond the audiofrequency range

TABLE 2-3
Set 3: Prefixes Related to Type

Prefix	Meaning	Example	Definition
a-, an-	without, absent	anemia	~~absence of blood~~ DEFICIENCY OF RED BLOOD CELLS
allo-	another, different form	allomorphic	assuming a different form
ambly-	dull	amblyopia	dull vision
andro-	male	androgen	male sex hormone
angi(o)-	vessel, duct, usually a blood vessel	angiospasm	contraction of a blood vessel
ankyl(o)-	crooked, bent, fused, stiff	ankylosed	fused joint
atel-	imperfect	atelectasis	imperfect expansion of lungs
auto-	self	autogenesis	starting with oneself
bacter-	bacteria	bacteroid	resembling a bacterium
bi(o)-	life	biochemistry	chemistry of living matter
brady-	slow	bradycardia	slow heart
cac(o)-	bad, ill	cacogeusia	bad taste
co-, com-, con-	with, together	congenital	form with
cry(o)-	cold	cryosurgery	destruction of tissue by application of cold
crypt(o)-	hidden	cryptorchidism	undescended testicle
dys-	difficult	dysmenorrhea	difficult menses
eu-	good, normal	euthanasia	good death
eury-	broad, wide	eurycephalic	flat head
glyco-, gluco-	sugar, sweet	glycolysis	breakdown of sugar
gyn-, gyneco-	female	gynecology	study of the female
haplo-	single, simple	haploderma	simple skin inflammation
hetero-	other, different	heterosexual	other sex
homeo-	unchanged	homeostasis	state of equilibrium
homo-	same	homosexual	same sex

TABLE 2-3
Set 3: Prefixes Related to Type *(continued)*

Prefix	Meaning	Example	Definition
hydra-, hydro-	water	hydrocele	watery hernia
idio-	peculiar to the individual, distinct	idiopathic	disease with no apparent external cause
iso-	equal, same	isopia	equal vision in both eyes
mal-	bad	malabsorption	impaired absorption
neo-	new, strange	neonatal	newborn
non-	not	noninfectious	not able to spread
normo-	normal	normovolemia	normal blood volume
ortho-	straight, erect, correct, normal	orthodontic	straight teeth
oxy-	sharp, acute	oxytocia	rapid labor
pachy-	thick	pachycheilia, pachyderma	thick lips, thickening skin
paleo-	old	paleopathology	study of ancient bodies
path(o)-	disease, suffering	pathogenic	capable of producing disease
phage(o)-	eat, consume	phagocyte	cell that can ingest
platy-	broad, wide	platypellic, platycephalic	wide hips, flat cranial vault
plic(o)-	fold	plication	a folding
poikilo-	varied	poikilocyte	irregularly shaped blood cell
pseudo-	false	pseudocyst	false cyst
sclero-	hard	sclerosis	hardening of tissue
steno-	contracted, narrow	stenosis	condition of being narrowed
stereo-	solid, firmly established, three-dimensional	stereotype	firmly established attitude
tachy-	fast	tachycardia	fast heart
terato-	malformed, monster	teratoid	resembling a monster
therap-	treatment	therapeutic	having a healing effect
thermo-	heat, warmth	thermometer	a device to measure heat
toxic-	poison	toxicosis	disease caused by a poison
trachy-	rough	trachyphonia	rough voice
xero-	dry	xerocheilia	dry lips

TABLE 2-4
Set 4: Prefixes Describing Direction

Prefix	Meaning	Example	Definition
ab-	away from	abduct	move away from
ad-	to, toward	adduct	move toward
clin(o)-	slope forward or slope away from	clinocephaly	sloping or flatness of the top of the head
de-	away, not, down	dehydrate	take water away from
dextro-	right	dextrogastria	stomach on the right side of body
dia-	apart, separate	diastasis	a separation of normal joined parts
e-	out	enucleate	remove from
ex-	away from, out, completely	exhale	breathe out
in-, im-	in, inside, within; not	immerse, injection	dip into, forcing into
ir-	against, into, toward	irradiate	emit rays into
levo-	left	levoduction	movement to the left
opisth-	backward	opisthognathism	receding lower jaw
pro-, proso-	forward, anterior	proptosis	forward-bulging
re-	back, again	reflex	bend back
retro-	behind, backward	retrograde	going backward
sinistr(o)-	left	sinistrocular	stronger vision in the left eye

Recall from Chapter 1 that a vowel may be added to a word root to make it a combining form and easier to pronounce.

Vowels are also added to prefixes to make them combining forms. The final *o* in many prefixes is the combining form vowel, though in many other cases it is part of the prefix.

The prefixes are presented in the basic form or in their combining form.

Some prefixes that end in consonants have spelling variations. For example, *in-*, meaning "not," may also be spelled *im-* as in "immeasurable" and *il-* as in "illegal." The final consonant of a prefix may change to match the beginning consonant of the root word it is added to. There are not many of these types of prefixes.

TABLE 2-5
Set 5: Prefixes Describing Number or Quantity

Prefix	Meaning	Example	Definition
ambi-, amphi-	both	ambidextrous, amphibious	using both hands, living on both land and sea
bi-	two	bifurcation	two branches
centi-	100	centimeter	$\frac{1}{100}$ meter
deca-	10	decaliter	10 liters
deci-	$\frac{1}{10}$	deciliter	$\frac{1}{10}$ liter
demi-	one-half	demibain	half a bath (sitz bath)
di-, dis-	twice, doubly	dioxide	two oxygen molecules
diplo-	double	diplopia	double vision
hemi-	one-half	hemiplegia	half-paralyzed state
holo-	whole, all	holography	three-dimensional picture
milli-	1000	millimeter	$\frac{1}{1000}$ meter
mono-	one	mononuclear	one nucleus
multi-	many	multigravida	many pregancies
null(i)-	none	nullipara	woman with no children
pan-	all	panphobia	fear of everything
pleo-	many, more	pleomorphic	having many shapes
plur(i)-	many, more	pluriglandular	several glands
poly-	many	polycystic	many cysts
quadr(i)-	four	quadriplegia	having four extremities paralyzed
semi-	one-half	semicircular	half-circle
tetra-	four	tetrabrachus	having four arms
tri-	three	triplets	three offspring at one birth
uni-	one	unilateral	one side

TABLE 2-6
Set 6: Prefixes Related to Size and Amount

Prefix	Meaning	Example	Definition
aniso-	unequal	anisocytosis	inequality in cell size
brachy-	short	brachycephalic	short head
brevi-	short, slow	brevicollis	shortness of the neck
lepto-	small, slender, soft	leptophonia	weak voice
macro-, mega-	large	macrorhinia, megacolon	large nose, large colon
micro-	small	microtia	small ears
mio-	less, smaller	miosis	smallness of the pupil
olig(o)-	little, small, scanty, deficient	oliguria	small amount of urine
per-	excessive; through, by means of	peracute; perforate	very acute; pierce through

TABLE 2-7
Set 7: Prefixes Denoting Color

Prefix	Meaning	Example	Definition
alba-	white	albino	lacking color, appearing white
chloro-	green	chloroplast	green body found in cells
chromo-	color	chromocyte	colored cell
cirrh-	yellow	cirrhosis	disease causing yellowing of the liver
cyano-	blue	cyanosis	bluish discoloration of the skin
erythro-	red	erythropoiesis	formation of red blood cells
leuko-	white	leukocyte	white blood cell
lute-	yellow	luteinizing hormone	hormone causing yellow areas in the ovary
melano-	black	melanoblast	melanin-forming cell
nigro-	black	substantia nigra	black area in the brain
rube-	red	rubedo	redness of skin
xantho-	yellow	xanthoma	yellow growth

PRETEST/ POSTTEST FOR CHAPTER 2

1. The following prefixes are related to position regarding time and place. Match column A with column B. Items in column B may be used more than once.

Column A	Column B
1. ______ ana-	A. beyond, over, between, change
2. ______ ante-	B. night
3. ______ cata-	C. together, union
4. ______ kata-	D. up, back again
5. ______ gen-	E. before
6. ______ meta-	F. first
7. ______ noct(i)-	G. down, through
8. ______ nyct(o)-	H. end
9. ______ post-	I. after
10. ______ pre-	J. beginning, origin
11. ______ prim-	K. third
12. ______ prot(o)-	
13. ______ sym-	
14. ______ syn-	
15. ______ telo-	
16. ______ ter(t)-	

2. The following two sets of matching columns are related to prefixes describing position in relation to other parts. In each set match column A with column B. Items in column B may be used more than once.

Set 1

Column A	Column B
1. ______ acro-	A. around
2. ______ anti-	B. on, upon, over
3. ______ apo-	C. separation, derivation from
	D. outside of, in addition to, beyond

4. _____ circum-	E. within
5. _____ contra-	F. above, excessive, beyond
6. _____ dorso-	G. extremity, tip
7. _____ ecto-	H. below, under
8. _____ endo-	I. opposite, against
9. _____ eso-	J. back
10. _____ epi-	K. before, in front of
11. _____ extra-	L. outside, misplaced
12. _____ fore-	M. against
13. _____ hyper-	
14. _____ hypo-	

Set 2

Column A	Column B
1. _____ infra-	A. near
2. _____ inter-	B. against
3. _____ intra-	C. around
4. _____ juxta-	D. excessive, extreme
5. _____ medi-, meso-	E. between parts
6. _____ ob-	F. beside, beyond
7. _____ para-	G. for, in front of, before
8. _____ peri-	H. below
9. _____ ultra-	I. excessive
10. _____ pro-	J. within a part
11. _____ schisto-	K. beneath
12. _____ sub-	L. middle
13. _____ super-	M. above, over
14. _____ supra-	N. distant, far
15. _____ tele-	O. split, divided
16. _____ trans-	P. across, through

3. The following three sets of matching columns are related to describing type. In each set, match column A with column B. Items in column B may be used more than once.

Set 1

Column A	Column B
1. _____ a-, an-	A. dull
2. _____ allo-	B. self
3. _____ ambly-	C. bacteria
4. _____ andro-	D. without
5. _____ angi(o)-	E. bad, ill
6. _____ ankyl(o)-	F. another, different from
7. _____ atel-	G. slow
8. _____ auto-	H. crooked, bent, fused
9. _____ bacter-	I. cold
10. _____ bi(o)-	J. with
11. _____ brady-	K. hidden
12. _____ cac(o)-	L. male
13. _____ co-, com-, con-	M. difficult, abnormal
14. _____ cry(o)-	N. vessel, duct
15. _____ crypt(o)-	O. life
16. _____ dys-	P. imperfect

Set 2

Column A	Column B
1. _____ eu-	A. other, different
2. _____ eury-	B. good, normal
3. _____ glyco-, gluco-	C. female
4. _____ gyn-	D. bad
5. _____ haplo-	E. not
6. _____ hetero-	F. single, simple
7. _____ homeo-	G. normal
8. _____ homo-	H. peculiar to the individual
	I. sugar, sweet
	J. new, strange
	K. sharp
	L. unchanged

Column A	Column B
9. ____ hydra-, hydro-	M. water
10. ____ idio-	N. same
11. ____ iso-	O. equal, same
12. ____ mal-	P. broad, wide
13. ____ neo-	Q. straight, erect
14. ____ non-	
15. ____ norm(o)-	
16. ____ ortho-	
17. ____ oxy-	

Set 3

Column A	Column B
1. ____ pachy-	A. disease
2. ____ paleo-	B. fast
3. ____ path(o)-	C. malformed, monster
4. ____ phage(o)-	D. eat, consume
5. ____ platy-	E. rough
6. ____ plic(o)-	F. broad
7. ____ poikilo-	G. solid, firmly established
8. ____ pseudo-	H. thick
9. ____ sclero-	I. treatment
10. ____ steno-	J. old
11. ____ stereo-	K. heat, warmth
12. ____ tachy-	L. false
13. ____ terato-	M. hard
14. ____ therap-	N. varied
15. ____ thermo-	O. poison
16. ____ toxic-	P. contracted, narrow
17. ____ trachy-	Q. dry
18. ____ xero-	R. fold

4. The following prefixes are related to describing direction. Match column A with column B. There are many similarities in this set, but an item in column A should match each item in column B. There is only one correct answer.

Column A	Column B
1. _____ ab-	A. away, not, down
2. _____ ad-	B. forward, anterior
3. _____ clin(o)-	C. slope
4. _____ de-	D. through, between
5. _____ dextro-	E. away from
6. _____ dia-	F. against, into, toward
7. _____ dis-	G. to, toward
8. _____ e-	H. backward
9. _____ ex-	I. right
10. _____ im-, in-	J. away from, out
11. _____ ir-	K. in, inside, within
12. _____ levo-, sinistro-	L. left
13. _____ opisth-	M. back, again
14. _____ pro-, proso-	N. apart, separate
15. _____ re-	O. behind, backward
16. _____ retro-	P. out

Two of these prefixes sometimes mean "completely." Which are they?

_______________ and _______________.

Three of these prefixes sometimes mean "not." Which are they?

_______________, _______________ and _______________.

5. The following prefixes are related to numbers and quantity. Fill in the meaning of the prefix.

Prefix	Meaning
1. demi-	_______________
2. mono-	_______________
3. pan-	_______________
4. ambi-, amphi-	_______________
5. pleo-	_______________

6. bi- ____________

7. holo- ____________

8. milli- ____________

9. di-, dis- ____________

10. plur(i)- ____________

11. tetra- ____________

12. semi- ____________

13. deca- ____________

14. null(i)- ____________

15. quadr(i)- ____________

16. poly- ____________

17. uni- ____________

18. tri- ____________

19. centi- ____________

20. diplo- ____________

21. hemi- ____________

22. multi- ____________

6. The following prefixes are related to size and amount. Fill in the meaning of the prefix.

1. brachy- ____________

2. lepto- ____________

3. micro- ____________

4. anis(o)- ____________

5. macro- ____________

6. olig(o)- ____________

7. brevis- ____________

8. mio- ____________

9. per- ____________

10. mega- ____________

7. The following prefixes denote color. Fill in the meaning of the prefix.

1. alba- ____________
2. xantho- ____________
3. chromo- ____________
4. nigro- ____________
5. leuko- ____________
6. rube- ____________
7. lute- ____________
8. cyano- ____________
9. erythro- ____________
10. melano- ____________
11. chloro- ____________
12. cirrh- ____________

PRETEST/ POSTTEST **ANSWERS** FOR CHAPTER **2**

1.
1. D **2.** E **3.** G **4.** G **5.** J **6.** A **7.** B **8.** B **9.** I **10.** E **11.** F **12.** F **13.** C **14.** C **15.** H **16.** K

2. Set 1
1. G **2.** M **3.** C **4.** A **5.** I **6.** J **7.** L **8.** E **9.** E **10.** B **11.** D **12.** K **13.** F **14.** H

Set 2
1. H or K **2.** E **3.** J **4.** A **5.** L **6.** B **7.** F **8.** C **9.** D **10.** G **11.** O **12.** H or K **13.** I or M **14.** M **15.** N **16.** P

3. Set 1
1. D **2.** F **3.** A **4.** L **5.** N **6.** H **7.** P **8.** B **9.** C **10.** O **11.** G **12.** E **13.** J **14.** I **15.** K **16.** M

Set 2

1. B	**4.** C	**7.** L	**10.** H	**12.** D	**14.** E	**16.** Q
2. P	**5.** F	**8.** N	**11.** O	**13.** J	**15.** G	**17.** K
3. I	**6.** A	**9.** M				

Set 3

1. H	**4.** D	**7.** N	**10.** P	**13.** C	**15.** K	**17.** E
2. J	**5.** F	**8.** L	**11.** G	**14.** I	**16.** O	**18.** Q
3. A	**6.** R	**9.** M	**12.** B			

4.

1. E*	**4.** A	**7.** N	**9.** J	**11.** F	**13.** H	**15.** M
2. G*	**5.** I	**8.** P	**10.** K	**12.** L	**14.** B	**16.** O
3. C	**6.** D					

dia-, ex-
im-, in-, de-

5.

1. one-half	**9.** twice, doubly	**16.** many
2. one	**10.** many, more	**17.** one
3. all	**11.** four	**18.** three
4. both	**12.** one-half	**19.** 100
5. many, more	**13.** 10	**20.** double
6. two	**14.** none	**21.** one-half
7. whole, all	**15.** four	**22.** many
8. 1000		

6.

1. short	**6.** little, small, scanty, deficient
2. small, slender, soft	**7.** short, slow
	8. less, smaller
3. small	**9.** excessive, through, by means of
4. unequal	**10.** large
5. large	

7.

1. white	**5.** white	**9.** red
2. yellow	**6.** red	**10.** black
3. color	**7.** yellow	**11.** green
4. black	**8.** blue	**12.** yellow

* To remember these, associate the "bump" on the *b* in *ab* as being *away* from the *a*, and the bump on the *d* in *ad* as being *toward* the *a*.

3 SUFFIXES

OBJECTIVES

At the end of this chapter you will be able to do the following:

1 Define suffix.
2 Describe eight functions of suffixes.
3 List and define suffixes for each function.

SUFFIX

A suffix is a word part that is added to the end of a word. It is added to a word root to change the meaning of the word and make it more specific.

Sets of Suffixes

For the purpose of study, suffixes have been divided into groups according to their function.

1 Suffixes that change a root word to a noun
2 Suffixes that change a root word to an adjective
3 Suffixes that denote a state or condition
4 Suffixes that indicate a surgical or diagnostic procedure
5 Diminutive suffixes that indicate smallness

There are three groups of word endings that are not true suffixes but that act like suffixes in that they make the meaning of the word more specific.

6 Suffixes that indicate a chemical compound
7 Suffixes that form plurals
8 Suffixes that form noun plurals

It is important to note that the final vowel or vowels of a root word or combining form of a root word may be omitted before a suffix beginning with a vowel.

TABLE 3-1
Set 1: Suffixes that Change a Root Word to a Noun

Suffix	Meaning	Example	Definition
-agogue	leading, inducing	galactagogue	agent that promotes flow of milk
-ance	quality or act of	resonance	quality or act of resounding
-cide	killer	germicide	killer of germs
-ectasia, -ectasis	dilation or expansion of	telangiectasis	dilation of capillaries
-form	structure, shape	ossiform	resembling the form of bone
-gen	production of	carcinogenesis	production of cancer
-ician, -ist	one charged with or skilled in	pediatrician	specialist in treating children's diseases
-ion	act of, state of, result of	incision	act of cutting or result of cutting
-meter	measure	thermometer	measurer of heat
-ology	science of	dermatology	science of skin and its diseases
-or	that which; one who	receptor; inventor	that which receives; one who invents
-phylaxis	protection	prophylaxis	for protection
-poiesis	production, formation of	hematopoiesis	production of blood cells
-sthenia	strength	asthenia	loss of strength
-ure	act, or the result of action	closure	result of a closing action

TABLE 3-2
Set 2: Suffixes that Change a Root Word to an Adjective

Suffix	Meaning	Example	Definition
-ac	pertaining to	celiac	pertaining to the abdominal region
-acy	that which is, pertaining to	fallacy	that which is false
-ad	toward, in the direction of	cephalad	toward the head
-al	pertaining to	digital	pertaining to the finger or toe
-an	pertaining to, related to, belonging to	ovarian	pertaining to the ovary
-ar	of, or related to, pertaining to	valvular	related to a valve

TABLE 3-2
Set 2: Suffixes that Change a Root Word to an Adjective *(continued)*

Suffix	Meaning	Example	Definition
-ary	related to, pertaining to	biliary	pertaining to bile
-ate	that which is acted on	separate	to keep apart
-facient	making or causing to become	febrifacient	causing a fever
-fugal	driving or traveling away from	centrifugal	moving away from the center
-ic	pertaining to	colonic	pertaining to the colon
-ile	having the qualities of or capability for	febrile	feverish
-ious	capable of, causing	infectious	capable of being transmitted
-ive	that which performs or tends toward	tardive disease	disease with late-appearing symptoms
-oid	like	ameboid	amoebalike
-ory	process of, pertaining to, function of	sensory	pertaining to the senses
-ose	full of, having the qualities of	comatose	having the qualities of a coma
-ous	pertaining to	venous	pertaining to a vein
-some	tendency, like	tiresome	tiring
-trophic	related to nutrition, growth, development	dystrophic	faulty nutrition
-tropic	turning toward, or changing	hydrotropic	turned toward water
-y	having the nature or quality of	gouty	goutlike

TABLE 3-3
Set 3: Suffixes that Denote a State or Condition

Suffix	Meaning	Example	Definition
-agra	severe pain, seizure	podagra	severe pain in the foot
-algia	pain	neuralgia	nerve pain
-atresia	abnormal closure	proctatresia	closed anus
-cele	swelling, tumor	cystocele	hernia of urinary bladder
-chezia, -chesia	discharge of foreign substance	hematochezia	passage of bloody stool
-cyst	bladderlike sac	hydrocyst	cyst containing water

TABLE 3-3
Set 3: Suffixes that Denote a State or Condition *(continued)*

Suffix	Meaning	Example	Definition
-dom	state of being	martyrdom	state of being a martyr
-dynia	pain	pleurodynia	pain on the side of the chest
-ema	swelling, distention	emphysema	distention of air sacs in lungs
-ful	full of, characterized by	stressful	causing stress
-hood	state, quality of, condition	childhood	state of being a child
-ia	a diseased condition	anuria	condition of lack of urine
-iasis	a diseased condition	cholelithiasis	condition of bile stones
-id	condition	flaccid	condition of softness
-ism	condition, act of, process of	dwarfism	a condition of being a dwarf
-itis	inflammation	phlebitis	inflammation of a vein
-ity	quality of, state of	obesity	state of being obese
-less	without, not capable of	odorless	without odor
-malacia	softening	osteomalacia	softening of bone
-ness	quality of, state of	illness	state of being ill
-oma	tumor	carcinoma	malignant tumor
-osis	action, state, process, condition	halitosis	condition of having bad breath
-pathy	suffering, disease	cardiopathy	heart disease
-penia	deficiency, lack	leukopenia	lack of white blood cells
-philia	love of	hemophilia	"love of blood," a blood disease
-phobia	fear of	claustrophobia	fear of confinement
-ptosis	dropping, or downward displacement	carpoptosis	wrist-drop
-rrhage, -rrhagia	bursting forth	hemorrhage	bursting forth of blood
-rrhea	flow, discharge	galactorrhea	excessive flow of milk
-rrhexis	rupture	splenorrhexis	rupture of the spleen
-ship	state of, quality of	hardship	state of being difficult to endure
-stasis	state of being at a standstill	hemostasis	stagnation of blood
-staxis	hemorrhage	epistaxis	hemorrhage from the nose, nosebleed

TABLE 3-3
Set 3: Suffixes that Denote a State or Condition *(continued)*

Suffix	Meaning	Example	Definition
-tion	act of, result of, process of	elongation	process of making longer
-tonia	stretching, putting under tension	hypertonia	excessive tension
-vert	turn	divert	turn aside

TABLE 3-4
Set 4: Suffixes that Indicate a Surgical or Diagnostic Procedure

Suffix	Meaning	Example	Definition
-centesis	puncture of a cavity	paracentesis	puncture of a space around an organ or within a cavity to remove fluid
-cis	cut	excise	cut out
-clasis, -clasia	breaking up	bacterioclasis	breaking up of bacteria
-cleisis	closure	colpocleisis	operation for closure of vagina
-desis	binding, fusion	tenodesis	fixation of loose tendon
-ectomy	excision, cutting out	laryngectomy	removal of larynx
-gram, -graphy	act or method of recording	radiography	process of taking an x-ray
-lysis	setting free, dissolution	adipolysis	decomposition of fats
-ostomy	creation of a mouth or opening	colostomy	creating a new opening between bowel and abdominal wall
-otomy	cutting into	tracheotomy	cut into the windpipe
-pexy	fixation	sigmoidopexy	fixation of large intestine
-plasty	molding or shaping	osteoplasty	plastic surgery on bone
-rrhaphy	closure of by suturing, repair	cystorrhaphy	suture of bladder
-scope, -scopy	looking at, examining	bronchoscope	instrument used to view inside breathing tubes
-sect	cut	dissect	cut into parts
-tome	instrument for cutting	craniotome	instrument for cutting into the skull
-tripsy	rubbing, crushing	neurotripsy	surgical crushing of a nerve

TABLE 3-5
Set 5: Diminutive Suffixes that Indicate Smallness*

Suffix	Example	Meaning
-cle	caruncle	small, fleshy growth
-cule	molecule	smallest part of an atom
-culum	tuberculum	small nodule or knot
-culus	calculus	small stone
-et	facet	small plane surface
-ium	bronchium	small bronchial tube
-ole	arteriole	minute artery
-olum	mesenteriolum	small mesentery
-olus	bronchiolus	smallest subdivision of bronchus

* Listed in singular form.

TABLE 3-6
Set 6: Chemical Compounds Indicated by a Word Ending

Suffix	Meaning	Chemical Example
-ase	enzyme	lipase
-ate	salt made from acid	sulfate
-ene	unsaturated compound	benzene
-ide	binary compound	oxide
-in, ine	halogen, alkaloid, or nitrogen base	quinine
-ol	oil	cholesterol
-ose	carbohydrate	fructose
-yl	matter, substance, radical	ethyl

TABLE 3-7
Set 7: Word Endings that Form Plurals*

Singular	Plural	Example
-a	-ae	lamina, laminae
-en	-ina	lumen, lumina
-ex	-ices	index, indices
-ies	-ietes	paries, parietes
-is	-es	psychosis, psychoses
-is	-ides	epididymis, epididymides

TABLE 3-7
Set 7: Word Endings that Form Plurals* *(continued)*

Singular	Plural	Example
-ma	-mata	trauma, traumata
-nx	-nges	phalanx, phalanges
-on	-a	criterion, criteria
-s	-tes	pons, pontes
-u	-ua	cornu, cornua
-um	-a	diverticulum, diverticula
-us	-i	bacillus, bacilli
-us	-era	viscus, viscera
-us	-ora	corpus, corpora
-x	-ces	calyx, calyces

* There are sometimes choices between an English plural form and a foreign plural form. The English plural is usually preferred.

TABLE 3-8
Set 8: Plural of Nouns

nouns ending in e	add a or ae	aperture/apertura venule(a)/venulae
nouns ending in os or us	add i	locus/loci
nouns ending in on or um	add es or a	bacterium/bacteria chalazion/chalazia

PRETEST/ POSTTEST FOR CHAPTER 3

1. The following suffixes change a root word to a noun. Some suffixes have more than one meaning. The suffix in column A must match all definitions in column B. There is only one correct answer.

Column A	Column B
1. _____ -agogue	A. killer
2. _____ -ance	B. act or result of action
	C. measure

Column A	Column B
3. _____ -cide	D. leading, inducing
4. _____ -ectasia	E. science of
5. _____ -form	F. quality or act of
6. _____ -gen	G. that which, one who
7. _____ -ician, -ist	H. act of, state of, result of
8. _____ -ion	I. protection
9. _____ -meter	J. dilation or expansion
10. _____ -ology	K. production of, formation of
11. _____ -or	L. strength
12. _____ -phylaxis	M. one charged with or skilled in
13. _____ -poiesis	N. structure, shape
14. _____ -sthenia	
15. _____ -ure	

2. The following suffixes change a root word to an adjective.

Set 1

Put an *X* next to the suffixes which have a meaning including "pertaining to."

_____ -ac	_____ -acy	_____ -ad
_____ -al	_____ -an	_____ -ar
_____ -ary	_____ -ate	_____ -ic
_____ -ile	_____ -ious	_____ -ive
_____ -oid	_____ -ory	_____ -ose
_____ -ous	_____ -some	

Set 2

Put an *X* following the correct meaning of the following suffixes. There may be more than one correct meaning.

1. -ac: in the direction of _____, pertaining to _____

2. -ad: toward _____, away _____, in the direction of _____

3. -an: pertaining to _____, causing _____

4. -ate: that which is acted upon _____, capable of _____

5. -facient: making _____, driving _____, causing _____
6. -fugal: driving away _____, driving to _____
7. -ious: capable of causing _____, preventing _____
8. -ive: pertaining to _____, tends toward _____
9. -oid: related to _____, tendency _____, like _____
10. -ose: full of _____, having the qualities of _____
11. -ous: pertaining to _____, function of _____
12. -some: tendency _____, like _____
13. -trophic: related to growth, nutrition _____, turning toward _____
14. -tropic: related to growth, nutrition _____, turning toward _____
15. -y: having the nature of _____, process of _____

3. The following suffixes denote a state or condition. Fill in the meaning of the suffix.

Set 1

1. -agra _______________
2. -algia _______________
3. -atresia _______________
4. -cele _______________
5. -chezia _______________
6. -cyst _______________
7. -dynia _______________
8. -ema _______________
9. -ia _______________
10. -iasis _______________
11. -itis _______________
12. -less _______________
13. -malacia _______________
14. -oma _______________
15. -osis _______________
16. -pathy _______________
17. -penia _______________
18. -philia _______________

19. -phobia ____________________

20. -ptosis ____________________

21. -rrhage ____________________

22. -rrhea ____________________

23. -rrhexis ____________________

24. -stasis ____________________

25. -staxis ____________________

26. -tion ____________________

27. -tonia ____________________

28. -vert ____________________

The following suffixes have similar meanings. Define the underlined suffix in the following list of words.

Set 2

1. stress<u>ful</u> ____________________

2. child<u>hood</u> ____________________

3. flacc<u>id</u> ____________________

4. dwarf<u>ism</u> ____________________

5. obes<u>ity</u> ____________________

6. ill<u>ness</u> ____________________

7. hard<u>ship</u> ____________________

4. The following suffixes indicate a diagnostic or surgical procedure. Match column A with column B. Items in column B may be used more than once.

Column A	Column B
1. _____ -centesis	A. cut
2. _____ -cis	B. setting free, dissolution
3. _____ -clasis	C. act or method of recording
4. _____ -cleisis	D. creation of a mouth or opening
5. _____ -desis	E. fixation
6. _____ -ectomy	F. an instrument for cutting
7. _____ -gram, -graphy	G. puncture of a cavity
8. _____ -lysis	H. looking at, examining
	I. closure
	J. binding, fusion
	K. cut into
	L. closure by suturing, repair

Column A	Column B
9. _____ -ostomy	M. rubbing, crushing
10. _____ -otomy	N. looking at, examining
11. _____ -pexy	O. to mold or shape
12. _____ -plasty	P. breaking up
13. _____ -rrhaphy	Q. excision, cutting out
14. _____ -scope, -scopy	
15. _____ -sect	
16. _____ -tome	
17. _____ -tripsy	

5. The following suffixes are diminutive suffixes. Fill in the blank: A diminutive suffix indicates _______________.

List nine diminutive suffixes.

1. _______ 4. _______ 7. _______
2. _______ 5. _______ 8. _______
3. _______ 6. _______ 9. _______

6. There are eight examples of suffixes indicating a chemical compound. List them.

1. _______ 4. _______ 7. _______
2. _______ 5. _______ 8. _______
3. _______ 6. _______

7. The following question relates to word endings that form plurals. The singular ending is listed. Write in the plural ending.

1. -a _______ 6. -ma _______ 10. -u _______
2. -en _______ 7. -nx _______ 11. -um _______
3. -ex _______ 8. -on _______ 12. -us _______
4. -ies _______ 9. -s _______ 13. -x _______
5. -is _______

8. If there is a choice between an English plural and a foreign plural, the English plural is preferred. True or false: _______________

PRETEST/ POSTTEST **ANSWERS** FOR CHAPTER **3**

1.

1. D	**4.** J	**6.** K	**8.** H	**10.** E	**12.** I	**14.** L
2. F	**5.** N	**7.** M	**9.** C	**11.** G	**13.** K	**15.** B
3. A						

2. Set 1

-ac, -acy, -al, -an, -ar, -ary, -ic, -ile, -ory, -ous

Set 2

1. pertaining to
2. toward, in the direction of
3. pertaining to
4. that which is acted upon
5. making, causing
6. driving away
7. capable of causing
8. tends toward
9. like
10. full of, having the qualities of
11. pertaining to
12. tendency, like
13. related to growth, nutrition*
14. turning toward*
15. having the nature of

3. Set 1

1. severe pain, seizure
2. pain
3. abnormal closure
4. swelling, tumor
5. discharge of foreign substance
6. bladderlike sac
7. pain
8. swelling, distention
9. a diseased condition
10. a diseased condition
11. inflammation
12. without, not capable of
13. softening
14. tumor

* Distinguish between -trophic and -tropic. The term meaning "growth" has grown one letter longer than the other (trophic).

15. a diseased condition
16. suffering, disease
17. deficiency, lack of
18. love of
19. fear of
20. dropping or downward displacement
21. bursting forth
22. flow, discharge
23. state of being at a standstill
24. rupture
25. act of, result of, process of
26. hemorrhage
27. stretching, putting under tension
28. turn

Set 2

1. full of, characterized by
2. state of, quality of, condition
3. condition
4. condition, act of, process of
5. state of, quality of
6. state of, quality of
7. state of, quality of

4.

1. G	**4.** I	**7.** C	**10.** K	**12.** O	**14.** H	**16.** F
2. A	**5.** J	**8.** B	**11.** E	**13.** L	**15.** A	**17.** M
3. P	**6.** Q	**9.** D				

5. smallness

1. -cle	**4.** -culus	**7.** -ole
2. -cule	**5.** -et	**8.** -olum
3. -culum	**6.** -ium	**9.** -olus

6.

1. -ase	**4.** -ide	**7.** -ose
2. -ate	**5.** -in, -ise	**8.** -yl
3. -ene	**6.** -ol	

7.

1. -ae	**6.** -mata	**10.** -ua
2. -ina	**7.** -nges	**11.** -a
3. -ices	**8.** -a	**12.** -i, -era, -ora
4. -ietes	**9.** -tes	**13.** -ces, -cis
5. -es, -ides		

8. True

4 THE STRUCTURE OF THE BODY

OBJECTIVES

At the end of this chapter you will be able to do the following:

1 Describe the structure of the body.
2 Identify root words related to the cell.
3 List and describe four types of body tissue.
4 Define an organ.
5 Name the body systems, and list the organs in each system.
6 Name the organs of special senses.
7 Name terms related to the physical structure of an organ or system of the body.
8 Identify selected root words related to the response of various tissues to disease.

THE STRUCTURE OF THE BODY

The human body is the most complex thing on earth. It is made of basic elements that go from simple to complex.

Cells form tissues.
Tissues form organs.
Organs form systems.
Systems form the body.

The cell is the simplest part of the body. It is a microscopic mass of protoplasm.

Cells

The word *cell* means "hollow vessel." The following terms are related to the word *cell:*

blast(o): a root word that means a stage in development of a cell.
blastocyte: a cell that is still developing.
cyt(o), cyte: root words meaning cell, as in *cyto*logy, the study of cells, or leuko*cyte,* a white blood cell.
plasm(o): the substance of a cell. Plasma means "formed or molded material."

protoplasm: the living substance of the cell.
clast: a root word that means either causing or undergoing a division into parts or something that breaks.
intracellular: inside (*intra*) the cell.
extracellular: outside (*extra*) the cell.
interstitial: the space (*stitial*) between (*inter*) the cells.

Tissues

A tissue is a collection of specialized cells that perform a special function. *Histo* is a root word denoting tissue. Histology is the study of tissue. *Morph* is a root word denoting shape. Morphology is the science of forms and structure of organized beings.

The primary tissues of the body are the following:

epithelial
connective
muscular
nervous

Epithelial tissue

The term *epithelial* may be broken down into three parts: *epi,* which is a prefix meaning "upon," *thele,* meaning "nipple," and *al,* a suffix that makes a word a noun. Defining this word literally from its parts, it means "covering of the nipple." The word in its correct usage means a tissue that is located on the surface of an organ or part of the body.

Epithelial tissue performs four basic functions depending on where it is located:

protection (skin)
absorption (lungs and small intestine)
secretion (glands)
excretion (kidneys and liver)

Terms related to the *shape* of epithelial tissue:

squamous: scaly or flat
cuboidal: resembling a cube
columnar: resembling a column or pillarlike shape

Terms related to the *arrangement* of epithelial tissue:

simple: tissue that is one cell layer thick.
stratified: tissue that is several layers thick.
transitional: a type of tissue that is several layers thick, is subject to change, and is easily stretched. This type of tissue lines the urinary system.

Terms related to the *location* of epithelial tissue:

endothelium: the tissue (*thelium*) lining the inner (*endo*) surfaces of the heart, blood vessels, and lymphatic system.

mesothelium: the middle layer of epithelial tissue. This tissue is part of the serous membrane, or tissue, which lines parts of the peritoneum, heart, and chest cavity.
glandular epithelium: the type of tissue that makes up the glands in the body.

Connective tissue

Connective tissue is the most abundant tissue in the body. It holds organs in place, holds the body together, and forms the framework of the body.

Connective tissue is often made up of fibers. A *fiber* is an elongated, threadlike structure. Root words meaning fiber are *fibro* and *ino.*

Connective tissue is typed according to its degree of firmness (loose and dense) and according to its type of specialized function.

Collagen is the main supportive substance of connective tissue. The term means a glue-producing [glue (*colla*), producing (*gen*)] substance.

Terms related to *loose* connective tissue:

areolar tissue: a tissue made of interlacing fibers. This is the basic supporting substance around organs, muscles, blood vessels, and nerves. There are small (*olar*) spaces (*are*) between the fibers; thus, the tissue is loose.
adipose tissue: also known as *fatty tissue.* This is made up of fat cells in areolar tissue.
reticular tissue: serves as the framework for the liver, lymphoid tissues, and bone marrow. The word *reticular* means "resembling a net."

Terms related to *dense* connective tissue:

dermis: the true skin. It is also called the *corium.*
tendon: a dense cord of stretchable (*tend*) connective fibers by which a muscle is attached to bones, cartilage, or skin.
aponeurosis: a white, ribbonlike, tendinous (*neuro*) band that comes off of (*apo*) a muscle and attaches to a structure that moves.
ligament: a dense fibrous tissue that connects or ties together (ligament) bones or cartilage.

Terms related to *specialized* connective tissue:

bone tissue: makes up the skeletal system.
cartilage tissue: of which there are three forms: hyaline, fibrous, and elastic; resembles gristle.
dentin: the specialized tissue that makes up teeth. *Dent* is a root word meaning "teeth."
hematopoietic tissue: the tissue that produces blood cells. *Hemato* means "blood," *poietic* refers to "producing"; thus, the word means producing blood. The red marrow of bones is composed of this tissue.
lymphoid tissue: the tissue in lymph nodes, the thymus gland, spleen, and tonsils.
membrane: a thin sheet of tissue, or a combination of tissues, which lines organs or connects parts of the body.

Terms related to membranous tissue:

meninges: the membranes covering the brain and spinal cord.
mucous membrane: a tissue combination that lines the digestive, respiratory, urinary, and reproductive tracts. These membranes produce mucus and are slippery. Root words meaning "mucous membrane" are *blenno* and *myx*.
reticuloendothelial tissue: more like a system than a tissue. It comprises an important network of tissues that act as an important body defense against infection.
serous membrane: a tissue combination that consists of the surface layers of the heart and chest cavity.
synovial membrane: the tissue that lines the synovial joints. It is found where joints come together (*syn*) (see Chapter 8).

Muscle tissue

Muscle tissue is involved in movement of the body and its parts. There are three types of muscular tissue:

voluntary muscle: called *striated* because it appears to be striped. Voluntary muscles are controlled by the individual. Most of these muscles are attached to the skeletal system.
involuntary muscle: called *smooth-muscle tissue* because it has a smooth texture. Involuntary muscles function automatically. Muscles in the circulatory, digestive, urinary, and reproductive systems are involuntary muscles.
cardiac muscle: the muscle of the heart.

Nervous tissue

Nervous tissue is involved in control, activation, stimulation, sense perception, plus other activities related to the activity of the body. Nerve cells are divided into two types:

neurons: specialized conducting cells of the nervous system.
neuroglial cells: the cells that form the tissue which makes up the supportive structure of the nervous system. *Neuro* means "nerve," and *glia* means "glue."

Organs

An organ is made of a collection of specialized tissues. An organ has a specific function(s), but does not act independently of other organs.

Organs make up systems. There are 10 general systems in the body. Each system comprises organs that collectively perform specific functions (see Table 4-1).

TABLE 4-1
Systems of the Body and Their Important Organs

System	Organs in the System
musculoskeletal	bones, ligaments, skeletal muscles, tendons, joints
nervous	brain, spinal cord, nerves
cardiovascular	heart, arteries, veins, capillaries
lymphatic	lymphatic vessels, lymph nodes, spleen, tonsils, thymus gland
hematologic (blood)	red blood cells, white blood cells, platelets, plasma
digestive	mouth, tongue, teeth, salivary glands, esophagus, stomach, small and large intestines, liver, gallbladder, pancreas
respiratory	nasal cavity, larynx, trachea, bronchi, lungs, diaphragm, pharynx
urinary	kidneys, ureters, urinary bladder, urethra
endocrine	endocrine glands: hypothalamus, hypophysis (pituitary), thyroid, thymus, parathyroid, pineal, adrenal, pancreas, gonads (ovary or testis)
reproductive	female: ovaries, uterine tubes (oviducts), uterus, vagina. Male: testes, penis, prostate gland, seminal vesicles, spermatic ducts
integumentary	skin, hair, nails, sebaceous glands, sweat glands, breasts
special sense organs	eyes (vision), ears (hearing), semicircular canals (balance)

Parts of organs

Organs are made from tissue. Some organs have similarities with other organs, and some are very unique. Following is a list of terms related to the parts of an organ. Not all organs have all of these parts.

Terms and root words related to the physical structure of an organ or system of the body:

ampulla: a dilated portion of a canal or duct, a small (*ulla*) area that resembles an oval-shaped storage jar (*ampu*)
aperture: an opening, as a hole in an organ
apex: the tip, or point, of an organ, usually of an organ with a more or less triangular shape
base: the part of an organ nearest its point of attachment

capsule: a membranous sac that resembles a small (*ule*) box (*caps*)
collum: a necklike part of a body or organ
corpus: a body or mass, usually relatively large in size
cortex: the outside part of a structure, the thick outer layer of a structure, usually on the outside surface of the medulla of an organ
duct: a tubelike or canal-like structure that transports fluid or air from one part to another
fiber: a threadlike element
fascia: a layer of connective tissue covering internal organs or parts
fascicle: a small bundle of tissue
foramen: an opening or hole in an organ or part of an organ
fundus: the base of an organ, the part of an organ opposite an aperture, or opening
gland: a specialized cell, group of cells, or organ that produces a secretion
hilum: the small place on an organ at which blood vessels, nerves, or ducts enter or leave
labium: a liplike part
lobe: a roundish projection or roundish division of an organ
meatus: an opening or channel
medulla: the center of an organ, on the inside of the cortex
node: a small mass of tissue
orifice: a mouthlike opening
papilla: any small (*illa*) nipplelike (*pap*) projection from a surface
sinus: a cavity, passageway, or channel; a curved space
splanchnic: pertaining to the viscera
stem: a supporting structure or part of an organ
tract: a definite region or area of the body, especially a group, series, or systems of related parts or organs
ventricle: a hollow space, a small (*icle*), bellylike (*ventr*) area in an organ
viscera: the organs in a cavity of the body, usually referring to the organs in the abdominal cavity

RESPONSE OF TISSUES TO DISEASE

Important

TABLE 4-2
Root Words, Words, or Combining Forms of Words Related to the Response of Various Tissues of the Body to Disease

Term	Meaning	Example or Definition
bol-	ball	embolism: a ball or clot of blood in (*em*) a blood vessel
carcin(o)-	cancer	carcinoma: a cancerous tumor (*oma*)
ede-	swelling	edema: abnormal collection of fluid in the tissues of the body
febr-	fever	febrile: a feverish condition
fiss-	split	fissure: a cleft, split, or groove that may or may not be normal
fistula	small pipe	an abnormal passage between two internal organs
hernia	protrusion	a protrusion of an organ or part of an organ

TABLE 4-2

Root Words, Words, or Combining Forms of Words Related to the Response of Various Tissues of the Body to Disease *(continued)*

Term	Meaning	Example or Definition
infect	contaminate	to contaminate with disease-producing germs
inflammation	burning	a condition in which there is a burning or a destruction of the cells of the body. This term is used because one of the classical signs of inflammation is the production of heat (calor) and redness (rubor). The other classical signs are pain (dolor) and swelling (tumor).
lesion	harm	an injury, wound, or area of disease
lip-	fat	lipoma: a tumor (*oma*) made of fat (*lip*)
lith-	stone, calculus	lithotomy: an incision (*otomy*) made to remove a stone (*lith*)
necro-	death	necrosis: a condition in which there is death of tissue
obesity	fatness	a condition in which there is excessive fat around the entire body, an excessive amount of adipose tissue
patho-	disease	pathology: the study (*ology*) of disease (*patho*)
phthi-	decay	phthisis: a wasting away of the body or part of the body
polyp	many feet	shortened form of the word *polypus*. A polyp is a growth, usually from mucous membranes, which has many projections, or feet.
pur-	pus	purulent: containing pus; suppurate: to discharge pus
pyo-	pus	pyocyst: a cyst containing pus
pyr-	fever	pyrexia: state of having a fever
scar	mark	the mark left by a healed wound; may be internal or external
stear-, steat-	fat	steatopygia: a condition in which there is excessive fat on the buttocks (*pygia*)
steno-	narrowing	stenosis: a narrowing condition
strict-	draw tight	constriction: a condition in which a vessel is narrowed, the walls of an organ are drawn together (*con*)
struct-	clogged	obstruction: a condition in which there is a clog in the normal passageway
tract-	draw, drag	contract; the condition in which parts of an organ are drawn (*tract*) together (*con*)
trauma	wound, injury	multiple trauma: a condition in which there is injury to more than one part of the body
tuber-	swelling	tuberculosis: a condition (*osis*) characterized by the appearance of small (*cul*) swellings (*tuber*)
tumor	swelling	a growth or swelling of tissue from a disease state. This is usually localized swelling.
ulcer	sore	a sore that is open on the surface of the body or on a wall of an internal organ

PRETEST/ POSTTEST FOR CHAPTER 4

1. The structure of the body is complex. The structure of the body from the simple to the complex is as follows:

   Cells form ________________.

   ________________ form ________________.

   ________________ form ________________.

   ________________ form the body.

2. The following terms are related to the cell. Match column A with column B.

Column A	Column B
1. _____ cell	A. space between the cells
2. _____ blast	B. outside the cell
3. _____ cyto, cyte	C. cell
4. _____ plasmo	D. formed material
5. _____ protoplasm	E. inside the cell
6. _____ clast	F. hollow vessel
7. _____ intracellular	G. developing stage
8. _____ extracellular	H. living substance
9. _____ interstitial	I. division or breaking

3. The following terms are related to tissues. Fill in the blanks.
   1. The root word for tissue is ________________.
   2. *Morph* is the root word meaning ________________.
   3. The type of tissue that covers the body surfaces is called ________________ tissue.
   4. The tissue that holds the body together is called ________________ tissue.
   5. The tissue of the body involved in movement is called ________________ tissue.
   6. The tissue that makes up the organs involved in control of the body is called ________________ tissue.

4. The functions of various types of epithelial tissue include the following examples.

Location	Function
1. skin	________________
2. lungs and small intestine	________________
3. glands	________________
4. kidneys and liver	________________

5. The following terms are related to epithelial tissue. Match column A with column B.

Column A	Column B
1. _____ squamous	A. one layer thick
2. _____ cuboidal	B. makes up glands of the body
3. _____ columnar	C. subject to change, stretchable
4. _____ simple	D. scaly or flat
5. _____ stratified	E. inner lining
6. _____ transitional	F. resembles a cube
7. _____ endothelium	G. middle layer
8. _____ mesothelium	H. several layers thick
9. _____ glandular	I. resembles a column

6. The following terms are related to connective tissue. Name the types of tissue.
   1. a loose connective tissue that is the basic supporting substance around organs, muscles, blood vessels, and nerves, known as ________________
   2. also known as fatty tissue ________________
   3. resembles a net and is the framework for the liver, lymphoid tissue, and bone marrow ________________
   4. referred to as the true skin ________________
   5. true skin, also known as the ________________

   A dense connective tissue that
   6. is a dense, stretchable cord ________________
   7. is a band that comes off of a tendon ________________
   8. ties bone or cartilage together ________________

The specialized tissue that

9. makes up the skeletal system ________________
10. resembles gristle ________________
11. makes up teeth ________________
12. produces blood cells ________________
13. makes up the lymph nodes, thymus gland, spleen, and tonsils

____

14. Two root words meaning fiber are ________ and ________.
15. The main supportive substance of connective tissue is called

________________.

7. Fill in the blanks:

1. A membrane is a thin sheet of ________________ that lines ________ or ________________ parts of the body.
2. The ________________ are the coverings of the brain and spinal cord.
3. A ________________ membrane produces mucus.
4. The reticuloendothelial tissue functions in the body's defense against

________________.

5. A ________________ membrane lines the heart and chest cavity.
6. The ________________ membrane is found where joints come together.
7. Two root words meaning mucus are ________________ and

________________.

8. The following terms are related to muscle tissue. The three types of muscle tissue are voluntary, involuntary, and cardiac. Indicate to which type of muscle the following statements relate by placing a *V* for voluntary muscle, an *I* for involuntary muscle, or a *C* for cardiac muscle in the space provided.

1. ____ also called striated
2. ____ the muscle of the heart
3. ____ also called skeletal
4. ____ also called smooth muscle
5. ____ muscles that function automatically

9. There are two types of nerve cells: ________________ and ________________.

10. Fill in the blanks: An organ is made of a collection of ________________. A system is made of a collection of ________________.

11. Following are a list of systems and a list of organs. Indicate in the space provided the letter corresponding to the system to which that organ belongs.

Systems

A. musculoskeletal	G. respiratory
B. nervous	H. urinary
C. cardiovascular	I. endocrine
D. lymphatic	J. reproductive
E. hematologic	K. integumentary
F. digestive	L. special sense organs

Some organs are considered a part of two systems. Indicate both systems.

1. _____ bronchi
2. _____ bones
3. _____ seminal vesicles
4. _____ skin
5. _____ capillaries
6. _____ nails
7. _____ ovaries
8. _____ spleen
9. _____ lungs
10. _____ ligaments
11. _____ prostate
12. _____ esophagus
13. _____ mouth
14. _____ nerves
15. _____ hypophysis
16. _____ blood cells
17. _____ arteries
18. _____ salivary glands
19. _____ lymph nodes
20. _____ thyroid
21. _____ veins
22. _____ testes
23. _____ nasal cavity
24. _____ pituitary
25. _____ ears
26. _____ tendon
27. _____ ureters
28. _____ spermatic ducts
29. _____ breasts
30. _____ adrenal glands
31. _____ pancreas
32. _____ tonsils
33. _____ gallbladder
34. _____ skeletal muscles
35. _____ penis
36. _____ gonads
37. _____ brain
38. _____ spinal cord

39. _____ thymus
40. _____ heart
41. _____ tongue
42. _____ hair
43. _____ larynx
44. _____ intestines
45. _____ teeth
46. _____ parathyroid glands
47. _____ trachea
48. _____ liver
49. _____ oviducts
50. _____ stomach
51. _____ urethra
52. _____ sebaceous glands
53. _____ diaphragm
54. _____ vagina
55. _____ semicircular canals
56. _____ urinary bladder
57. _____ sweat glands
58. _____ kidneys
59. _____ uterus
60. _____ eye

12. The following terms are related to the physical structure of an organ. Match column A with column B.

Set 1

Column A

1. _____ ampulla
2. _____ cervix
3. _____ duct
4. _____ foramen
5. _____ fundus
6. _____ hilum
7. _____ node
8. _____ sinus
9. _____ stem
10. _____ tract

Column B

A. a supporting structure
B. base, part of the organ opposite the opening
C. dilated portion that is like a small jar
D. cavity, passageway, curved space
E. an opening or hole
F. a necklike part
G. a definite region, series of related parts
H. tubelike structure that transports fluid or air
I. the place where blood vessels, nerves, or ducts enter
J. a small mass of tissue

Set 2

Column A

1. _____ aperture
2. _____ capsule
3. _____ collum
4. _____ cortex

Column B

A. necklike part
B. the middle or inside part
C. produces a secretion
D. an opening
E. membranous sac, a small box
F. the outside part, thick outer layer

5. _____ fascia	G. related to viscera or abdominal organs
6. _____ gland	H. layer of connective tissue
7. _____ meatus	I. small, bellylike space in an organ
8. _____ medulla	J. an opening or channel
9. _____ splanchnic	
10. _____ ventricle	

Set 3

Column A	**Column B**
1. _____ apex	A. a body or mass
2. _____ base	B. a roundish projection or division of an organ
3. _____ corpus	C. the tip or point of an organ
4. _____ fiber	D. a mouthlike opening
5. _____ fascicle	E. a small bundle of tissue
6. _____ labium	F. a liplike part
7. _____ lobe	G. a nipplelike projection from a surface
8. _____ orifice	H. the part of an organ nearest its attachment
9. _____ papilla	I. the organs of the body, usually the abdominal organs
10. _____ viscera	J. threadlike element

13. The following terms are related to the response of tissue to disease. Mark statement true, *T,* or false, *F.*

1. _____ An embolism is a clot of blood in a blood vessel.
2. _____ Carcinoma is a fat tumor.
3. _____ Edema means the same thing as tumor.
4. _____ *Febr-* and *pyr-* both mean fever.
5. _____ Fissure means cavity.
6. _____ A fistula is a normal passageway between two organs.
7. _____ A hernia means a protrusion.
8. _____ Infect and contaminate mean the same thing.
9. _____ A lesion is an area of disease.

14. Complete the following statements:

1. A lipoma is a ________ (*oma*) made of ________ (*lip*).
2. The root word *lith* means ________________.
3. Necrosis is a condition in which there is ________ of tissue.
4. Pathology is the study (*ology*) of ________ (*patho*).
5. *Phthi* means ________.
6. A polyp is a growth that has many ________________ or ________.
7. The root words for pus are ________ and ________.
8. A scar is the ________ left by a healed wound.
9. Root words for fat are ________, ________, or ________.
10. Stenosis of a part means that the opening into or through the part has been ________________.
11. Constriction is a condition in which the walls of a part have been ________________.
12. A clog in a normal passageway is called an ________________.
13. Contraction means the condition of having the walls of organs ________________.
14. Trauma means ________ or ________.
15. Tuberculosis is a condition in which there are small ________________.
16. Tumor means ________________ swelling.
17. An ulcer is a ________.
18. Obesity results from the excessive accumulation of ________________.
19. Inflammation refers to a burning or ________________ of cells.

PRETEST/ POSTTEST **ANSWERS** FOR CHAPTER 4

1. tissues; Tissues, organs; Organs, systems; Systems

2. **1.** F **2.** G **3.** C **4.** D **5.** H **6.** I **7.** E **8.** B **9.** A

3. **1.** histo
2. shape
3. epithelial
4. connective
5. muscular
6. nervous

4. **1.** protection
2. absorption
3. secretion
4. excretion

5. **1.** D
2. F
3. I
4. A
5. H
6. C
7. E
8. G
9. B

6. **1.** areolar
2. adipose
3. reticular
4. dermis
5. corion
6. tendon
7. aponeurosis
8. ligament
9. bone
10. cartilage
11. dentin
12. hematopoietic
13. lymphoid
14. ino, fiber
15. collagen

7. **1.** tissue, organs, connects
2. meninges
3. mucous
4. infection
5. serous
6. synovial
7. blenno, myx

8. **1.** V **2.** C **3.** V **4.** I **5.** I and C

9. neurons, neuroglial cells

10. tissues, organs

11.

1. G	**10.** A	**19.** D	**28.** J	**37.** B	**45.** F	**53.** G
2. A	**11.** J	**20.** I	**29.** K	**38.** B	**46.** I	**54.** J
3. J	**12.** F	**21.** C	**30.** I	**39.** D, I	**47.** G	**55.** L
4. K	**13.** F	**22.** I, J	**31.** F, I	**40.** C	**48.** F	**56.** H
5. C	**14.** B	**23.** G	**32.** D	**41.** F	**49.** J	**57.** K
6. K	**15.** I	**24.** I	**33.** F	**42.** K	**50.** F	**58.** H
7. I, J	**16.** E	**25.** L	**34.** A	**43.** G	**51.** H	**59.** J
8. D	**17.** C	**26.** A	**35.** J	**44.** F	**52.** K	**60.** L
9. G	**18.** F	**27.** H	**36.** I, J			

12. **Set 1**

1. C **2.** F **3.** H **4.** E **5.** B **6.** I **7.** J **8.** D **9.** A **10.** G

Set 2

1. D **2.** E **3.** A **4.** F **5.** H **6.** C **7.** J **8.** B **9.** G **10.** I

Set 3

1. C **2.** H **3.** A **4.** J **5.** E **6.** F **7.** B **8.** D **9.** G **10.** I

13. **1.** T **2.** F **3.** F **4.** T **5.** F **6.** F **7.** T **8.** T **9.** T

14.
1. tumor, fat
2. stone, calculus
3. death
4. disease
5. decay
6. projections, feet
7. pur-, pyo-
8. mark
9. stear-, steat-, lip-
10. narrowed
11. drawn together
12. obstruction
13. drawn together
14. wound, injury
15. swellings, tubers
16. localized
17. sore
18. fat or adipose tissue
19. destruction

5 THE BODY AS A WHOLE

OBJECTIVES

At the end of this chapter you will be able to do the following:

1. Describe the body as a whole.
2. Define terms related to the position of the body.
3. Define terms related to the surfaces or depth of parts of the body.
4. List and describe the major cavities of the body.
5. Identify the regions and quadrants of the abdomen.
6. Describe the anatomical division of the back surface of the body.
7. Identify terms associated with specific areas of the body, from head to toe.
8. Identify planes and directional aspects in reference to the body.
9. Describe the practice of medicine as it is related to the diagnosis and treatment of disease.
10. Analyze selected terms related to diseases that affect systems of the body.

THE BODY AS A WHOLE

The body as a whole is made up of systems. Some of the systems are concentrated in a particular part of the body, for example, the urinary system, while others reach out to all parts of the body, as the circulatory system does.

soma, somato: root words meaning the body, as distinguished from the mind
psycho: the root word meaning mind; example: psychosomatic, means mind-body-related
corpse: the body shortly after death

Positions of the Body

Terms related to the position of the body are the following:

anatomical position: the stance the body has when it is erect with the arms hanging to the side, palms facing forward
erect position: the body in a standing position

supine position: the body lying in a horizontal position with the face up
prone position: the body lying with the face down in a horizontal position
laterally recumbent position: the body lying horizontally on either the right or left side

Surface and Depth of Body Parts

Terms related to the surface and depth of parts of the body:

internal: the inside part of the body or inside surfaces of the body itself
external: the outside surface of the body
deep: a part that is situated far beneath the surface
superficial: a part that is situated close to the surface
parietal: the wall of a part of the body

Body Cavities

Terms related to body cavities (Figure 5-1):

cavum: hollow spaces
ventral cavities: cavities located in the front part of the body. There are three ventral cavities: thoracic, abdominal, and pelvic.
thoracic cavity: also known as the *chest.* It is that part of the body between the neck and the diaphragm. The three sections of the thoracic cavity are the *left pleural space,* the *mediastinum,* and the *right pleural space.* The pleural spaces contain the lungs. The mediastinum is the middle area of the cavity that contains the heart, large blood vessels, and esophagus.
abdominal cavity: also known as the *belly.* The term *venter* literally means "belly" or "abdomen." This is the part of the body between the diaphragm and the pelvic organs. Other terms related to the abdomen are *celiac* (abdominal), *laparo* (loin, flank), and *flank* (wide upper part of the abdomen over the hipbone). The abdominal cavity contains the stomach, small intestine, most of the large intestine, appendix, liver, gallbladder, pancreas, spleen, kidney, adrenal glands, upper portion of the ureters, and the peritoneum.
pelvic cavity: situated below the abdominal cavity. It contains some of the large intestine, the rectum, urinary bladder, and the internal reproductive organs.
dorsal cavities: located toward the back of the body.
cranial cavity: contains the brain and related structures.
vertebral cavity: contains the spinal cord and extends from the base of the cranial cavity to a level corresponding to the bottom edge of the abdominal cavity.
torso, trunk: terms related to the main part of the body to which the head and limbs are attached. The torso includes all of the ventral cavities and the vertebral cavity.

Abdominal Regions and Quadrants

The abdominal cavity is divided into regions and quadrants as shown in Table 5-1 and Figures 5-2 and 5-3.

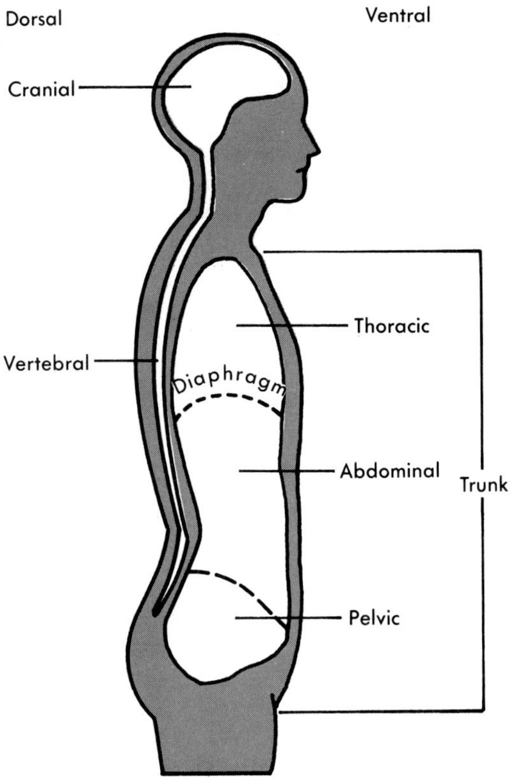

FIGURE 5-1
Body cavities.

Quadrants of the abdomen are named for the position they occupy. They are frequently referred to by initials only.

Posterior Regions of the Trunk

The *back* or posterior surface of the trunk is also divided into regions. The terms used to describe these regions are related to the names of the vertebrae in the spinal column. In descending order they are as follows:

cervical region: the neck (7 cervical vertebrae)
thoracic region: the chest (12 thoracic vertebrae)
lumbar region: the loin (5 lumbar vertebrae)
sacral region: the sacrum (5 sacral vertebrae that are fused into one bone)
coccyx: the tailbone (4 coccygeal vertebrae that are fused into one bone)

Specific Body Parts or Areas

There are terms and root words that denote specific parts of the body or specific areas of the body. These terms and root words appear in Table 5-2.

TABLE 5-1
Abdominal Regions

Region Number	Region Name	Definition
1	Right hypochondriac	The region on the right that is under (*hypo*) the ribs (*chondriac*)
2	Epigastric	The region over (*epi*) the stomach (*gastric*)
3	Left hypochondriac	The region on the left that is under (*hypo*) the ribs (*chondriac*)
4	Right flank	The region on the right that is near the lumbar vertebrae; the right loin area
5	Umbilical	The region near the umbilicus, which is also known as the navel, belly button, or omphalos
6	Left flank	The left loin area
7	Right inguinal	The region on the right that is located near the groin
8	Suprapubic	The region above (*supra*) the pubic bone.
9	Left inguinal	The region near the left groin

Body Planes and Directional Aspects

Terms related to planes (i.e., flat surfaces) and directional aspects of the body are listed below and in Figure 5-4.

Planes

coronal plane: the plane that cuts the body into front and back halves. Sometimes called the *frontal plane.*

midsagittal plane: divides the body into right and left equal halves. Sometimes called the *median plane.*

sagittal plane: any plane parallel to the midsagittal plane vertically dividing the body into right and left portions. The term *sagittal* refers to an arrow or arrowhead. Remember this plane by associating it with an arrow through the body.

transverse plane: a plane cutting crosswise through the body. It is situated at right angles to the long axis of the body. Sometimes called the *horizontal plane.* It divides the body into top and bottom parts.

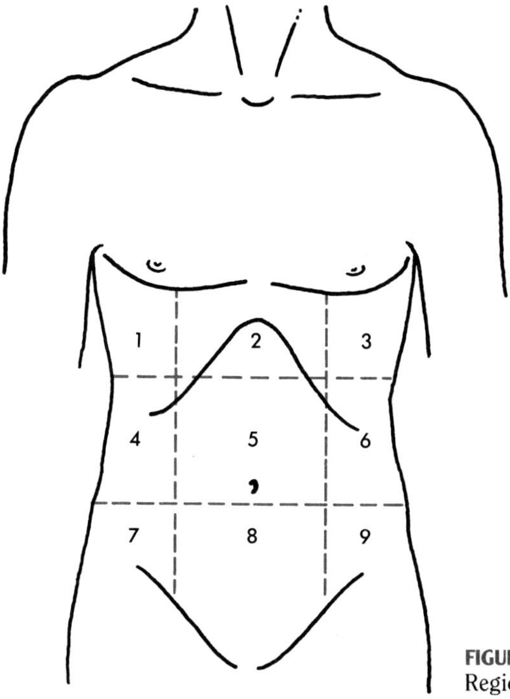

FIGURE 5-2
Regions of the abdomen.

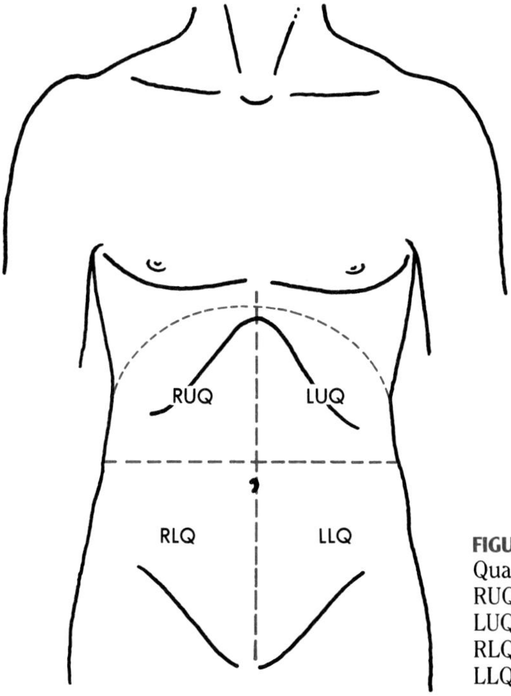

FIGURE 5-3
Quadrants of the abdomen.
RUQ = right upper quadrant,
LUQ = left upper quadrant,
RLQ = right lower quadrant,
LLQ = left lower quadrant.

TABLE 5-2
Terms and Root Words for Specific Areas of the Body

Area	Term	Description
head	vertex	top of the head
	caput-	head
face	facies	face
	mento-	chin
	genio-	chin
	gnatho-	jaw
neck	cervix	neck
	nucha	nape, back part of neck
chest	stetho-	chest
	thoraco-	
extremities	melos-	limb, arm, or leg
shoulder and upper extremity	omo-	shoulder
	axilla	armpit
	brachium	upper arm from shoulder to elbow
	cubitus	elbow
	carpo-	wrist
	chiro-, cheiro-	hand
	manus	hand
	dactyl-	fingers; may also refer to toe
	digit	fingers; may also refer to toe
	pollex	thumb
groin and lower extremities	inguinal	bottom, the juncture of the thighs and abdomen, the groin
	pygo-, pygia-	buttocks, rump
	crural	thigh, the leg from the hip to the knee
	genu-	knee
	popliteal	area in back of the knee
	crus	shin, leg from knee to foot
	talus	ankle
	ped-, pedia-, pedo-, pes, pod	foot
	tarso-	instep
	hallux	big toe, great toe

Directional aspects

medial: pertaining to the middle or midline of the body
cephalad: toward (*ad*) the head (*cephal*)
caudad: toward (*ad*) the tail (*caud*)
superior: situated above or directed upward
inferior: situated below or directed downward
proximal: refers to a point nearest the center or to a part closer to another part
distal: situated away from the center of a structure, distal (distant); refers to a point farther from another

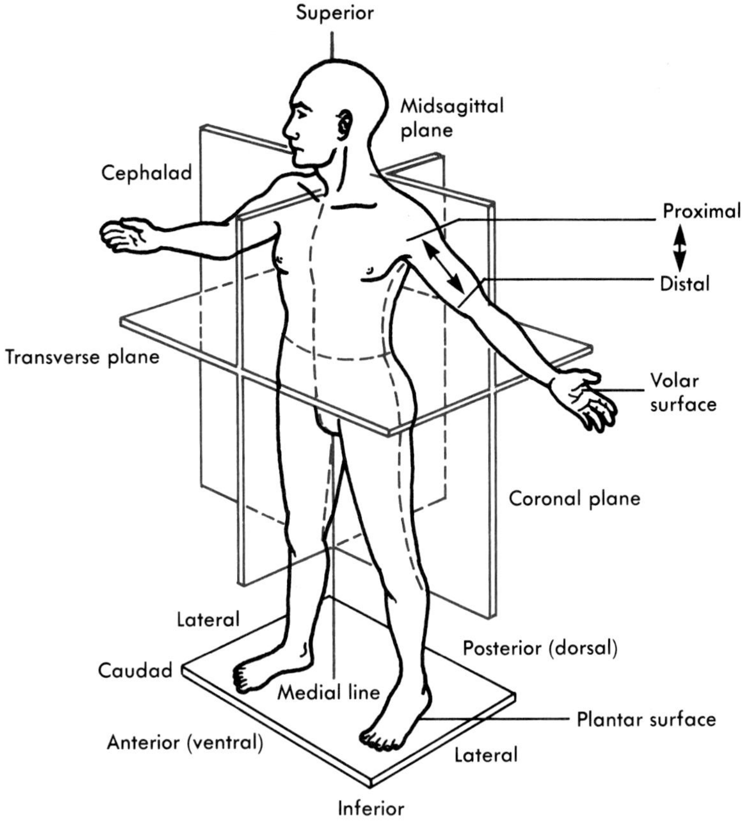

FIGURE 5-4
Planes and directional aspects of the body.

peripheral: peri (around), *pheral* (bear), bearing around; the circumference or an area away from the center
anterior, ventral: the front (*ante*) surface of the body or part
posterior, dorsal: the back (*post*) surface of the body or part
lateral: pertains to a side of the body or a point away from the midline
volar: refers to the palm side of the hand; also called *palmar*
plantar: refers to the sole side of the foot
varus: bent inward, angulation of a part of the body toward the midline
valgus: bent outward (associate *val* with "wall"), bent toward the wall
dextral (*dextro*): right
sinistral (*sinistro*): left; *levo* also used for left

CLINICAL MEDICINE

Terms related to medicine deal with the diagnosis and treatment of disease. The actual practice of medicine in the diagnosis and treatment of disease is referred to as *clinical medicine.*

The term *clinic* refers to the "sick bed" or "bedside"; thus the term *clinical* pertains to care given at the bedside. Modern medical practice also involves persons who are not well but who are able to walk around: these are *ambulatory patients.*

Diagnosis of Disease

The first step in the practice of clinical medicine is the diagnosis of disease. A diagnosis is made following a complete examination of the body and mind and the taking of a complete medical history. Terms related to the examination of the mind are found in Chapter 22.

Physical examination

The examination of the body as a whole includes the following aspects and is called a *complete physical examination:*

inspection: the act of (*tion*) looking into (*inspect*) or looking at the patient, either directly or indirectly through various instruments. For example, an ophthalmoscope is an instrument for viewing the inside of the eye (*ophthalmo*).

palpation: the act of (*tion*) touching (*palpat*) or feeling specific areas of the patient's body. The body is palpated for irregularities in size, firmness, lumps, or other physical findings evaluated by touch.

auscultation: the act of (*tion*) listening (*ausculta*) to the sounds produced by internal organs as they are functioning or to sound produced in response to electronic devices. A stethoscope is an instrument for listening to the sounds in the chest (*stetho*). It is also used to listen to many other areas of the body. The term auscula- means "little ear."

percussion: the act of (*ion*) striking (*percuss*) various parts of the body to determine the quality of the sounds produced, the reflexes or reaction of nerves, or the existence of tenderness.

various measurements: vital signs, measured to complete the total evaluation of the person's state of health. The vital signs measured are the temperature, pulse, respiratory rate, and blood pressure. They are commonly abbreviated as T, P, R, and BP, respectively.

The purpose of a physical examination is to find signs of disease.

Medical history

The medical history is a body of information collected to learn of past events that might relate to the patient's health or illness. A medical history includes the following information:

family history
history of present illness, if illness is present
presenting symptoms of chief complaint
past history
social history

The purpose of taking a medical history is to evaluate symptoms of a disease and to gather information about possible problems.

The information gathered from the physical examination and medical history is recorded in one place. This is called the *health record.* The patient's physician, evaluating all of the information, makes a diagnosis and plans the method of treatment.

Diagnosis terminology

Terms related to the diagnosis of disease conditions of the body are the following:

acute: sharp. An acute condition is one that is brief and severe.

ambulatory: able to walk. The sick person is not confined to a sickbed or clinic but is capable (*ory*) of walking about (*ambulat*).

anomaly: irregularity, a deviation from normal.

atrophy: a wasting away of the body or of an organ or part. Term means lack (*a*) of nutrition to a part or organ that causes it to waste away.

benign: good. A disease that is not malignant.

chronic: "time-related." A condition that lasts a long time.

clinic: a sick bed or area where sick persons are confined, or an area where persons go for the diagnosis and treatment of disease.

clinical: related to examination in a clinic, as in the first-hand observation of a disease, resulting in diagnosis and treatment.

diagnosis: identification of a disease, having complete (*dia*) knowledge (*gnosis*) of the process of a disease.

malignant: bad. A condition that becomes progressively worse and may result in death.

metastatic: "next place." A disease that spreads from one place (*static*) to the next (*meta*) place.

prognosis: to know beforehand, having knowledge (*gnosis*) of the course of a disease beforehand [before (*pro*)]. A prediction of the course of a disease process.

sign: an observable occurrence that indicates a disease state. Example: fever is a sign of infection.

symptom: "fall with." An indication of something that occurs, or falls, with a particular disease process. Example: chest pain is a symptom of heart disease.

syndrome: "run together." A group of signs and symptoms that usually occur, or run, together. Example: respiratory distress syndrome, a group of signs and symptoms that result from respiratory distress.

systemic: involving systems. A systemic disease affects the body as a whole.

Treatment of Disease

The term commonly used for the treatment of disease is *therapy.* Therapeutics is the phase of medicine that deals with the treatment of disease. Therapy means healing, and all forms of treatment deal with some form of healing.

Two general categories of treatment in the field of medicine are *surgery* and *internal medicine.*

Surgical therapy involves the art and practice of treating disease, injuries, and deformities by operation or by the application of devices either internally or externally. The person giving this type of treatment is called a *surgeon.*

Internal medicine deals with the treatment of diseases that are treated with drugs. This category of treatment is commonly called *medical therapy.* The person giving this type of treatment is called an *internist.*

There are many specialties of these two categories. See the appendix listing the medical and surgical specialties.

Terms related to the practice of clinical medicine

drug: a chemical substance administered to a person to treat disease. A root word meaning "drug" is *pharmo*

internist: a physician who deals with (*ist*) internal (*intern*) medicine

internal medicine: the branch of medicine dealing with the treatment of disease with drugs or medication

operation: the act of (*tion*) performing a treatment using instruments

surgeon: a physician who deals with surgery; a physician who works with his or her hands

surgery: the branch of medicine dealing with the treatment of disease by operation or application of devices

therapeutics: the practice in medicine of treating disease

therapy: healing

Selected terms related to diseases

agenesis: condition in which a natural body structure was not (*a*) produced (*genesis*).

bacterial: a disease caused by bacteria.

cancer: a disease in which the natural course leads to death. The astrological sign for cancer is the crab. A cancer is a malignant, invasive growth that spreads out like the legs of a crab..

congenital: condition or defect that a child is born (*genital*) with (*con*).

degenerative: disease characterized by a breakdown in the structure of a part.

endemic: disease that is occurring in (*en*) a particular group of people (*demic*).

epidemic: disease that is spread over (*epi*) a large number of people (*demic*) in a particular area.

exacerbation: condition in which a disease becomes increasingly severe. The disease comes out (*ex*) in a harsh (*acer*) way.

fungal: disease caused by fungus.

helminthic: condition caused by disease-producing worms (*helminth).*

iatrogenic: disease that is a side effect of the treatment prescribed by a physician (*iatro*).

idiopathic: a disease (*pathic*) that is peculiar (*idio*) to that one person. A disease of unknown cause.

infectious: disease that makes its way into (*in*) a person. A disease that is spread from one person to another.
neoplastic: disease in which new (*neo*) cells are formed (*plastic*). This type of disease is referred to as *cancer.*
nosocomial: disease (*noso*) that originates in a hospital or other institution designed to care for (*comial*) sick people.
palliation: treatment that is directed at the symptoms of the disease, rather than at curing the disease. The symptoms are covered (palliate) rather than cured.
pandemic: disease that is spread over all (*pan*) the people (*demic*). A widespread disease.
parasitic: disease caused by a parasite such as a protozoan.
sepsis: presence in the blood of organisms or poisons from those organisms capable of producing a breakdown (*sepsis*) of body tissues.
trauma: a wound (*trauma*) either to the body or to the mind.
viral: a disease caused by a virus.

PRETEST/ POSTTEST FOR CHAPTER 5

1. The root words for body are ________, ________, and ________. The root word for mind is ________.

2. The following terms are related to the position of the body. Match column A with column B.

Column A	Column B
1. _____ anatomical	A. the body in a standing position
2. _____ erect	B. the body lying horizontally on either the right or left side
3. _____ supine	C. the body standing straight with arms to the side and palms facing forward
4. _____ prone	D. the body lying horizontally with face up
5. _____ laterally recumbent	E. the body lying face down

3. The following terms are related to the surface and depth of parts of the body. Match column A with column B.

Column A	Column B
1. ____ internal	A. inside part or surface
2. ____ external	B. far beneath the surface
3. ____ deep	C. walls of a part
4. ____ superficial	D. outside part or surface
5. ____ parietal	E. close to the surface

4. The following terms are related to the cavities of the body. Fill in the blanks.

   1. The root word for cavity is cavus which means ________ ________.
   2. The ventral cavities are located in the ________ part of the body.
   3. The thoracic cavity is also known as the ________ cavity. It is made of the right and left ________ spaces and the ________________. It contains the ________, ________, ________________, and ________________.
   4. The abdominal cavity is also known as the ________. Other names or root words for abdomen are ________ and ________.
   5. The pelvic cavity is situated below the ________ cavity. It contains ________________, ________, ________________, and ________________.
   6. The dorsal cavities are located in the ________ part of the body.
   7. The cranial cavity contains the ________.
   8. The vertebral cavity contains the ________________.
   9. The terms ________ and ________ are related to the main part of the body.

5. The following terms are related to the regions of the abdominal cavity. Fill in the blanks.

   1. The epigastric region is ________ the ________.
   2. The inguinal regions are located near the ________.
   3. The suprapubic region is ________ the ________ bone.
   4. The flank regions are near the ________ vertebrae.
   5. The hypochondriac region is ________ the ________.

6. The following terms are related to the quadrants of the abdomen. Write the terms abbreviated with the following letters.

R U Q ____________________

L U Q ____________________

R L Q ____________________

L L Q ____________________

7. The following terms are related to the back of the trunk. List the regions of the back from the neck to the tail bone.

1. ____________

2. ____________

3. ____________

4. ____________

5. ____________

8. The following terms are related to specific areas of the body. Identify the areas these terms are related to.

Term	Area	Term	Area
1. facies	________	**16.** stetho-	________
2. nucha	________	**17.** capt-	________
3. omo-	________	**18.** hallux	________
4. pollex	________	**19.** genu-	________
5. vertex	________	**20.** digit	________
6. inguinal	________	**21.** brachium	________
7. crural	________	**22.** melos-	________
8. manus	________	**23.** gnatho-	________
9. axilla	________	**24.** dactyl-	________
10. cervix	________	**25.** mento-	________
11. talus	________	**26.** carpo-	________
12. tarso-	________	**27.** genio-	________
13. chiro-	________	**28.** cubitus	________
14. crus-	________	**29.** cheiro-	________
15. popliteal	________	**30.** pygia-	________

9. The following terms are related to the planes of the body. Match column A with column B (some terms may be used more than once).

Column A	Column B
1. _____ coronal plane	A. divides the body into right and left sections
2. _____ sagittal plane	B. divides the body into top and bottom sections
3. _____ horizontal plane	C. cuts the body into front and back sections
4. _____ frontal plane	
5. _____ median plane	
6. _____ transverse plane	

10. The following is a list of terms in sets as related to directional aspects of the body. Identify the direction indicated by the terms.

Term	Direction
1. superior	______________________
inferior	______________________
2. medial	______________________
lateral	______________________
peripheral	______________________
3. cephalad	______________________
caudad	______________________
4. proximal	______________________
distal	______________________
5. ventral	______________________
dorsal	______________________
6. volar	______________________
plantar	______________________
7. varus	______________________
valgus	______________________
8. dextral	______________________
sinistral	______________________
levo	______________________
9. anterior	______________________
posterior	______________________

11. The actual diagnosis and treatment of diseases is referred to as ______________. A clinic is a place where persons go for ______________ of diseases. Ambulatory refers to the ability of a sick person to ______________.

12. The following terms are related to the diagnosis and treatment of disease. The term physical refers to the __________. The physical exam includes the following:

    1. ______________
    2. ______________
    3. ______________
    4. ______________
    5. ______________

13. Vital signs include the following signs:

    1. ______________
    2. ______________
    3. ______________
    4. ______________

14. The purpose of a physical examination is to find __________ of disease. The purpose of the recording of a medical history is to evaluate ______________ of a disease.

15. The following are clinical terms related to the diagnosis of disease conditions. Match column A with column B.

Column A	Column B
1. _____ acute	A. to know beforehand
2. _____ anomaly	B. leads to a favorable recovery
3. _____ benign	C. falls with particular disease process
4. _____ chronic	D. complete knowledge of a disease
5. _____ diagnosis	E. signs and symptoms run together
6. _____ malignant	F. irregular, deviation from normal
7. _____ metastatic	G. brief, severe condition
8. _____ prognosis	H. becoming progressively worse and may result in death
9. _____ sign	I. involves the whole body
	J. a condition that lasts a long time
	K. an observable occurrence
	L. a disease that spreads from one place to another
	M. a wasting away of an organ or part

10. ____ symptom
11. ____ syndrome
12. ____ systemic
13. ____ atrophy

16. The following terms are related to the treatment of disease. Match column A with column B.

Column A	Column B
1. ____ drug	A. branch of medicine dealing with the treatment of disease with drugs
2. ____ internist	B. a chemical substance
3. ____ internal medicine	C. a physician who works with his or her hands
4. ____ operation	D. the act of treating disease with instruments
5. ____ surgeon	E. root word meaning drug
6. ____ surgery	F. treating disease
7. ____ therapeutics	G. a physician who deals with internal medicine
8. ____ therapy	H. the branch of medicine dealing with the treatment of diseases by operation or the application of devices
9. ____ pharmo	I. healing

17. The following sets of terms are related to disease. Using the list of words complete the following statements:

Set 1

agenesis	infectious
cancer	neoplastic
congenital	sepsis
degenerative	trauma
exacerbation	

1. A ____________ condition means that the child is born with the disease.
2. A disease that is spread from one person to another is said to be ____________.
3. The term that means new growth is ____________.
4. A condition in which a disease is becoming increasingly severe is known as ____________.
5. The presence in the blood of organisms capable of producing a breakdown of tissue is called ____________.

6. The breakdown in the structure of a part is called a ______________ disease.

7. The congenital absence of a body structure is called ______________.

8. A wound to the body or mind is called ______________.

9. A disease that can be fatal is referred to as ______________.

Set 2
Write in the cause of the following types of disease.

bacterial: ______________

fungal: ______________

helminthic: ______________

parasitic: ______________

viral: ______________

Set 3
Match column A with column B. Choose the one best answer.

Column A	Column B
1. ____ endemic	A. disease of unknown cause
2. ____ epidemic	B. disease occurring in a particular group of people
3. ____ pandemic	C. disease that is the side effect of treatment prescribed by a physician
4. ____ iatrogenic	D. disease that originates while a person is in the hospital
5. ____ idiopathic	E. disease spread over a large group of people in a particular area
6. ____ nosocomial	F. widespread disease

PRETEST/ POSTTEST **ANSWERS** FOR CHAPTER **5**

1. soma, somato, corpse, psycho

2. **1.** C **2.** A **3.** D **4.** E **5.** B

3. **1.** A **2.** D **3.** B **4.** E **5.** C

4. **1.** hollow spaces
   2. front
   3. chest, pleural, mediastinum, heart, lungs, large blood vessels, esophagus
   6. back
   7. brain
   8. spinal cord
   9. torso, trunk

4. belly, celiac, laparo
5. abdominal, large intestine, rectum, urinary bladder, reproductive organs

5.
1. over, stomach
2. groin
3. above, pubic
4. lumbar
5. under, ribs

6. right upper quadrant, left upper quadrant, right lower quadrant, left lower quadrant

7.
1. cervical
2. thoracic
3. lumbar
4. sacral
5. coccyx

8.
1. face
2. nape of the neck
3. shoulder
4. thumb
5. top of the head
6. groin
7. thigh
8. hand
9. armpit
10. neck
11. ankle
12. instep
13. hand
14. skin
15. back of the knee
16. chest
17. head
18. great toe
19. knee
20. finger or toe
21. upper arm
22. limb, arm, or leg
23. jaw
24. finger or toe
25. chin
26. wrist
27. chin
28. elbow
29. hand
30. buttocks

9. **1.** C **2.** A **3.** B **4.** C **5.** A **6.** B

10.
1. above or directed upward
   below or directed downward
2. pertaining to the middle
   pertaining to the sides
   bearing around the circumference
3. toward the head
   toward the tail
4. closest to
   farthest away
5. front
   back
6. palm of hand
   sole of foot
7. bent inward
   bent outward
8. right
   left
   left
9. in front of
   in back of

11. clinical medicine, diagnosis and treatment, walk around

12. body

1. inspection
2. palpation
3. percussion
4. auscultation
5. various measurements

13. **1.** temperature
2. pulse
3. respiratory rate
4. blood pressure

14. signs, symptoms

15. **1.** G **2.** F **3.** B **4.** J **5.** D **6.** H **7.** L **8.** A **9.** K **10.** C **11.** E **12.** I **13.** M

16. **1.** B **2.** G **3.** A **4.** D **5.** C **6.** H **7.** F **8.** I **9.** E

17. **Set 1**

1. congenital
2. infectious
3. neoplastic
4. exacerbation
5. sepsis
6. degenerative
7. agenesis
8. trauma
9. cancer

Set 2

bacteria, fungus, worms, parasite, virus

Set 3

1. B **2.** E **3.** F **4.** C **5.** A **6.** D

PART TWO

6 THE SKELETAL SYSTEM

OBJECTIVES

At the end of this chapter you will be able to do the following:

1. List and describe the mechanical and biological functions of the skeletal system.
2. List the components of the skeletal system.
3. Define terms related to the descriptive anatomy and bones.
4. Describe cartilage and ligaments.
5. Name the major bones of the skeletal system.
6. State the meaning of the names of various bones of the body.
7. Describe the relationship of the skeletal system with other systems of the body.
8. Analyze selected diagnostic terms, including terms related to signs and symptoms.
9. Analyze selected terms related to disease conditions.
10. Analyze selected terms related to the treatment of disease conditions.

FUNCTIONS OF THE SKELETAL SYSTEM

There are five functions of the skeletal system. Three functions are mechanical and two are biological. (See Table 6-1.)

CONSTITUENTS OF THE SKELETAL SYSTEM

The skeletal system consists of three elements:

bones
cartilage
ligaments

Bone

Bone is a dense connective tissue made up mostly of calcium and phosphate; *os-*, *ossa-*, *oste-*, and *osteo-* are all combining forms that have the meaning "bone."

TABLE 6-1
Functions of the Skeletal System

Function	Parts of the Skeletal System That Carry on This Function
	Mechanical Functions
framework for the body	bones, cartilage, ligaments
levers for muscles	appendicular skeleton: made of bones that are levers for the action of muscles* pectoral girdle: the shoulders and arms pelvic girdle: the hips and legs
protection	axial skeleton: made of bones surrounding body cavities cranial and facial bones: protect the brain vertebral column: protects the spinal cord ribs, costal cartilages, and sternum: protect the organs in the chest, including the lungs and heart pelvis: protects the organs in the pelvic cavity
	Biological Functions
production of blood	bone marrow
storage of calcium and phosphate	matrix of bone

* A lever is a relatively rigid structure to which movable muscles are attached to allow for movement of areas of the body.

A fibrous membrane called *periosteum* (*peri* = around, *osteum* = bone) covers the bones on all surfaces except at moving joints. *Articular cartilage* covers the bones at these joints. Periosteum contains blood vessels that penetrate into the underlying bone.

A bone consists of three rings of tissue:

compact bone: the hard external surface.
cancellous, or *spongy bone:* the internal ring.
medullary canal: the center (*medius* = middle, *ulla* = small) of bone that contains the bone marrow. Bone marrow has relative proportions of red marrow and yellow, or fatty, marrow depending on an individual's age and condition. Blood cells are produced by cells in the bone marrow. *Myel(o)-* is the combining form meaning "marrow."

Terms related to bone cells:

osteoblasts: cells that form (*blast*) bone (*osteo*)
osteoclasts: cells that break down (*clast*) bone (*osteo*)
osteocytes: bone cells

Osteocytes are constantly being formed. The process of bone cell production is referred to as *ossification*.

Descriptive anatomy of bones

There are many terms used to describe the anatomy of bones themselves. Following are groups of selected terms that you should learn.

Terms related to *shapes* of bones:

long bones: limbs.
short bones: hands and feet.
flat bones: skull and ribs.
irregular bones: spinal column and skull.
sesamoid bones: patella (knee cap): *Sesamoid* means "resembling a sesame seed."

Terms related to *parts* of bones:

body: broadest or longest part of a bone.
diaphysis: the shaft of long cylindrical bone. The root word *physis* means "that which grows." The part of the bone that grows *(physis)* between *(dia)* the ends.
epiphysis: ends of long bones. The part of the bone that grows (*physis*) upon (*epi*) the bone.
epiphyseal line: growth center for elongation of bone. This is found between the shaft and the ends of bone.
metaphysis: wider part of bone next to (*meta*) the epiphysis.
neck: narrow part of a bone near the head of the bone.

Terms related to *depressions, openings,* or *surfaces* of bone:

alveolus: small saclike dilatation, such as is found in the jawbone for the teeth
aditus: entrance to *(ad)* a cavity
antrum: a cavity or chamber within a bone
foramen: a hole through a bone
fossa: a hollow place, pit, cavity, or depression
glenoid: a depression, particularly in the scapula (shoulder blade)
lamina: a thin, flat area
meatus: a tube-shaped opening
sinus: a cavity or spongelike area in a bone
sulcus: a groove, trench, furrow, or depression

Terms related to *projections* or *processes* that fit into joints:

apophyseal: any outgrowth of bone. *Apo* means "away from."
process: a projection large enough to be grasped with the fingers.
condyle: a rounded, knucklelike projection.
head: a rounded projection beyond the neck of the bone.
malleolus: a rounded process such as at the medial and lateral sides of the ankles. Malleolus means small *(olus)* hammer *(malles).*

Terms related to *projections* or *processes* to which muscles attach:

crest: a ridge
line: a prominent area
spine: (spinous process) a sharp projection

tuberosity: a rounded projection (*tuber*)
tubercle: a small, rounded projection *(tuber)*

Selected terms related to other projections from *bones:*

capitulum: a small eminence on a bone. The term means small *(ulum)* head *(capit)*
epicondyle: an eminence on a bone above the condyle.
eminence: a prominence on the surface of a bone.
olecranon: the head *(cran)* of the bone at the elbow.
protuberance: a swellinglike area on a bone that can be felt.
ramus: a small projection that comes off of a larger structure in a branchlike fashion.
styloid: a long, pointed process that resembles a pole.
trochlea: a pulleylike structure.

Selected terms related to *attachments** of bones:

articulation: a connection between bones; a joint.
joint: a place where bones join.
insertion: a place of attachment of a muscle to the bone it moves. This exists only on a movable bone.
origin: a place of attachment of a muscle to a bone that is the lever for the specific muscle.

Names of *specific processes*:

acromion: the process at the tip (*acro*) of the shoulder (*om*).
coracoid: the process of the scapula that is like (*oid*) a raven's beak (*cora*).
coronoid: the process of the mandible shaped like (*oid*) a crow's beak (*coron*).
mastoid: the breastlike [breast (*mast*), like (*oid*)] projection of the temporal bone.
odontoid: the tooth-shaped [tooth (*odent*), shaped (*oid*)] process of the axis, which is the second cervical vertebra.
trochanter: a very large process on the side of the femur.
xiphoid: the swordlike [sword (*xiph*), like (*oid*)] process of the lower end of the sternum.

Cartilage

There are two types of cartilage in the skeletal system.

Hyaline cartilage, which is very elastic, cushiony, and slippery, makes up the articular surfaces at the joints, the cartilage between the ribs, at the nose, larynx, and trachea, and the fetal skeleton. It has a pearly, bluish color. *Hyaline* means "glass."

White fibrocartilage, which is also elastic, flexible, and tough, is interarticular fibrocartilage found in joints such as the knee. The connecting fibrocartilage is a cartilage that is only slightly mobile. It is found between the vertebrae, referred to as *disks,* and between the pubic bones, the *symphysis pubis.*

* See Chapter 8.

Ligaments

Where the bones of the skeleton join, there is a joint or articulation. Movable joints are covered by cartilage and are held together by ligaments.

Ligaments are made of white fibrous tissue. They are pliant, flexible, strong, and tough.

Terms related to ligaments will be covered in Chapter 8.

THE SKELETAL SYSTEM

Figures 6-1 and 6-2 show the major bones of the skeletal system. Study the terms related to the names of the bones.

One way to study the names of the bones is to look at the figure and starting at the top of the picture of the skeleton, say the name of the bone aloud. Locate and touch the bone on your own body and repeat the name of the bone. Do this until you can readily indicate the names of the bones in your own skeleton without the help of the diagram. Making the association of names of bones with the bones in your body will help you remember the names.

Following the diagrams are tables listing groups of bones. Use these tables to study the names of bones not shown in the diagram.

Groups of Bones

Bones may be put into groupings according to the region of the body they are in.

Following is a list of bone groupings to be used to study the names of bones:

group 1: bones of the skull
group 2: bones of the trunk
group 3: bones of the pectoral girdle
group 4: bones of the pelvic girdle

Group 1: Bones of the skull

skull: the group of bones making up the shell (*skull*) of the head.

cranium: the part of the skull enclosing the brain.

frontal: pertaining to (*al*) the bone in the front.

occipital: pertaining to (*al*) the bone in the back of the head (*occiput*).

parietal: pertaining to (*al*) the bones that make up the walls (*parietis*) of the skull.

temporal: pertaining to (*al*) the bones at the side, or temple, of the skull.

sphenoid: the wedge-shaped [wedge (*sphen*), shaped (*oid*)] bone at the base of the cranium.

ethmoid: the sievelike [sieve(*ethm*), like (*oid*)] bone at the base of the cranium (not shown in Figures 6-1 or 6-2).

facial bones: pertaining to (*al*) the bones making up the face.

nasal: pertaining (*al*) to the bone at the nose (*nas*).

zygomatic bones: the bones that are yoked (*zygoma*) into an arch. This bone has a malar (cheek) surface that is the cheekbone.

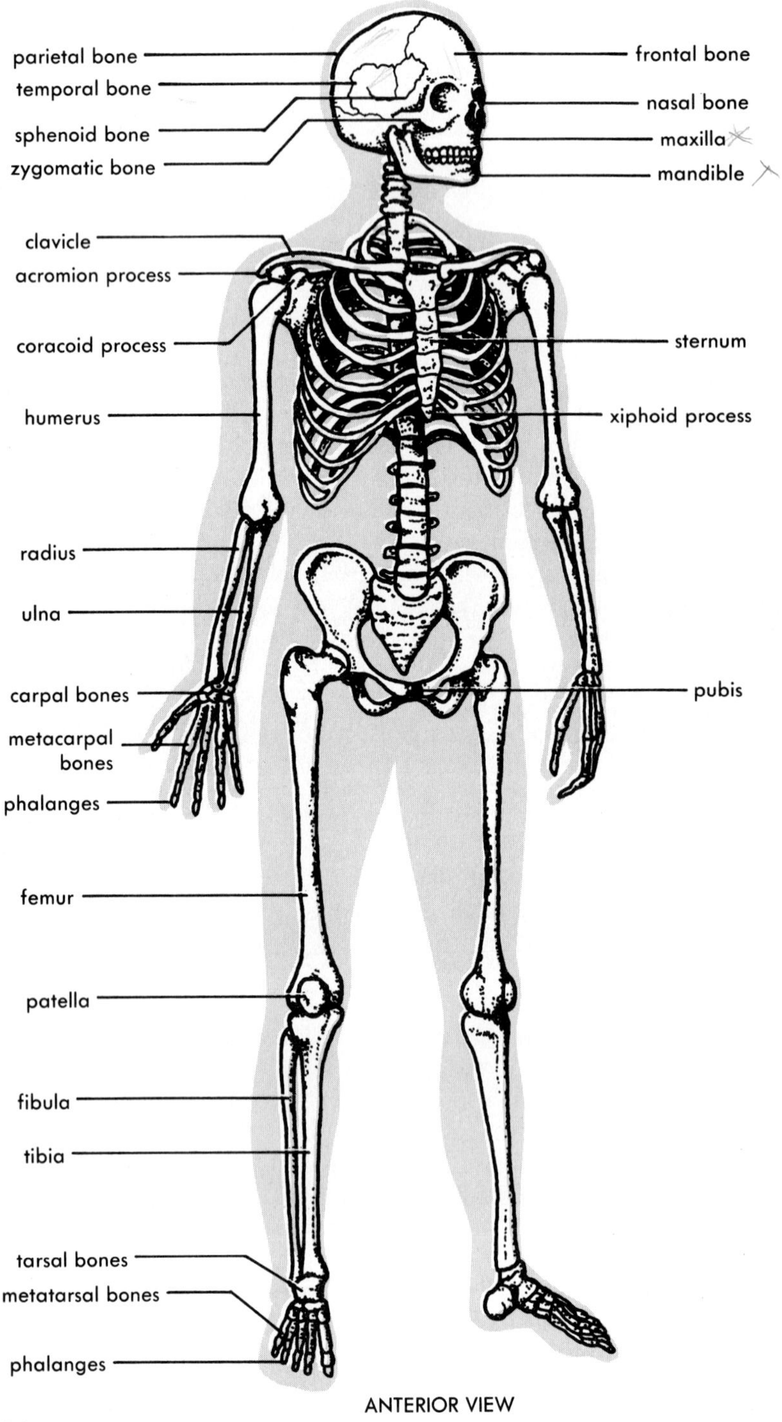

FIGURE 6-1
Anterior view of the human skeletal system.

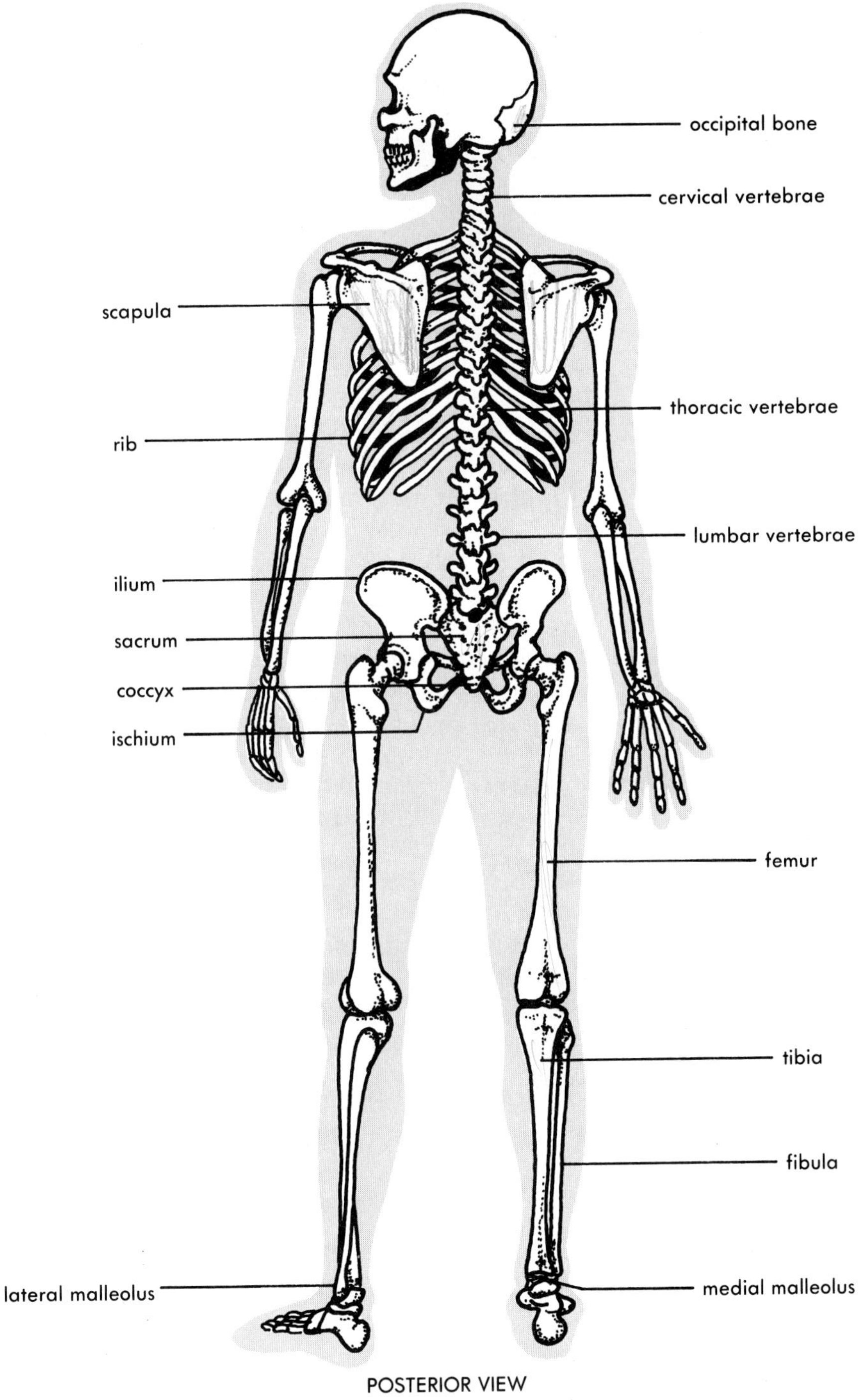

FIGURE 6-2
Posterior view of the human skeletal system.

turbinates (*conchae*): the bones in the nose that look like shells (*conchae*) or turbans (not shown in Figures 6-1 or 6-2).
palatine: the bone at the roof (*palate*) of the mouth (not shown in figures).
vomer: the bone resembling a plowshare (*vomer*) that forms part of the nasal septum (not shown in Figures 6-1 or 6-2).
hyoid: the bone shaped like (*oid*) the Greek letter upsilon (υ) (not shown).
maxilla: the bone of the upper jaw. The term literally means little (*illa*) cheek (*max,* variation of *mala*).
mandible: the bone of the lower jaw which moves to permit chewing (*mandere,* to chew).

Group 2: Bones of the trunk

vertebrae: there are 26 separate vertebrae in the backbone of an adult. The name vertebrae comes from the word to turn *(vert)*. A combining form that means vertebrae is *spondylo-*. The vertebrae are subdivided as follows:

cervical vertebrae: there are seven cervical vertebrae. These are the bones of the neck (*cervix*). C1 is the first cervical vertebra and is also called the *atlas* or *atlanto*. This vertebra holds the head. C2 is the second vertebra and is called the *axis* on which the atlas sits to allow the head to turn. C3 to C6 make up the neck. C7 is the *vertebra prominens,* which is at the base of the neck. It is called *prominens* because it can be felt.

thoracic vertebrae: the 12 vertebrae in the back thorax or chest cavity.

lumbar vertebrae: the five vertebrae of the lumbar (loin) region. These are the largest and strongest vertebrae.

sacral vertebrae (*sacrum*): the five fused vertebrae of the sacrum, usually counted as single vertebra in the adult. The name means "sacred"; this was a bone used in sacrificial ceremonies. It is triangular in shape and can be remembered by associating it with "sacred trinity."

coccygeal vertebrae (*coccyx*): a bone made of four fused vertebrae that resembles the bill of a cuckoo (*coccyx*) bird.

Ribs: there are 12 ribs. Ribs are the bones that form the thoracic cavity, or chest wall. *True ribs* are the seven ribs that are directly attached to the sternum. *False ribs* are the five ribs that are not directly attached to the sternum. Three are attached by cartilage, and two are unattached to the sternum. These two are attached only to the thoracic vertebrae in back and are sometimes called the "floating ribs."

Sternum: the bone that makes up the anterior border of the thoracic cavity. It is also called the *breast bone.* It is made of three parts:

manubrium: which is the uppermost portion. The word means "handle," and the manubrium appears to be the handle of the sternum.

body: main part of the sternum.

ziphoid process: the lower swordlike [sword (xiph), like (oid)] projection from the sternum.

Group 3: Bones of the pectoral girdle

The pectoral (*pector* = chest) (*al* = pertaining to) girdle is the bony arch that attaches the upper arm to the axial skeleton at the chest.

clavicle: the bone of the shoulder called the "collarbone." It resembles a key (*clavicle*).

scapula: the other bone of the shoulder. Also called the *shoulder blade* because of its triangular, bladelike appearance. It has, among other projections, the acromion process and the coracoid process.

humerus: the long single bone in the upper arm. Sometimes referred to as the *brachium.* This bone is commonly called the "funnybone"; associate *humerus* with humor.

ulna: the larger of the two bones in the forearm. It is on the small-finger side.

radius: the smaller of the bones in the forearm. It is on the thumb side of the arm and allows the arm to move in a radial (*radius*) motion.

carpal: the bones in the wrist. There are eight carpal bones in two rows.

metacarpal bones: the bones that are next (*meta*) to the wrist (*carpal*) bones. There are five of these bones in each hand, four in the palm of the hand and one at the base of the thumb.

phalanges: the bones of the thumb and fingers. The term means "line of soldiers" (*phalanx*). There are 14 in each hand; 3 in each finger and 2 in the thumb. There are also phalanges in the foot.

Group 4: Bones of the pelvic girdle

pelvis: sometimes called the *innominate bone,* or the bone without (*in*) a name (*nominate*). The word *pelvis* means "basin." The pelvis is made of three bones:

- *ilium:* the large, superior portion of the hip. This is also called the *os coxa,* or the bone (*os*) of the hip (*coxa*).
- *ischium:* the inferior, dorsal part of the hip. The bone you sit on.
- *pubis:* the anterior bone of the hip at the base of the trunk. The term pubis leads to terms such as puberty, the evidence of which is the appearance of hair over the pubic bone.
- *symphysis pubis:* the area where the two pubic bones (pubis) grow (*physis*) together (*sym*).

femur: the thighbone. This is the longest and strongest bone of the body. A large process near the head of this bone is called the *greater trochanter. Trochanter* means "runner." The femur is the bone which takes the greatest strain when a person runs.

patella: the kneecap. It gets its name from its resemblance to a small (*ella*) shallow dish (*pat*). The patella is also the largest of the sesamoid bones.

tibia: a pipe-shaped bone that is the larger, inner bone of the lower leg. Also called the *shinbone.*

fibula: the smaller (*ula*) outer bone of the lower part of the leg.

tarsal bones: the bones of the ankle. There are seven tarsal bones in each ankle, the largest of which is the *calcaneus,* or heelbone. Also called the *os calcis.*

metatarsal bones: the bones of the foot next to (*meta*) the ankle (*tarsal*) bones. There are five in each foot, one to each of the toes.

phalanges: the small bones in the toe that correspond to the phalanges (*phalanx*) of the fingers. There are two phalanges in the great toe, and three in each of the smaller toes.

DISEASES OF THE SKELETAL SYSTEM

Disease conditions of the skeletal system are closely associated with conditions of the muscular and articular systems. They may also be associated with conditions of the nervous system.

The following terms related to diseases of the skeletal system may occasionally include word roots related to conditions of the articular system.

Selected Diagnostic Terms

This will be an analysis of selected diagnostic terms, including terms related to signs and symptoms of disease conditions of the skeletal system.

bone biopsy: the excision of a small piece of bone for microscopic examination
bone marrow test: the insertion of a needle through the bone into the medullary canal (*marrow*) to take a sample of bone marrow
coccygodynia: a condition in which there is pain (*dynia*) in the tailbone (*coccyx*)
crepitation: the grating sound (*crepitus*) at the site of a bone fracture or at other sites where bones rub together
monostotic: pertaining (*ic*) to one (*mon*) bone (*ostot*)
polyostotic: pertaining (*ic*) to many (*poly*) bones

Selected Terms of Disease Conditions

This section is an analysis of selected terms related to disease conditions of the skeletal system.

achondroplasia: a condition (*ia*) in which there is a lack of (*a*) growth (*plas*) of the ends of long bones that are covered with cartilage (*chondr*)
aseptic necrosis of the hip: a condition (*osis*) in which there is destruction and death (*necr*) of bone cells in the hip joint that are not (*a*) associated with infection (*septic*)
avascular necrosis of the hip: a condition (*osis*) in which there is destruction and death (*necr*) of bone cells in the hip joint as a result of the lack (*a*) of blood vessels (*vascular*) that supply blood and nourishment
bunion: a turniplike (*bunion*) protrusion on the inner surface of the foot near the joint of the big toe
callus: a new, hard (*callus*) bone formation at the site of a bone fracture
cervical rib: a congenital overdevelopment of the costal (*rib*) projection of the seventh cervical vertebrae. The overgrown projection resembles a rib.

chondroma: a tumor (*oma*) that arises from cartilage (*chondr*)
coxa plana: a disease condition in which the head of the femur, which is part of the hip (*coxa*) joint, becomes flattened (*plana*)
dwarfism: a condition in which a person is smaller than normal
exostosis: a condition (*osis*) in which there is excessive (*ex*) formation of bone (*ost*) making a protuberance on the bone
fibrous dysplasia: abnormal (*dys*) formation (*plasia*) in which fibrous tissue (*fibrous*) replaces bone tissue
fracture: a condition in which there is a break in a bone
multiple myeloma: multiple tumors (*oma*) of the bone marrow (*myel*) that replace normal bone cells
myositis ossificans: the formation (*ficans*) of bone (*ossi*) in a muscle (*myo*) that has been inflammed (*itis*)
osteitis deformans: inflammation (*itis*) of bone (*oste*) that results in deformity (*deformans*) of bony structures
osteoarthritis: inflammation (*itis*) of the bone (*osteo*) at the joint (*arthr*)
osteochondritis: inflammation (*itis*) of bone (*osteo*) and cartilage (*chondr*)
osteochondroma: a tumor (*oma*) of the bone and the cartilage (*chondr*) covering the bone
osteochondrosis: a group of disease conditions (*osis*) involving growth centers of bone (*osteo*) and the articular cartilage (*chondr*), e.g., coxa plana, listed earlier
osteoclasia: a condition (*ia*) in which bone (*osteo*) is destroyed (*clas*)
osteodystrophies: a group of diseases in which there is a disturbance (*dys*) in the growth (*trophy*) of bone (*osteo*)
osteogenesis imperfecta: a disease in which the production (*genesis*) of bone (*osteo*) is imperfect (*imperfecta*)
osteogenic sarcoma: a tumor (*oma*) of connective tissue (*sarc*) arising (*genic*) in bone (*osteo*)
osteoma: a tumor (*oma*) of bone (*osteo*)
osteomalacia: a condition in which the bones (*osteo*) become softened (*malacia*)
osteomyelitis: a condition in which the bone (*osteo*) and bone marrow (*myel*) are inflammed (*itis*)
osteopenia: a condition in which there is a decrease (*penia*) in the bone (*osteo*) mass of bony structures
osteoporosis: a condition (*osis*) in which the bone (*osteo*) becomes porous (*por*)
sequestrum: a section of bone that has become necrotic and has separated (*sequestrum*) from the healthy bone
spondylitis: an inflammation (*itis*) of the spine (*spodyl*)
syndactylism: a condition in which the fingers or toes (*dactyl*) have grown together (*syn*)

Selected Terms of Treatment

This section will analyze selected terms related to the treatment of conditions of the skeletal system.

ablation: the surgical removal of a part of a bone.
alignment: the act of putting bones back in the natural position.
amputation: the removal of a part of the body; the cutting off of a part of the body, especially the cutting off of an extremity.
carpectomy: the removal of the wrist bones.
condylectomy: removal of a condyle.
disarticulation: the process (*ion*) in which the joint (*articula*) is taken apart (*dis*) and the limb is cut off at the joint.
diskectomy: the removal of the intervertebral cartilage (*disk).*
fixation: the use of metal devices to hold (*fix*) a fractured bone in its set position.
grafting: the placement of bone fragments from a normal or donor site in a diseased site.
manipulation: the skilled treatment or handling of a part of the body, such as a fractured bone or dislocated joint.
osteoclasis: the surgical fracture or breaking (*clasis*) of bone to bring about a change in alignment.
osteoplasty: the reconstruction or repair (*plasty*) of a bone (*osteo).*
osteotomy: the surgical procedure in which bone (*oste*) is cut into (*otomy).*
osteotripsy: the procedure of crushing (*tripsy*) a part of bone (*osteo*).
prosthetic devices: specially designed equipment (*devices*) put (*pros*) in the place (*thesis*) of a missing part of the body.
reduction: the nonsurgical manipulation done to return (*reduce*) fractured bones to their normal alignment. This is a *closed reduction.* An *open reduction* involves the surgical procedure done to reduce a fractured bone.
replantation: the reattaching of a limb that has been severed.
saucerization: creation of a saucerlike depression in a bone.
scapulopexy: the shoulder blade (*scapula*) is fixed (*pexy),* or made immovable, by attaching it to the ribs.
sequestrectomy: the removal of (*ectomy*) a portion of dead bone (*sequestrum).*
spinal fusion: the joining (*fusion*) together of two or more vertebrae.

PRETEST/ POSTTEST FOR CHAPTER 6

1. There are three mechanical and two biological functions of the skeletal system. List them.

Mechanical	Biological
1. ______________	1. ______________
2. ______________	2. ______________
3. ______________	

2. What are the three parts of the skeletal system?

   1. ______________ 2. ______________ 3. ______________

3. List four combining forms meaning bone.

   1. ________ 2. ________ 3. ________ 4. ________

4. The following terms are related to bone structure. Match column A with column B.

Column A	Column B
1. _____ compact bone	A. a bone cell
2. _____ cancellous	B. marrow
3. _____ medullary canal	C. cells that form bone
4. _____ bone marrow	D. produces blood cells
5. _____ myelo-	E. internal ring, spongy bone
6. _____ osteoblasts	F. process of bone-cell production
7. _____ osteoclasts	G. center of bone
8. _____ osteocytes	H. hard external surface
9. _____ ossification	I. cells that break down bone

5. The following terms are related to the descriptive anatomy of bones. There are eight sets of terms.

   Set 1: Terms related to *shapes* of bones
   List the five shapes of bones:

   1. ______________
   2. ______________

3. ____________________

4. ____________________

5. ____________________

Set 2: Terms related to *parts* of bones
Match column A with column B. There are two answers to a few items in column A.

Column A	Column B
1. _____ body	A. the shaft
2. _____ diaphysis	B. the part that grows on the bone
	C. the part that grows between the ends of bone
3. _____ epiphysis	D. narrow part near the head
4. _____ epiphyseal line	E. broadest or longest part of a bone
	F. growth center for elongation of bone
5. _____ metaphysis	G. the ends of long bone
6. _____ neck	H. wide part next to the epiphysis

Set 3: Terms related to *depressions, openings,* or *surfaces* of bone
Write in the meaning of the term.

1. alveolus ____________________
2. aditus ____________________
3. antrum ____________________
4. foramen ____________________
5. fossa ____________________
6. glenoid ____________________
7. lamina ____________________
8. meatus ____________________
9. sinus ____________________
10. sulcus ____________________

Set 4: Terms related to *projections* or *processes* that fit into joints
Write the meaning of the term.

1. apophyseal ____________________
2. process ____________________
3. condyle ____________________
4. head ____________________
5. malleolus ____________________

Set 5: Terms related to *projections* to which *muscles* attach
Write the meaning of the term.

1. crest ____________
2. line ____________
3. spine (spinous process) ____________
4. tuberosity ____________
5. tubercle ____________

Set 6: Terms related to *other projections* from bones
Write the meaning of the term.

1. capitulum ____________
2. epicondyle ____________
3. eminence ____________
4. olecranon ____________
5. protuberance ____________
6. ramus ____________
7. styloid ____________
8. trochlea ____________

Set 7: Terms related to *attachments* of bone
Write in the meaning of the term.

1. articulation ____________
2. joint ____________
3. insertion ____________
4. origin ____________

Set 8: Terms related to names of *specific processes*
Write in the meaning of the term.

1. acromion ____________
2. coracoid ____________
3. coronoid ____________
4. mastoid ____________
5. odontoid ____________
6. trochanter ____________
7. xiphoid ____________

6. Name the two types of cartilage found in the skeletal system.

1. ____________________
2. ____________________

7. Fill in the blank: Movable joints are covered by cartilage and are held together by ____________________.

8. Label the major bones of the skeletal system as shown in Figures 6-3 and 6-4.

9. The following are bones of the skull. Match column A with column B.

Column A	Column B
1. _____ skull	A. bone in back of skull
2. _____ cranium	B. pertaining to the face
3. _____ frontal	C. sievelike bone
4. _____ occipital	D. resembles turbans or shells
5. _____ parietal	E. upper jaw
6. _____ temporal	F. shell of the head
7. _____ sphenoid	G. the yoked bones
8. _____ ethmoid	H. bone in front of skull
9. _____ facial	I. resembles a plowshare
10. _____ nasal	J. wedge-shaped bone
11. _____ zygomatic	K. cheekbones
12. _____ malar surface	L. resembles Greek letter upsilon
13. _____ turbinates or conchae	M. enclosing the brain
14. _____ palatine	N. pertaining to the nose
15. _____ vomer	O. bones at the temples
16. _____ hyoid	P. lower jaw
17. _____ maxilla	Q. roof of the mouth
18. _____ mandible	R. walls of the skull

10. The following are bones of the trunk. Match column A with column B.

Column A	Column B
1. _____ vertebrae	A. vertebra holding the head
2. _____ spondylo-	B. vertebrae of the loin
	C. bones of the chest wall

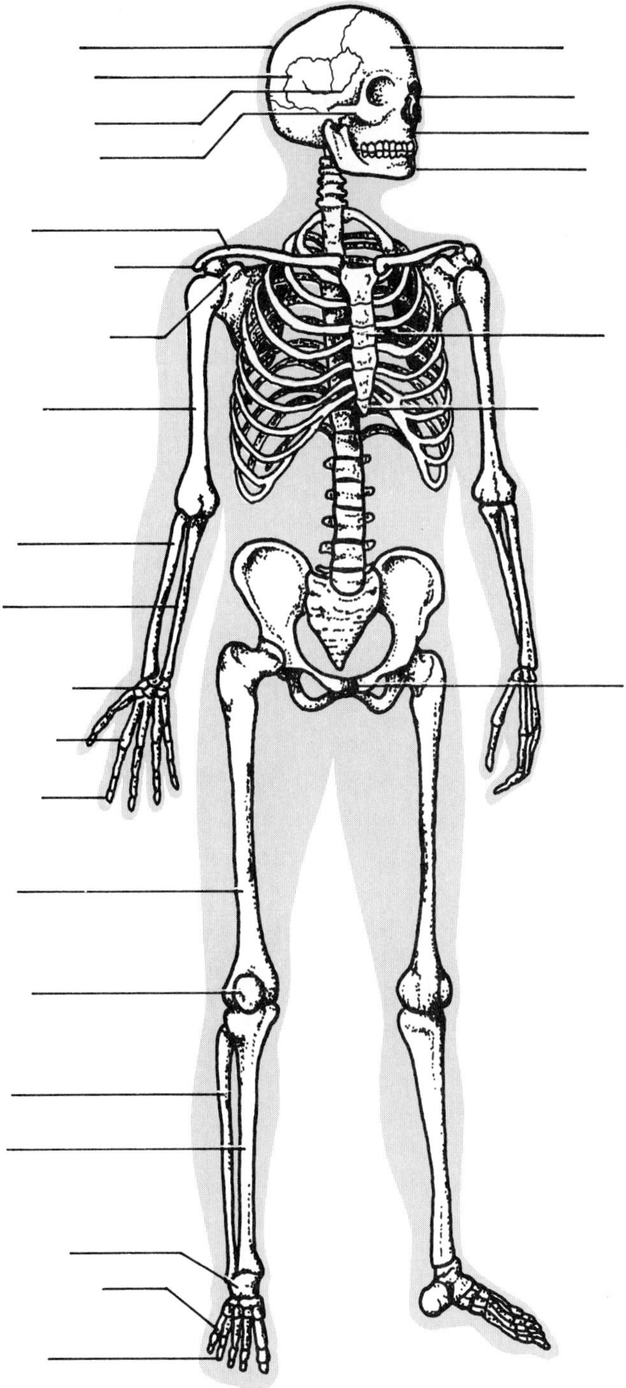

FIGURE 6-3
Anterior view of the human skeletal system.

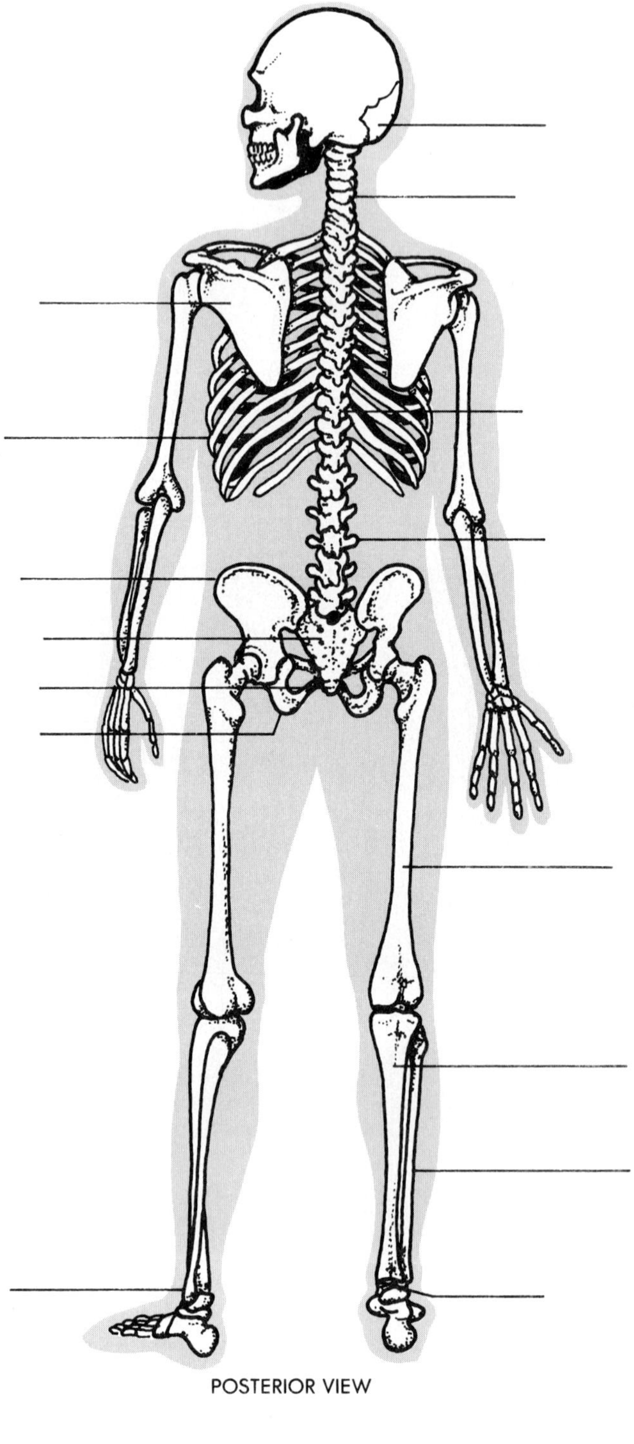

FIGURE 6-4
Posterior view of the human skeletal system.

Column A	Column B
3. ____ cervical vertebrae	D. vertebra that allows head to turn
4. ____ atlas	E. swordlike projection from the sternum
5. ____ axis	F. vertebrae of the back and chest
6. ____ prominens	G. means "to turn"
7. ____ thoracic vertebrae	H. the breastbone
8. ____ lumbar vertebrae	I. bones of the neck
9. ____ sacral vertebrae	J. cervical vertebrae that may be felt
10. ____ coccygeal vertebrae	K. the handle or upper part of the sternum
11. ____ ribs	L. five fused vertebrae
12. ____ sternum	M. combining form meaning vertebrae
13. ____ manubrium	N. tailbone
14. ____ xiphoid process	

11. The following bones are found in the pectoral girdle; the shoulder and upper extremity. Match column A with column B. There are two answers for some items in column A.

Column A	Column B
1. ____ clavicle	A. single bone of the upper arm
2. ____ scapula	B. bones in fingers and thumb
3. ____ humerus	C. small bone in the forearm on the thumb side
4. ____ ulna	D. larger bone in the forearm
5. ____ radius	E. bones of the wrist
6. ____ carpal bones	F. the collarbone
7. ____ metacarpal bones	G. shoulder blade
8. ____ phalanges	H. the brachium
	I. bones in the hand
	J. resembles a key
	K. allows the arm to turn

12. The following bones are found in the pelvic girdle: the pelvis and lower extremities. Match column A with column B.

Set 1: The pelvis

Column A	Column B
1. ____ pelvis	A. anterior bone at the base of the trunk
2. ____ innominate	B. place where the pubic bones grow together
	C. shaped like a basin

Column A	Column B
3. _____ ilium	D. superior portion of the hip
4. _____ ischium	E. means "without a name"
5. _____ os coxa	F. the "bone of the hip"
6. _____ pubis	G. inferior portion of the hip
7. _____ symphysis pubis	

Set 2: The lower extremity. In this set there are two correct answers for one of the items in column A.

Column A	Column B
1. _____ femur	A. knee cap
2. _____ trochanter	B. large process on the femur
3. _____ patella	C. anklebone
4. _____ tibia	D. thighbone
5. _____ fibula	E. bones of the toes
6. _____ tarsal bones	F. shinbone
7. _____ metatarsal bones	G. outer, thinner bone of the lower leg
8. _____ phalanges	H. bones of the foot
9. _____ os calcis or calcaneous bone	I. inner, larger bone of the lower leg
	J. heelbone

13. Fill in the blanks: Diseases of the skeletal system are closely related to diseases of the __________ system and __________ system. They may also be associated with diseases of the __________ system.

14. The following list relates to diagnostic terms and signs and symptoms. Match column A with column B.

Column A	Column B
1. _____ bone biopsy	A. grating sound
2. _____ bone marrow test	B. involving many bones
3. _____ coccygodynia	C. pain in the tailbone
4. _____ crepitation	D. involving only one bone
5. _____ monostotic	E. excision of a small piece of bone for examination
6. _____ polyostotic	F. examination of medullary canal contents

15. The following sets of items are related to disease conditions of the skeletal system. Match column A with column B.

Set 1

Column A

1. _____ achondroplasia
2. _____ aseptic necrosis
3. _____ avascular necrosis
4. _____ bunion
5. _____ callus
6. _____ cervical rib
7. _____ chondroma
8. _____ coxa plana
9. _____ dwarfism
10. _____ exostosis
11. _____ fibrous dysplasia
12. _____ fracture
13. _____ multiple myeloma
14. _____ myositis ossificans
15. _____ osteitis deformans

Column B

A. tumor from cartilage
B. excessive bone formation
C. hip disease in which the head of femur is flattened
D. formation of bone cells in muscle
E. cell destruction from lack of blood vessels to supply blood
F. turniplike protrusion
G. new bone forms at fracture site
H. small person
I. cell destructs without infection
J. fibrous tissue replaces bone tissue
K. lack of growth of the ends of long bones
L. break in a bone
M. many bone marrow tumors
N. bone inflammation results in deformity
O. riblike growth from the seventh cervical vertebra

Set 2

Column A

1. _____ osteoarthritis
2. _____ osteochondritis
3. _____ osteochondroma
4. _____ osteochondrosis
5. _____ osteoclasia
6. _____ osteodystrophies
7. _____ osteogenesis imperfecta
8. _____ osteogenic sarcoma
9. _____ osteoma

Column B

A. imperfect production of bone
B. connective tissue tumor arising in bone
C. inflammation of bone and cartilage
D. group of diseases in which there is disturbance in growth
E. decrease in bone mass
F. condition in which bone is destroyed
G. bone tumor
H. inflammation of bone at joint
I. bone and marrow inflamed
J. softened bones
K. tumor of bone and cartilage covering the bone

Column A	Column B
10. _____ osteomalacia	L. porous bones
11. _____ osteomyelitis	M. group of diseases of the growth centers of bone and articular cartilage
12. _____ osteopenia	
13. _____ osteoporosis	

Set 3
Fill in the blanks:

1. Sequestrum is a condition in which a section of bone has become necrotic and has ____________________ from the healthy bone structure.
2. Spondylitis means ____________________ of the __________.
3. In syndactylism, the ____________________ have ____________________.

16. The following sets of terms are related to the treatment of bone diseases. Match column A with column B.

Set 1

Column A	Column B
1. _____ ablation	A. removal of wrist bones
2. _____ alignment	B. placement of bone fragments from a normal site in a diseased site
3. _____ amputation	C. removal of a condyle
4. _____ carpectomy	D. cutting off part of the body
5. _____ condylectomy	E. use of metal devices to hold a fracture in position
6. _____ disarticulation	F. surgical removal of a part
7. _____ diskectomy	G. removal of intervertebral cartilage
8. _____ fixation	H. putting things in a natural or straight line
9. _____ grafting	I. skilled handling of a part of the body
10. _____ manipulation	J. the joint taken apart, and the limb taken off

Set 2

Column A	Column B
1. _____ osteoclasis	A. reconstruction, repair of bone
2. _____ osteoplasty	B. creation of a saucerlike depression in a bone
3. _____ osteotomy	C. equipment put in the place of a missing part of the body
4. _____ osteotripsy	D. removal of portion of dead bone

Column A	Column B
5. _____ prosthetic devices	E. reattachment of severed limb
6. _____ reduction	F. surgical breaking of bone
7. _____ replantation	G. cutting into bone
8. _____ saucerization	H. action to return bone to its natural position
9. _____ scapulopexy	I. two or more vertebrae joined together
10. _____ sequestrectomy	J. the shoulder blade fixed into position
11. _____ spinal fusion	K. crushing of bone

PRETEST/ POSTTEST **ANSWERS** FOR CHAPTER **6**

1. **1.** framework for the body
   2. levers for muscles
   3. protection
   1. production of blood
   2. calcium phosphate and storage

2. **1.** bones **2.** cartilage **3.** ligaments

3. **1.** os- **2.** ossa- **3.** oste- **4.** osteo-

4. **1.** H **2.** E **3.** G **4.** D **5.** B **6.** C **7.** I **8.** A **9.** F

5. **Set 1**
   1. long
   2. short
   3. flat
   4. irregular
   5. sesamoid

   Set 2
   1. E **2.** A, C **3.** B, G **4.** F **5.** H **6.** D

   Set 3
   1. small saclike dilation
   2. entrance to a cavity
   3. cavity or chamber
   4. hole through a bone
   5. hollow place, pit, cavity
   6. depression in the scapula
   7. thin flat area
   8. tube-shaped opening
   9. cavity or spongelike area
   10. groove, trench, furrow

Set 4
1. any outgrowth from bone
2. projection large enough to be grasped
3. knucklelike, rounded projection
4. rounded projection beyond neck of bone
5. rounded, small, hammerlike process

Set 5
1. ridge
2. prominent area
3. sharp projection
4. rounded projection
5. small, rounded projection

Set 6
1. small, headlike eminence
2. eminence above the condyle
3. prominence on surface of a bone
4. head of the bone at the elbow
5. swellinglike area that can be felt
6. branchlike structure
7. long, polelike process
8. pulleylike structure

Set 7
1. connection between bones, a joint
2. place where bones join
3. place muscle attaches to the bone it moves
4. place of attachment of muscle to the bone which is the lever for the specific muscle

Set 8
1. process at tip of the shoulder
2. process of scapula, resembles raven's beak
3. process of mandible, resembles crow's beak
4. breastlike projection of temporal bone
5. tooth-shaped process of the axis
6. large process on side of femur
7. swordlike process of lower end sternum

6. **1.** hyaline cartilage
2. white fibrocartilage

7. ligaments

8. Refer to Figures 6-1 and 6-2.

9.

1. F	**4.** A	**7.** J	**10.** N	**13.** D	**15.** I	**17.** E
2. M	**5.** R	**8.** C	**11.** G	**14.** Q	**16.** L	**18.** P
3. H	**6.** O	**9.** B	**12.** K			

10. **1.** G **2.** M **3.** I **4.** A **5.** D **6.** J **7.** F **8.** B **9.** L **10.** N **11.** C **12.** H **13.** K **14.** E

11. **1.** F, J **2.** G **3.** A, H **4.** D **5.** C, K **6.** E **7.** I **8.** B

12. **Set 1**

1. C **2.** E **3.** D* **4.** G* **5.** F **6.** A **7.** B

Set 2

1. D **2.** B **3.** A **4.** F†, I‡ **5.** G† **6.** C **7.** H **8.** E **9.** J

13. muscular, articular, nervous

14. **1.** E **2.** F **3.** C **4.** A **5.** D 6. B

15. **Set 1**

1. K **2.** I **3.** E **4.** F **5.** G **6.** O **7.** A **8.** C **9.** H **10.** B **11.** J **12.** L **13.** M **14.** D **15.** N

Set 2

1. H **2.** C **3.** K **4.** M **5.** F **6.** D **7.** A **8.** B **9.** G **10.** J **11.** I **12.** E **13.** L

Set 3

1. separated
2. inflammation, spine or vertebrae
3. toes or fingers, grown together

16. **Set 1**

1. F **2.** H **3.** D **4.** A **5.** C **6.** J **7.** G **8.** E **9.** B **10.** I

Set 2

1. F **2.** A **3.** G **4.** K **5.** C **6.** H **7.** E **8.** B **9.** J **10.** D **11.** I

---

* To remember the difference between these terms, think that the ischium has an *h* that resembles a chair. You sit on a chair. Thus, the ischium is the bone on which you sit.

† To remember these terms, think that the suffix ula means small. The fibula is smaller than the tibia.

‡ The tibia, being large, is called the shinbone because it can be felt in the shin.

7 THE MUSCULAR SYSTEM

OBJECTIVES

At the end of this chapter you will be able to do the following:

1 Define muscle.
2 List three types of muscle in the body.
3 Name the parts of a skeletal muscle.
4 Define *tendon* and *aponeurosis.*
5 Define terms related to the action of muscles.
6 Describe the agonist, antagonist, and synergist relationship of muscles.
7 Define terms used in naming muscles.
8 Identify and name selected muscles of the skeletal system.
9 Analyze diagnostic terms related to muscle disorders, including signs and symptoms.
10 Analyze terms related to disease conditions of muscles.
11 Analyze terms related to the treatment of muscle disorders.

MUSCLE TISSUE

Muscle tissue is found in many organs of the body. Muscle tissue also makes up muscles that are themselves organs. These muscles give the body shape and produce movement.

Terms related to muscles:

muscle: this term means little (*cle*) mouse (*mus*); possibly so called because of the appearance of some muscles, or the rippling action of some muscles.
myo-: a combining form meaning "muscle."

There are three types of muscle in the body, smooth, cardiac, and skeletal muscle.

Smooth Muscle

This type of muscle is located in the viscera, in the walls of arteries and veins, and in the digestive, respiratory, reproductive, and urinary systems.

Terms related to smooth muscle:

involuntary: the action of these muscles is not (*in*) consciously controlled (*voluntary*). The actions are automatic.
leio-: a combining form meaning "smooth."
unstriated: muscle not (*un*) striped (*striated*) in microscopic appearance.

Cardiac Muscle

The muscle of the heart.

Terms related to cardiac muscle:

cardio-: combining form meaning "heart."
myocardio-: combining form meaning "muscle (*myo*) of the heart."

Skeletal Muscle

The muscles attached to the skeleton.

Terms related to skeletal muscles:

creat-: a combining form meaning "flesh."
rhabdo-: a combining form meaning "striated."
striated: these muscles appear striped (*striated*) under the microscope.
voluntary: the actions of these muscles are consciously (*voluntary*) controlled.

SKELETAL MUSCLE

The information in this chapter deals with skeletal muscles. Each skeletal muscle is made up of sections. It has two ends, which are attached to other structures, and a belly.

Terms related to sections of a muscle:

origin: the end of a muscle that is attached to the bone which does not move when the muscle contracts
belly: the long extension of the body of the muscle
insertion: the end of a muscle attached to the bone which moves when the muscle contracts

Muscles are held together by a sheath of connective tissue called *fascia.*

Terms related to fascia:

fascia: a layer of thin, fibrous tissue between muscles or enclosing muscles (*fascial sheath*)
fascicle: a small (*cle*) bundle (*fasci*) of muscle fibers

Muscles are attached to other muscles and to bones by tendons and aponeuroses, which are bands of tissue continuous with muscle and bone.

Terms related to muscle attachment:

tendon: a band of cordlike, strong, nonelastic fibrous tissue. It is a stretched (*tendo*) end of a muscle. Example: *tendocalcaneus,* the tendon (*tendo*) attached to the heelbone (*calcaneus*). This is the largest tendon in the body and is also known as the *Achilles tendon.*

aponeurosis: a wide, flat, thin band of tissue formed by the expansion of a tendon. It develops from (*apo*) the tendon (*neuro* here means tendon) and is continuous with it.

ACTION OF SKELETAL MUSCLE

Muscles cause and permit motion by the action of contraction and relaxation.

Contraction refers to the reduction in size or the shortening of a muscle. When one muscle contracts, another opposite muscle is stretched and put in a state of tension.

Relaxation occurs when there is a reduction of tension and thus a return to the size of the resting muscle.

Muscles work in pairs of agonists and antagonists.

Agonists are muscles responsible for the primary desired movement. The agonist is the prime mover.

Antagonists are the muscles that oppose the action of the agonists.

Synergists are muscles that assist the agonist by holding a part of the body steady and thus giving leverage.

The agonist-antagonist-synergist relationship permits the skeletal muscles to work in a purposeful manner and gives fluidity to motion. This is referred to as *coordination.*

Terms related to the action of muscles:

agonist: a contracting (*agony* = struggle) muscle, the prime mover
antagonist: a muscle that works against (*ant*) a contracting muscle (*agonist*)
coordination: the movement of the body in which the muscles work together (*co*) with order (*ordinat*)
kine: a root word meaning "motion"
relaxation: the loosening or stretching out (*laxa*) again (*re*) of a tightened or contracted muscle
sthen: a combining form meaning "strength"
synergist: a muscle that works (*ergist*) with (*syn*) another muscle
tone (tonus): the ability of a muscle to hold a partial steady contraction, which gives the muscle firmness

NAMES OF SKELETAL MUSCLES

There are over 400 skeletal muscles in the body. There are only 200 names because there are similar muscles on the right and left sides of the body. For example, the deltoid muscle is the triangular muscle of the shoulder, and there is a right deltoid muscle and a left deltoid muscle.

Most names of muscles indicate one or more of the variations listed in Table 7-1.

Most muscles come in pairs. Often if there is a muscle that extends a part, there is also a muscle that flexes that part. As an example, flexor carpi ulnaris flexes the wrist, and extensor carpi ulnaris extends the wrist.

TABLE 7-1
Terms Used to Name Muscles

Variation	Root Word	Meaning
Size	maximus	largest
	minimus	smallest
	major	larger
	minor	smaller
	longus	long
	brevis	short
	vastus	great, large, vast
	gracilis	slender, delicate
Shape	cuneiform	wedge-shaped
	deltoid	triangular
	fusiform	spindle-shaped
	latus	broad
	lumbricale	wormlike
	penniform	featherlike, pennate
	platy-	flat
	pterygoid	winglike
	pyramidal	cone-shaped
	quadrilateral	four-sided
	rhomboid	four-sided with opposite sides parallel
	serratus	sawlike edge
	teres	long and round
	trapezoid	four-sided with two parallel sides
Fiber arrangement	bipennate	muscle fibers joining a central tendon from both sides in a featherlike fashion
	unipennate	muscle fibers joining a central tendon from one side
	curved	fibers in a bent arrangement
	oblique	a somewhat slanted or angled arrangement
	parallel	fibers that extend in the same direction and do not cross or separate
	rectus	straight
	transversus	lying across
Action	adductor	muscle moving a part toward the midline
	abductor	muscle moving a part away from the midline
	flexor	muscle that bends a part
	extensor	muscle that straightens a part
	levator	muscle that raises a part
	depressor	muscle that lowers a part
	tensor	muscle that tightens a part
Number of divisions of a muscle	triceps	muscle having three (*tri*) heads (*ceps*)
	biceps	muscle having two (*bi*) heads (*ceps*)
	quadriceps	muscle having four (*quadri*) heads (*ceps*)
	digastric	muscle with two (*di*) bellies (*gastric*)
Points of attachment (selected examples)	sternocleidomastoid	muscle attached to the sternum, the collarbone (*cleido*), and the mastoid process of the temporal bone
	peroneus longus	long muscle attached to the fibula (*peroneus*)

(*Continued.*)

TABLE 7-1
Terms Used to Name Muscles *(continued)*

Variation	Root Word	Meaning
Location (selected examples)	intercostal	between (*inter*) the ribs (*costal*)
	tibialis posterior	behind the tibia
	epicranial	upon (*epi*) the skull (*cranium*)
	medial pterygoid	wing-shaped (*pterygoid*) muscle toward the midline (*medial*)
	subclavius	muscle under (*sub*) the clavicle (*clavius*)
	extensor digitorum profundus	deeply (*profundus*) situated muscle that extends (*extensor*) the finger (*digitorum*)
Miscellaneous		
Muscles named according to the specific body areas they control, cf. Chapter 5, objective 7		
(Selected examples)	orbicularis oris	muscle that encircles the mouth (*oris*)
	palmaris longus	long (*longus*) muscle of the palm of the hand
	extensor pollicis brevis	short (*brevis*) muscle that extends the thumb (*pollicis*)
	iliopsoas	muscle from the ilium and loin (*psoas*)
Muscle names with unusual associations		
(Selected examples)	sartorius	muscle that is stretched when a person sits tailor-fashion (*sartorial*)
	masseter	muscle which aids in chewing (*masseter*)

Hints on How to Learn the Names of the Skeletal Muscles

Look at the figures (Figures 7-1 and 7-2) showing the major skeletal muscles. Say the name of the muscle out loud. Refer to your medical dictionary to help you correctly pronounce the difficult names.

Following each illustration is a listing of the muscles indicated in that illustration. The name of the muscle has been analyzed in these tables (Tables 7-2 and 7-3).

The illustrations do not show all of the muscles of the body. Not all variations of the terms in Tables 7-2 and 7-3 are included in this selected list. If you learn the names of bones and the terms listed in Tables 7-2 and 7-3, you should be able to understand the names of muscles not listed.

TABLE 7-2
Analysis of Names of Muscles Listed in Figure 7-1 in Descending Order

Anterior View—Right Anatomical Side
temporalis: muscle over the temporal (*temporalis*) bone
masseter: muscle of chewing (*masseter*) or mastication
sternocleidomastoid: muscle attached to the breastbone (*sterno*), the collarbone (*cleido*), and the mastoid (*mastoid*) process of the temporal bone

TABLE 7-2
Analysis of Names of Muscles Listed in Figure 7-1 in Descending Order *(continued)*

Anterior View—Right Anatomical Side

deltoid: triangular (*deltoid*) muscle of the shoulder

serratus anterior: sawtooth-shaped [sawtooth (*seratus*)] muscle in front of (anterior) the shoulder

triceps brachii: three-headed [three (*tri*), headed (*ceps*)] muscle of the arm (*brachii*)

pronator teres: long, round (*teres*) muscle that turns the palm downward into a prone (*pronator*) position

flexor carpi radialis: muscle that flexes (*flexor*) the wrist (*carpi*) toward the radius (*radialis*)

palmaris longus: long (*longus*) muscle of the palm (*palmaris*) of the hand

flexor carpi ulnaris: muscle that flexes (*flexor*) the wrist (*carpi*) and hand and is attached to the ulna

tensor fascia lata: muscle that tenses (*tensor*) the fascia of the thigh (*fascia lata*)

pectineus: muscle from the pubic (*pectineus*) bone

gracilis: slender (*gracilis*) muscle of the thigh

vastus lateralis: large (*vastus*) part of the quadriceps muscle on the lateral (*lateralis*) side of the leg. The quadriceps muscle is a muscle with four (*quadri*) heads (*ceps*).

peroneus longus: long (*longus*) muscle attached to the fibula (*peroneus*)

tibialis anterior: muscle in front (*anterior*) of the tibia (*tibialis*)

extensor hallucis longus: long (*longus*) muscle that extends (*extensor*) the great toe (*hallucis*)

Anterior View—Left Anatomical Side

frontalis: muscle over the frontal bone

orbicularis oculi: muscle circling (*orbicularis*) the eye (*oculi*)

orbicularis oris: muscle circling (*orbicularis*) the mouth (*oris*)

trapezius: four-sided, trapezoid-shaped (*trapezius*) muscle of the shoulder

pectoralis major: large (*major*) muscle of the chest (*pectoralis*)

biceps brachii: muscle with two (*bi*) heads (*ceps*) in the arm (*brachii*)

brachioradialis: muscle that extends from the upper arm (*brachii*) to the radius (*radialis*)

external oblique: outermost (*external*) muscle that is at an angle (*oblique*) from the ribs to the hip

rectus abdominis: muscle that extends in a straight (*rectus*) line upward across the abdomen (*abdominis*); the center border of the left and right rectus abdominis muscles is the *linea alba,* or the white (*alba*) line (*linea*) at the midline of the abdomen

iliopsoas: muscle that is formed from the iliacus and psoas major muscles. The iliacus muscle extends from the iliac bone (*iliacus*); the *psoas major* muscle is the large (*major*) muscle of the loin (*psoas*)

adductor longus: long (*longus*) muscle that moves the leg toward (*adductor*) the midline

rectus femoris: part of the quadriceps muscle that is straight (*rectus*) and lies near the femur (*femoris*)

sartorius: muscle of the leg that enables a person to sit in a cross-legged tailor's (*sartorial*) position

vastus medialis: large (*vastus*) part of the quadriceps muscle that is toward the midline (*medialis*)

gastrocnemius: muscle that makes up the belly (*gastroc*) of the lower leg (*nemius*)

soleus: muscle that resembles a flat fish (*sole*)

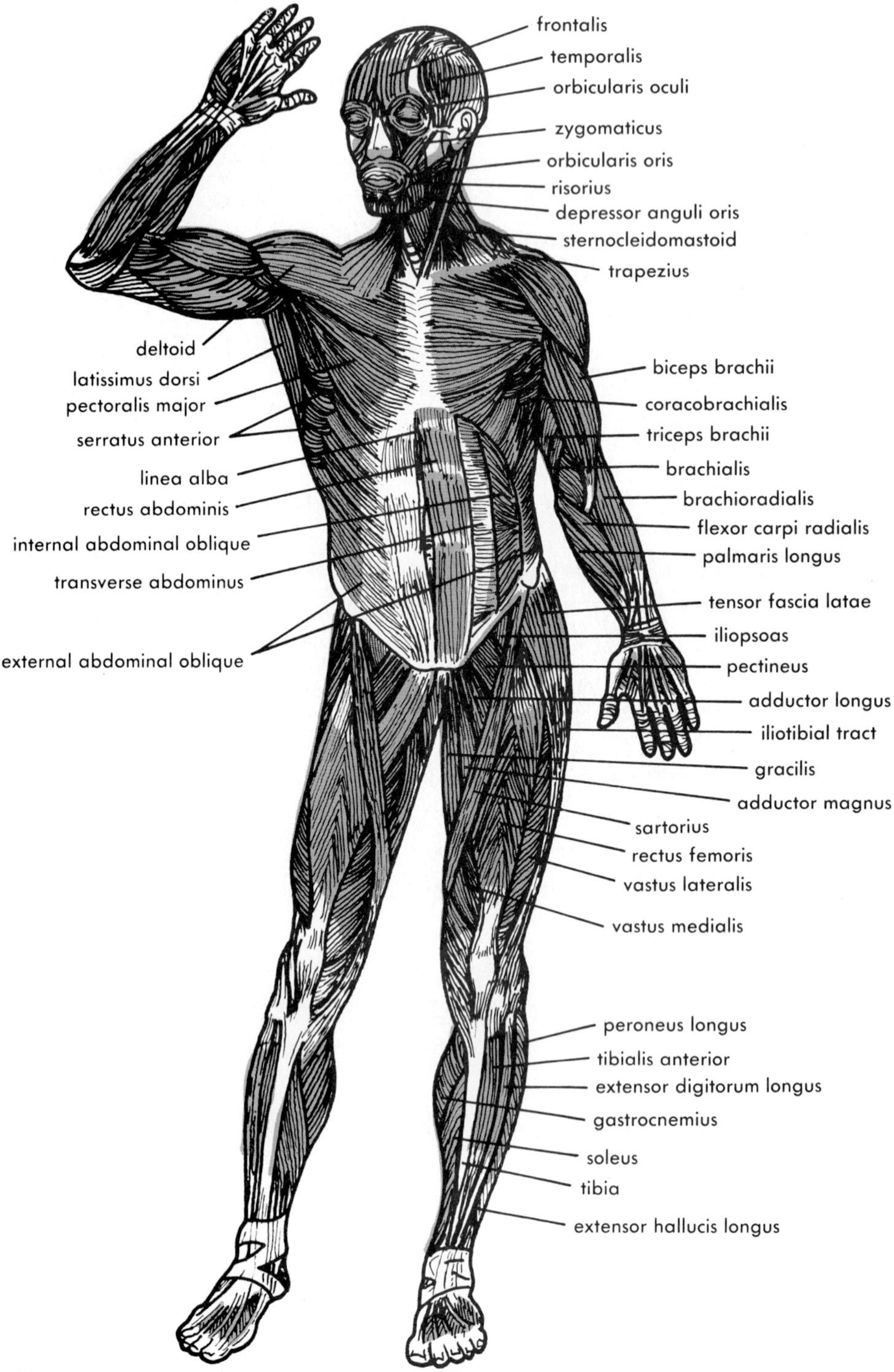

FIGURE 7-1
Anterior view of the muscular system.

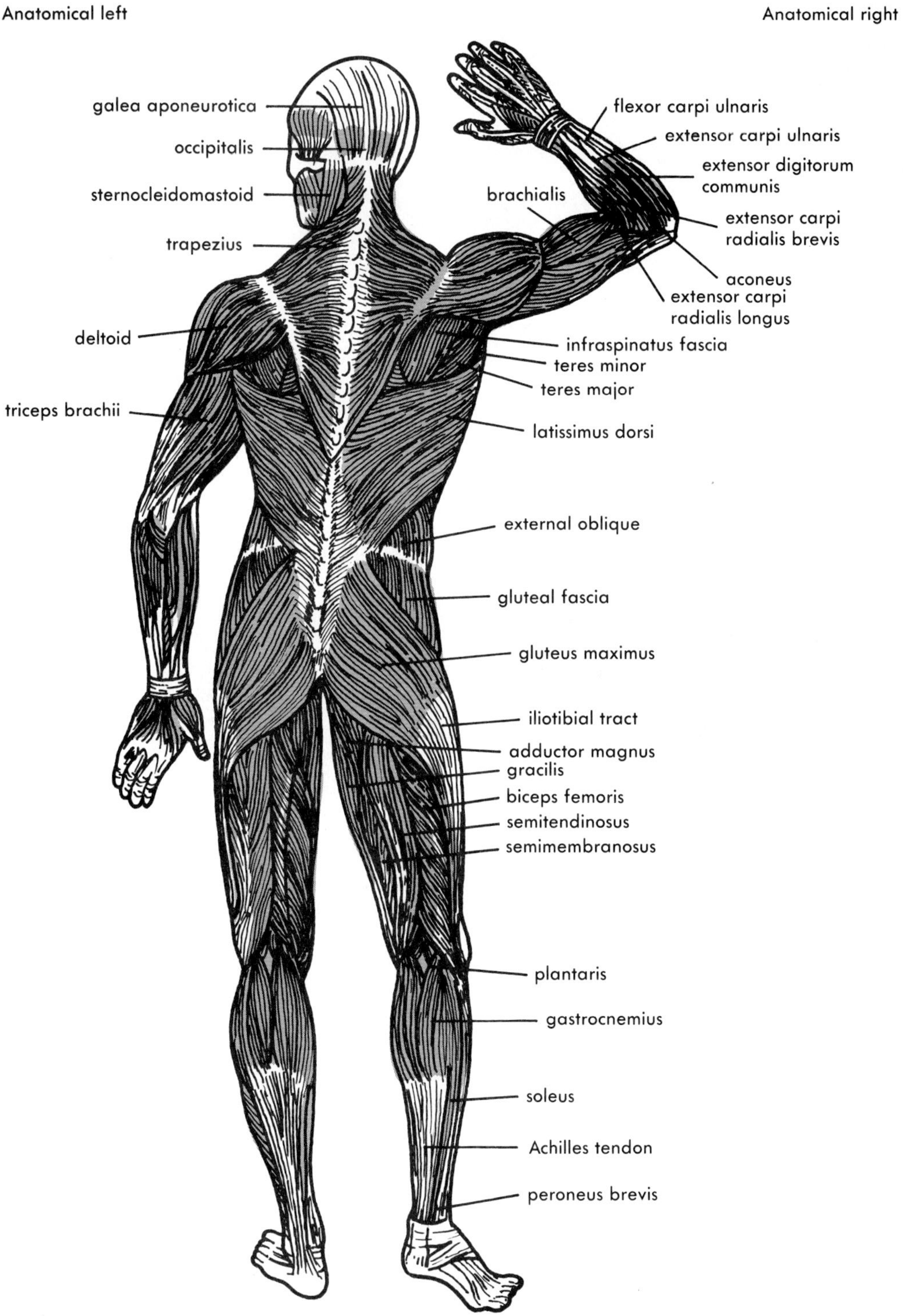

FIGURE 7-2
Posterior view of the muscular system.

DISORDERS OF THE MUSCULAR SYSTEM

Disorders of the muscular system may occur because of problems in skeletal muscle tissue itself, or they may be associated with diseases of the nervous system, which affect the purposeful movement of the skeletal muscles, or disorders of the circulatory system, which supplies blood to the muscle.

Diagnostic Terms of Muscular Conditions

Analysis of diagnostic terms related to conditions of muscles, including signs and symptoms:

asthenia: condition (*ia*) in which there is a lack (*a*) of strength (*sthen*); weakness.
calisthenics: exercise of muscles that results in beautiful (*cali*) strength (*sthen*).
clonic spasm: series of rapidly repeated (*clonic*) muscular contractions (*spasm*).
clonus: alternating muscular contraction and relaxation in rapid succession when a muscle is passively stretched.
contracture: shortening (*contracture*) of muscular tissue. A flexion contracture is a shortening of a muscle that results in the bending (*flexion*) of a part.
cramp: painful, prolonged spasmodic muscular contraction.
fasciculation: visible muscular action (*ation*) of a small bundle (*fascicul*) of muscles.
hyperkinesia: condition (*ia*) characterized by excessive (*hyper*) movement (*kines*).
hypotonia: condition (*ia*) of decreased (*hypo*) muscle tone (*ton*).
myalgia: muscle (*my*) pain (*algia*).
rigidity: condition in which there is stiffness and inflexibility.
rigor: condition in which there is hardness of a muscle.
spasm: sudden violent muscle contraction.
tone: normal degree of tension in muscle.
tonic spasm: prolonged (*tonic*) excessive contraction (*spasm*).
tremor: trembling or quivering of muscles.
torticollis: condition in which the neck (*collis*) is twisted (*torti*). Also called *wryneck*.

Selected Terms of Muscular Disease Conditions

Analysis of selected terms related to disease conditions of muscles:

fibromyositis: inflammation (*itis*) of the muscle (*myo*) and fibrous tissue (*fibro*).
hemiplegia: paralysis (*plegia*) of one-half (*hemi*) of the body, either right or left side.
myasthenia gravis: muscle (*my*) weakness (*asthenia*) of a very grave (*gravis*) type.
muscle atrophy: condition of muscle in which there is a lack of (*a*) growth (*trophy*), and the muscle shrinks.
muscle hypertrophy: condition of muscle in which there is an excessive (*hyper*) growth (*trophy*) or enlargement of muscle.

TABLE 7-3
Analysis of Names of Muscles Listed in Figure 7-2 in Descending Order

Posterior View—Right Anatomical Side

trapezius: see Table 7-2

deltoid: see Table 7-2

triceps brachii: see Table 7-2

extensor digitorum communis: muscle that extends (*extensor*) all (*communis*) of the fingers (*digitorum*)

extensor carpi ulnaris: muscle that extends (*extensor*) the wrist (*carpi*) and hand and is attached to the ulna (*ulnaris*)

abductor pollicis longus: long (*longus*) muscle which moves the thumb away (*abductor*) from the hand.

extensor pollicis brevis: short (*brevis*) muscle which extends (*extensor*) the thumb (*pollicis*)

adductor magnus: large (*magnus*) muscle which moves the leg toward (*adductor*) the midline

semitendinosus: muscle made up partly (*semi*) of tendinous tissue; this is one of the so-called hamstring muscles.

semimembranosus: muscle made up partly (*semi*) of membranous tissue. Also one of the hamstring muscles.

gastrocnemius: see Table 7-2

Posterior View—Left Anatomical Side

sternocleidomastoid: see Table 7-2

teres minor: a small (*minor*) long, round (*teres*) muscle that moves the arm

teres major: a larger (*major*) long, round (*teres*) muscle that moves the arm

latissimus dorsi: the broadest (*latissimus*) muscle of the back (*dorsi*)

external oblique: see Table 7-2

flexor carpi ulnaris: see Table 7-2

gluteus medius: the muscle of the buttocks (*gluteus*) that lies in the middle (*medius*) between the other gluteus muscles

gluteus maximus: the largest (*maximus*) muscle of the buttocks (*gluteus*)

biceps femoris: muscle with two (*bi*) heads (*ceps*), one of which attaches to the femur (*femoris*)

plantaris: muscle that flexes the foot (*plantaris*) and leg

peroneus longus: see Table 7-2

soleus: see Table 7-2

muscular dystrophy: condition of muscle in which there is a weakening, degeneration, or abnormal (*dys*) development (*trophy*) of muscle.

paraplegia: paralysis (*plegia*) of the lower extremities. *Para* is used loosely in this term but may be remembered by associating with the word *parallel;* thus, the term may be defined as "paralysis of the lower extremities downward from a line that is parallel to the floor."

paralysis: loosening (*lysis*) of the muscle beside (*para*) a part; thus, an inability to use the part.

pes planus: flat (*planus*) foot (*pes*).

polymyositis: inflammation (*itis*) of many (*poly*) muscles (*myo*).

rhabdomyolysis: condition in which there is a breakdown (*lysis*) of striated (*rhabdo*) muscle (*myo*).

Selected Terms of Muscular Disease Treatment

Analysis of selected terms related to the treatment of disease conditions of muscles:

myectomy: removal (*ectomy*) of a muscle (*my*) or part of a muscle
myoneurectomy: removal (*ectomy*) of the nerves (*neur*) to a specific muscle (*myo*)
myomectomy: removal (*ectomy*) of a muscle (*my*) tumor (*om*)
myoplasty: plastic surgery (*plasty*) on a muscle (*myo*)
myorrhaphy: repair of a muscle (*myo*) by suturing (*rrhaphy*)
myotomy: incision (*otomy*) into a muscle (*myo*)
physiotherapy: treatment (*therapy*) of muscle weakness by physical (*physio*) methods such as massage, heat, or exercise
traction: application of a pulling force (*traction*) to stretch a contracted muscle

PRETEST/ POSTTEST FOR CHAPTER 7

1. Fill in the blank:

The combining form of the word *muscle* is ________________.

2. There are three types of muscle tissue in the body:

A smooth muscle B cardiac muscle C skeletal muscle

In the spaces below indicate the letter, either A, B, or C, corresponding to the type of muscle to which the term is related:

1. _____ involuntary

2. _____ heart

3. _____ leio-

4. _____ striated

5. _____ rhabdo-

6. _____ voluntary

7. _____ myocardio-

8. _____ creat-

9. _____ unstriated

3. The following terms are related to parts and attachments of skeletal muscles. Match column A with column B.

Column A	Column B
1. _____ origin	A. small bundle of muscle fibers
2. _____ belly	B. the end of a muscle attached to the bone that moves
3. _____ insertion	C. stretched end of a muscle
4. _____ fascicle	D. end of the muscle attached to bone that does not move
5. _____ fascia	E. layer of thin fibrous tissue between muscles and enclosing muscles
6. _____ tendon	F. wide, flat band of tissue continuous with a tendon
7. _____ aponeurosis	G. long extension of a muscle

4. The following terms are related to the actions of contraction and relaxation of muscles. Match column A with column B.

Column A	Column B
1. _____ agonist	A. muscle that works against a contracting muscle
2. _____ antagonist	B. root word meaning motion
3. _____ contraction	C. contracting muscle, the prime mover
4. _____ coordination	D. root word meaning strength
5. _____ kine-	E. loosening of a muscle
6. _____ relaxation	F. ability to hold a partial steady contraction
7. _____ sthen-	G. reduction in length of a muscle
8. _____ synergist	H. muscle that works with other muscles
9. _____ tone	I. movement in which the muscles move together

5. The following sets of terms are related to variations in characteristics used to name muscles. In each set match column A with column B. There is only one correct answer.

Set 1: Variation in size

Column A	Column B
1. _____ maximus	A. slender, delicate
2. _____ minimus	B. smallest
3. _____ major	C. great, large
4. _____ minor	D. largest
5. _____ longus	E. larger
6. _____ brevis	F. long
7. _____ vastus	G. short
8. _____ gracilis	H. smaller

Set 2: Variation in shape

Column A	Column B
1. _____ cuneiform	A. winglike
2. _____ deltoid	B. featherlike, pennate
3. _____ fusiform	C. long and round
4. _____ latus	D. wormlike
5. _____ lumbrical	E. four-sided
6. _____ penniform	F. wedge-shaped
7. _____ platy-	G. four-sided with opposite sides parallel
8. _____ pterygoid	H. flat
9. _____ pyramidal	I. sawlike edge
10. _____ quadrilateral	J. spindle-shaped
11. _____ rhomboid	K. four-sided with two parallel and two nonparallel sides
12. _____ serratus	L. broad
13. _____ teres	M. cone-shaped
14. _____ trapezoid	N. triangular

Set 3: Variation in fiber arrangement

Column A	Column B
1. _____ bipennate	A. lying across
2. _____ unipennate	B. joining a tendon from both sides
3. _____ multipennate	C. slanted or angled arrangement
	D. joining a tendon from one side

Column A	Column B
4. _____ curved	E. extend in same direction and don't cross
5. _____ oblique	F. joining many tendons
6. _____ parallel	G. bent arrangement
7. _____ rectus	H. straight
8. _____ transversus	

Set 4: Variation in action

Column A	Column B
1. _____ adductor	A. muscle that raises
2. _____ abductor	B. muscle that straightens
3. _____ flexor	C. muscle that tightens a part
4. _____ extensor	D. muscle that moves a part away from midline
5. _____ levator	E. muscle that lowers a part
6. _____ depressor	F. muscle that moves a part toward midline
7. _____ tensor	G. muscle that bends a part

Set 5: Numbers of divisions

Column A	Column B
1. _____ triceps	A. muscle with three heads
2. _____ biceps	B. muscle with two bellies
3. _____ quadriceps	C. muscle with four heads
4. _____ digastric	D. muscle with two heads

6. In the following figures (Figures 7-3 and 7-4) identify the muscles:

7. The following diagnostic terms are related to conditions of the muscular system. Match column A with column B.

Column A	Column B
1. _____ asthenia	A. excessive movement
2. _____ calisthenics	B. normal degree of tension in muscle
3. _____ clonic spasm	C. twisted neck
4. _____ clonus	D. painful prolonged spasmodic muscle contraction
5. _____ contracture	E. shortening of muscle tissue
6. _____ cramp	F. rapidly repeated muscular contraction
	G. stiffness and inflexibility
	H. decreased muscle tone

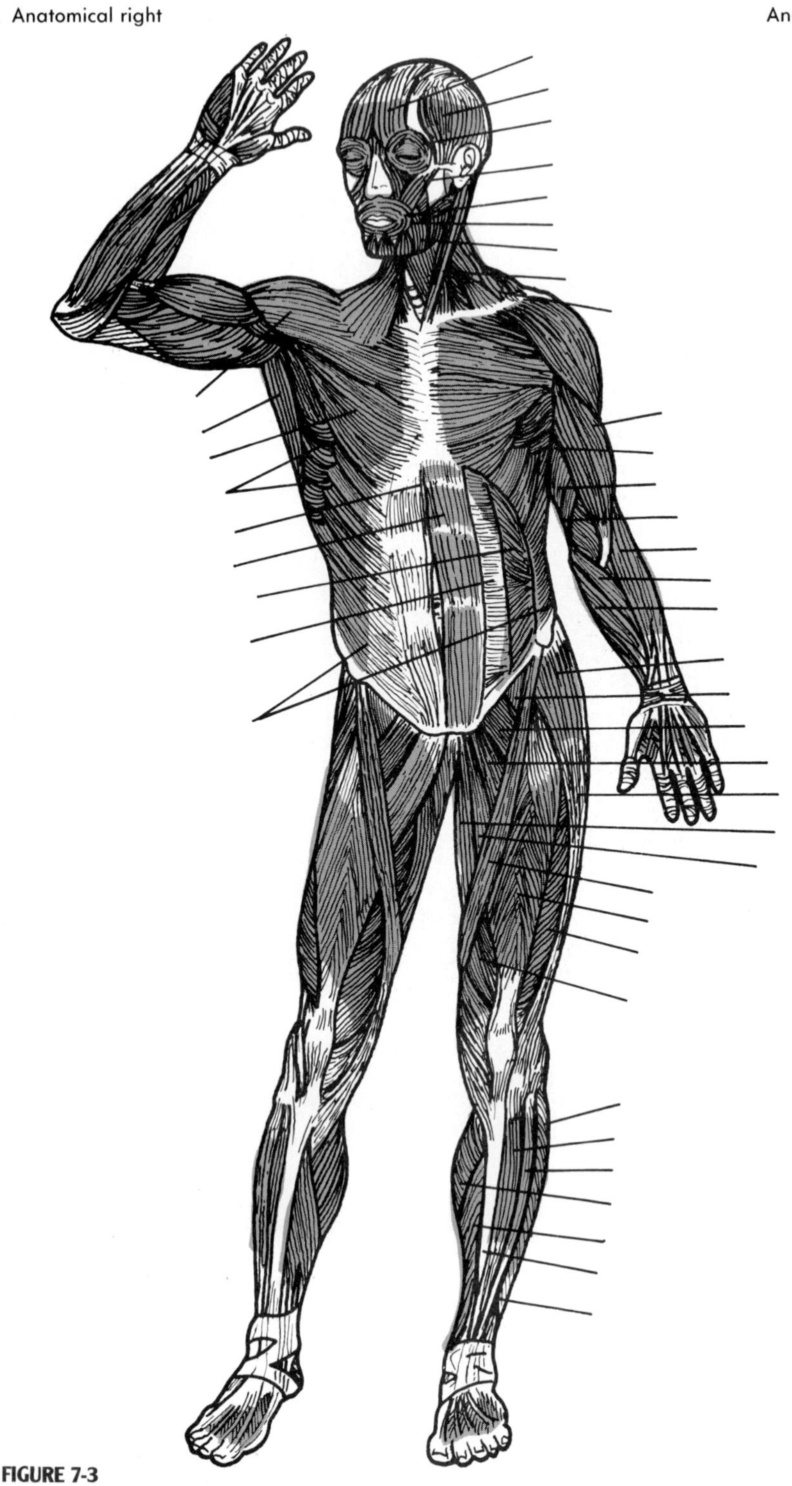

FIGURE 7-3
Anterior view of the muscular system.

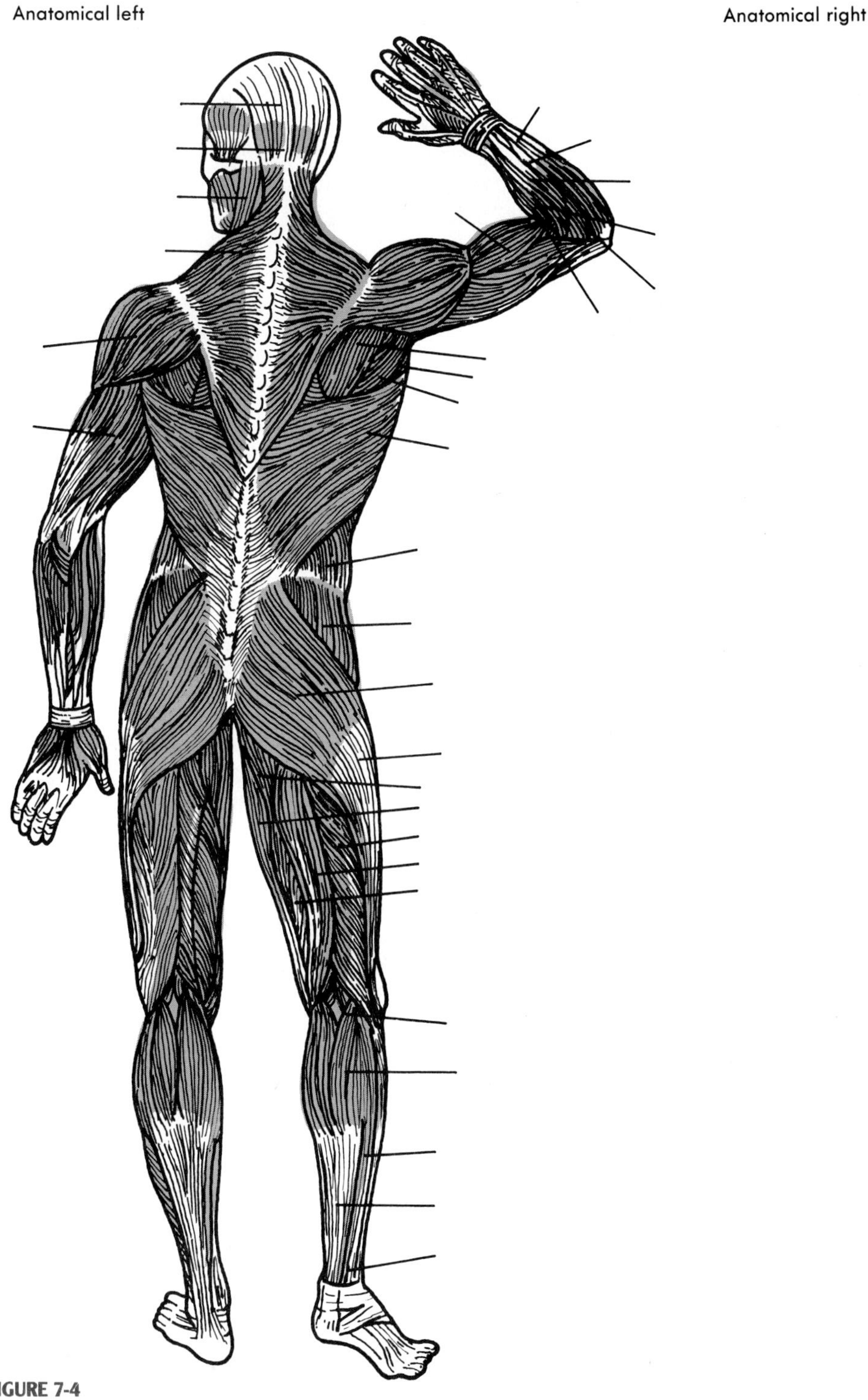

FIGURE 7-4
Posterior view of the muscular system.

Column A	Column B
7. ______ fasciculation	I. beautiful strength
8. ______ hyperkinesia	J. visible action of a small bundle of muscles
9. ______ hypotonia	K. sudden violent muscle contraction
10. ______ myalgia	L. pain in muscle
11. ______ rigidity	M. hardness in muscle
12. ______ rigor	N. lack of strength
13. ______ spasm	O. alternating muscle contraction and relaxation
14. ______ tone	P. prolonged excessive contraction
15. ______ tonic spasm	Q. trembling or quivering of muscles
16. ______ tremor	
17. ______ torticollis	

8. The following terms are related to disease conditions of the muscular system. Match column A with column B.

Column A	Column B
1. ______ fibromyositis	A. muscle weakness of a grave type
2. ______ hemiplegia	B. abnormal development of muscles
3. ______ myasthenia gravis	C. inflammation of many muscles
4. ______ muscle atrophy	D. excessive growth, muscle enlargement
5. ______ muscle hypertrophy	E. flat foot
6. ______ muscular dystrophy	F. breakdown of striated muscle
7. ______ paraplegia	G. inflammation of muscle and fibrous tissue
8. ______ paralysis	H. paralysis of left or right half of the body
9. ______ pes planus	I. lack of growth, muscle shrinks
10. ______ polymyositis	J. paralysis of the lower extremities
11. ______ rhabdomyolysis	K. inability to use a part

9. The following terms are related to the treatment of muscle disorders. Match column A with column B.

Column A	Column B
1. ______ myectomy	A. removal of muscle tumor
2. ______ myoneurectomy	B. plastic surgery on a muscle
	C. treatment by physical methods

Column A	Column B
3. _____ myomectomy	D. removal of muscle
4. _____ myoplasty	E. application of a pulling force on a muscle
5. _____ myorrhaphy	F. removal of a nerve to a muscle
6. _____ myotomy	G. incision into a muscle
7. _____ physiotherapy	H. repair of a muscle
8. _____ traction	

PRETEST/ POSTTEST **ANSWERS** FOR CHAPTER **7**

1. myo-

2. **1.** A **2.** B **3.** A **4.** B,C **5.** C **6.** C **7.** B **8.** C **9.** A

3. **1.** D* **2.** G **3.** B* **4.** A **5.** E **6.** C **7.** F

4. **1.** C **2.** A **3.** G **4.** I **5.** B **6.** E **7.** D **8.** H **9.** F

5. **Set 1**
1. D **2.** B **3.** E **4.** H **5.** F **6.** G **7.** C **8.** A

Set 2
1. F **2.** N **3.** J **4.** L **5.** D **6.** B **7.** H **8.** A **9.** M **10.** E **11.** G† **12.** I **13.** C **14.** K†

Set 3
1. B **2.** D **3.** F **4.** G **5.** C **6.** E **7.** H **8.** A

Set 4
1. F **2.** D **3.** G **4.** B **5.** A **6.** E **7.** C

Set 5
1. A **2.** D **3.** C **4.** B

---

* To learn to differentiate origin and insertion, associate the term *insertion* with a hook. The muscle inserts a hook into a bone and moves that bone.

† To learn to distinguish rhomboid and trapezoid, associate trapezoid with a flattop tent in which you can be trapped.

6. Refer to Figures 7-1 and 7-2.

7. **1.** N **2.** I **3.** F **4.** O **5.** E **6.** D **7.** J **8.** A **9.** H **10.** L **11.** G **12.** M **13.** K **14.** B **15.** P **16.** Q **17.** C

8. **1.** G **2.** H **3.** A **4.** I **5.** D **6.** B **7.** J **8.** K **9.** E **10.** C **11.** F

9. **1.** D **2.** F **3.** A **4.** B **5.** H **6.** G **7.** C **8.** E

8 THE ARTICULAR SYSTEM

OBJECTIVES

At the end of this chapter you will be able to do the following:

1. Describe the function of joints in the musculoskeletal system.
2. List three classifications of joints, and describe the degree of motion of each.
3. Define the terms related to the diarthrodial (synovial) joints.
4. Define terms related to the range of motion that is permitted by the diarthrodial joints.
5. Define and describe *bursae.*
6. Analyze terms related to pathological conditions of the articular system.
7. Analyze terms related to surgical and diagnostic procedures pertaining to joints.

FUNCTION OF JOINTS

Joints are places where bones come together, where limbs are attached, and where motion of the skeletal system occurs.

Some joints are rigid, and some allow a great degree of flexibility.

Functions of joints:

1. to allow motion of the musculoskeletal system
2. to bear weight
3. to hold the skeleton together

Terms related to the articular system:

articulation: a joint, the joining of bones
arth-, arthro-: combining forms meaning "joints"
flexibility: the capability (*ibility*) of being bent (*flex*)

TYPES OF JOINTS

There are three types of joints in the body, which are classified according to their degree of mobility: *synarthrodial, amphiarthrodial,* and *diarthrodial.*

Synarthrodial Joints

These are joints (*arthr*) that do not permit movement because the bones are joined together (*syn*). An example is the *suture*, a joint in which the bones appear to be sewn (suture) together. This is the type of joint that joins the bones in the skull.

Examples:

coronal suture: the junction of the frontal bone and the two parietal bones. The line that a crown (*corona*) sits on. This lies on the "coronal plane."

sagittal suture: the line between the two parietal bones. This line resembles a straight arrow (*sagitt*) the point of which is the frontal fontanel, which is the soft spot in an infant's skull. The sagittal suture lies on the sagittal plane.

Amphiarthrodial Joints

These are joints that permit only slight motion of the bones on both sides (*amphi*) of the joint. An example is the *symphysis*, in which bones are joined by a disk of cartilage and appear to have grown (*physis*) together (*sym*).

Examples:

symphysis pubis: the union of the two pubic bones

sacroiliac symphysis: the area of the union of the sacral vertebrae to the pelvic bone (ilium)

Diarthrodial Joints

These are joints that are freely or completely (*dia*) movable. They are the most common joints in the body. They are surrounded by a capsule that extends around the opposing end of the bones that form the joints. The capsule acts as a small box (*capsule*) of connective tissue through which the bones protrude.

Parts of the diarthrodial joint:

articular cartilage: provides a smooth, gliding surface on the ends of opposing bones.

articular disks: fibrocartilage pads between the articular cartilages in some joints.

ligaments: bonds or ties (*ligament*) that connect bones. Ligaments are sometimes named for the bones or bony processes to which they attach, and sometimes for their shape.

synovial fluid: a lubricating substance found where bones come together (*syn*). The fluid is similar to the white of an egg (*ovial*). Diarthrodial joints are also called *synovial joints*.

tendon: a cord or band of dense, tough fiber that connects a muscle with a bone or part. A tendon is stretched (*tendo*) between a muscle and the part to which it is attached. A tendon is sometimes named for the muscle and bone it is attached to. Example: *calcaneal tendon,* the tendon attached to the heel (*calcaneal*). Also known as the *Achilles tendon.*

Types of movement permitted by diarthrodial joints

flexion: bending
extension: straightening or stretching
abduction: movement away (*ab*) from the midline
adduction: movement toward (*ad*) the midline
pronation: turning of the palm downward
supination: turning of the palm upward
eversion: turning (*version*) of the sole of the foot away from (*e*) the midline
inversion: turning (*version*) of the sole of the foot inward (*in*)
plantar flexion: bending of the plantar surface of the sole of the foot downward
rotation: rolling to the side
internal rotation: rolling toward the midline
external rotation: rolling away from the midline
circumduction: making a circle; the ability to move the limb in a circular manner
protraction: thrusting a part of the body forward (*pro*)
retraction: pulling a part of the body backward (*re*)
elevation: raising a part of the body
depression: lowering a part of the body
opposition: the act of placing part of the body opposite another, as in placing the tip of the thumb opposite the tips of the fingers

Classification of Diarthrodial joints

Diarthrodial or synovial joints are classified according to the range of motion permitted. (See Tables 8-1 and 8-2.)

TABLE 8-1
Classification of Diarthrodial Joints

Type	Motion Permitted	Example
ball and socket	Widest range of motion, freely movable	hip
hinge	Flexion and extension in one direction. One bone hangs (*hinge*) from the other bone.	knee
pivot	Rotation, turning as a key in a lock	between the first and second cervical vertebrae, atlas, and axis
condyloid	Circumduction or motion in two directions. The joint allows flexion, extension, abduction, and adduction. A condyle of one bone fits into a cavity of the other bone.	wrist
saddle	All movement except turning or pivoting	thumb
gliding	Gliding or sliding motion	intercarpal joints, the joints between the bones of the wrist

TABLE 8-2
Diarthrodial Joints from Head to Toe

Joint	Type	Description
temporomandibular	condyloid	joint located where the lower jaw attaches to the head at the temporal bone
atlantoaxial	pivot	joint located between the first cervical vertebra and the second cervical vertebra; where the atlas (*atlanto*) turns on the axis (*axial*)
intervertebral	gliding	joint that allows flexion and extension of the backbone
costovertebral	gliding	joints where ribs (*costo*) and vertebra come together
sternoclavicular	gliding	joint of the sternum and clavicle (collarbone)
acromioclavicular	gliding	joint of the shoulder between the acromion process of the scapula and the clavicle
shoulder	ball and socket	joint of the humerus (ball) and glenoid (socketlike) cavity of the scapula
radioulnar	pivot	joint at the proximal ends of the radius (*radio*) and ulna (*ulnar*)
radiocarpal	condyloid	joint at the wrist where the radius and carpal bones join
intercarpal	gliding	joints between (*inter*) the wrist bones (*carpal*)
first carpometacarpal	saddle	joint of the thumb between the carpal bones and the metacarpal bone
2d-5th carpometacarpal	condyloid	joints between the carpal and metacarpal bones of the hand
metacarpophalangeal	condyloid	joints between the metacarpal bones and the first phalanx of the fingers
interphalangeal	hinge	joints between (*inter*) the phalanges of the fingers and also the toes
hip	ball and socket	joint of the head of the femur and the acetabulum, or socket of the ilium [named because it looks like a small (*ulum*) vinegar (*acetab*) jar]
knee	hinge	joint where the end of the femur, the patella, and the end of the tibia meet
tibiofibular	gliding	joint where the fibula joins the tibia
intertarsal	gliding	joints between (*inter*) the anklebones (*tarsal*)

(*Continued.*)

TABLE 8-2
Diathrodial Joints from Head to Toe *(continued)*

Joint	Type	Description
tarsometatarsal	gliding	joints between the tarsal and metatarsal bones
metatarsophalangeal	condyloid	joints between the metatarsal bones and proximal phalangeal bones where the toes are attached to the foot

BURSAE

Bursae are closed sacs or saclike structures (*bursa*) usually close to joint cavities, with a lining similar to the synovial membrane lining of a true joint. Some bursae are continuous with the lining of a joint.

The function of a bursa is to lubricate an area between tendons, ligaments, and bones where friction would otherwise develop.

Terms related to bursae:

subcutaneous bursa: found under (*sub*) the skin (*cutaneous*) between the skin and underlying bony processes
subfascial bursa: found under (*sub*) the fascia
subtendinous bursa: found under (*sub*) tendons where one tendon overlies another tendon or bony projection

PATHOLOGICAL CONDITIONS OF THE ARTICULAR SYSTEM

Disease conditions and methods of treatment of joint diseases are closely associated with disease of the skeletal system, the muscular system, and the nervous system.

Joint diseases listed here most often are associated with the diarthrodial joints.

Diagnostic Terms of Articular System Disease

Analysis of diagnostic terms including terms related to signs and symptoms of diseases of the articular system:

arthrogram: x-ray picture (*ogram*) of a joint (*arthr*) taken after the injection of radiopaque dye into the joint.
diastasis: separation, a standing (*stasis*) apart (*dia*), a separated joint.
dislocation: condition where a structure is apart (*dis*) from its normal location.
luxate: to put a joint out of position.
genu valgum: the leg points outward (*valgum*) from the knee (*genu*). Also called "knock-kneed."

genu varum: the lower legs point inward (*varum*) below the knee (*genu*). Also called "bowlegged." Knees are abnormally separated.
hallux malleus: condition that results in the hammer (*malleus*) appearance of the great toe (*hallux*).
pes planus: condition in which the foot (*pes*) is flat (*planus*).
slipped disk: protrusion of the cartilage (*disk*) between the vertebrae.
spinal curvature: condition in which the curve of the spine is exaggerated beyond the limits of the natural curves of the spine.
scoliosis: condition (*osis*) in which there is a lateral, or sideways, bending (*scoli*) of the spine.
kyphosis: condition (*osis*) in which the thoracic portion of the spine is abnormally curved, resulting in a hunched (*kypho*) back. This condition is referred to as "hunchback."
lordosis: condition (*osis*) in which the lumbar portion of the spine is curved inward or backward (*lord*). This condition is referred to as "hollow-back" or as "swayback."
spondylolisthesis: forward slipping (*listhesis*) of a vertebra (*spondylo*).
sprain: injury of joint ligaments without dislocation.
subluxation: degree of dislocation (*luxation*) less than (*sub*) a total dislocation. An incomplete or partial dislocation.
talipes: term that indicates an abnormality in the ankle (*tali*) and the foot (*pes*). It commonly refers to a "clubfoot."
talipes calcaneus: condition in which the foot touches the floor only at the heel bone (*calcaneus*).
talipes equinas: the foot is shaped like a horse's (*equinas*) hoof.
talipes valgus: joints of the foot are turned outward (*valgus*).
talipes varus: joints of the foot are turned inward (*varus*).

Selected Terms of Joint and Bursae Disease Conditions

Analysis of selected terms related to disease conditions of joints and bursae:

ankylosis: condition (*osis*) in which the joint becomes crooked (*ankyl*).
arthritis: inflammation (*itis*) of the joints (*arthr*).
bursitis: inflammation (*itis*) of the bursa (*burs*).
coxa vara: femur at the joint of the hip (*coxa*) turns inward (*varus, vara*).
degenerative joint disease: disease of joints that results from a deterioration of tissue in the joint.
ganglion: a benign cyst (*ganglion*), usually of a tendon at the wrist or ankle.
gout: joint disease caused by accumulation of drops (*gout* = variation of guttae drops) of a substance in and around a joint.
rheumatoid arthritis: an inflammation (*itis*) in a joint (*arthr*). The term *rheum* is from ancient theory of diseases, being caused by a change in the flow (*rheum*) of body fluids.
tendonitis: inflammation (*itis*) of a tendon (*tendon*).
tenosynovitis: tendon (*teno*) and synovial (*synov*) membrane are inflamed (*itis*).

Terms Related to Treatment for Joint Diseases

arthrodesis: the surgical fusion (*desis*) of a joint (*arthr*).
arthroplasty: the surgical repair of a joint.
capsulorrhaphy: repair (*rrhaphy*) of a joint capsule (*capsul*) to control dislocations.
diskectomy: removal (*ectomy*) of a vertebral cartilage (*disk*).
ganglionectomy: removal (*ectomy*) of a benign cyst (*ganglion*).
meniscectomy: removal of the crescent-shaped (*menisc*) cartilage, usually at the knee.
osteoarthrotomy: incision (*otomy*) into the bone (*oste*) at the joint (*arthr*).
phalangectomy: removal (*ectomy*) of a phalanx of finger or toe.
range of motion exercises: activity done to move all joints in their normal range of motion.
reduction: the act (*ion*) of putting (*duct*) a bone back (*re*) into its normal position in a joint.
spinal fusion: surgical procedure to bind (*fuse*) together some vertebrae (*spinal*).
synovectomy: removal (*ectomy*) of a synovial (*synov*) membrane in a joint.

PRETEST/ POSTTEST FOR CHAPTER 8

1. The functions of joints of the body are:
   1. ____________________
   2. ____________________
   3. ____________________
2. The following terms are related to joints. Define them.
   1. articulation: ____________________
   2. arthr-, arthro-: ____________________
   3. flexibility: ____________________
   4. joint: ____________________
3. The following statements are related to types of joints. Indicate by letter the type of joint which fits the description.
   A = synarthrodial B = amphiarthrodial C = diarthrodial
   1. ____ joints surrounded by a capsule
   2. ____ bones appearing to be sewn together

3. _____ symphysis pubis, for example
4. _____ most common type of joint in the body
5. _____ joints that permit only slight motion
6. _____ sagittal suture, for example
7. _____ freely movable joints
8. _____ joints that do not permit motion
9. _____ also called synovial joints

4. The following terms are related to diarthrodial joints. Match column A with column B.

Column A	Column B
1. _____ ligaments	A. pads between cartilage
2. _____ tendons	B. lubricates the joint
3. _____ articular cartilage	C. connects muscle to bone
4. _____ articular disks	D. bonds or ties connecting bones
5. _____ synovial fluid	E. smooth, gliding surface

5. The following terms are related to motion permitted by diarthrodial joints. Match column A with column B.

Column A	Column B
1. _____ flexion	A. turning the palm downward
2. _____ extension	B. turning the sole of the foot inward
3. _____ abduction	C. placing a part opposite another part
4. _____ adduction	D. straightening or stretching
5. _____ pronation	E. turning the palm upward
6. _____ supination	F. bending the foot downward
7. _____ eversion	G. movement away
8. _____ inversion	H. turning the sole of the foot away from the midline
9. _____ plantar flexion	I. lowering a part of the body
10. _____ rotation	J. bending
11. _____ circumduction	K. pulling a part backward
12. _____ protraction	L. movement toward
13. _____ retraction	M. making a circle
	N. raising a part of the body
	O. thrusting a part forward
	P. rolling to the side

Column A

14. _____ elevation

15. _____ depression

16. _____ opposition

6. Diarthrodial joints are classified according to the range of motion permitted. Give at least one example of each type of joint.

Type of Joint	Example
1. ball and socket	1.
2. hinge	2.
3. pivot	3.
4. condyloid	4.
5. saddle	5.
6. gliding	6.

7. Fill in the blanks:

Bursae are closed ________________ structures that function to ________________ an area between the tendons, ligaments, and bones.

Subcutaneous bursae are found ________________.

Subfascial bursae are found ________________.

Subtendinous bursae are found ________________.

8. The following diagnostic terms are related to joint diseases. Match column A with column B.

Column A	Column B
1. _____ arthrogram	A. flat foot
2. _____ diastasis	B. protrusion of cartilage between the vertebrae
3. _____ dislocation	C. abnormality in the ankle and foot
4. _____ luxate	D. structure apart from its normal location
5. _____ genu valgus	E. normal curves exaggerated
6. _____ genu varus	F. incomplete dislocation
7. _____ hallux malleus	G. x-ray picture of a joint after the injection of a radiopaque dye
8. _____ pes planus	H. injury of joint ligaments without dislocation
9. _____ slipped disk	I. separation
	J. forward slipping of a vertebra

Column A	Column B
10. ____ spinal curvature	K. joint put out of position
11. ____ spondylolisthesis	L. legs point outward, knock-kneed
12. ____ sprain	M. hammer toe
13. ____ subluxation	N. legs point inward, bowlegged
14. ____ talipes	

9. There are variations in the condition known as talipes. Describe the following:
   1. talipes calcaneous: ____________
   2. talipes equinas: ____________
   3. talipes valgus: ____________
   4. talipes varus: ____________

10. Describe the following spinal curvatures:
    1. scoliosis: ____________
    2. kyphosis: ____________
    3. lordosis: ____________

11. The following terms are related to disease conditions of the articular system. Match column A with column B.

Column A	Column B
1. ____ ankylosis	A. inflammation of a joint
2. ____ arthritis	B. deterioration of a joint
3. ____ bursitis	C. inflammation of a tendon
4. ____ coxa vara	D. crooked joint
5. ____ degenerative joint disease	E. joint at the hip turning inward
6. ____ tendonitis	F. inflammation of a bursa
7. ____ tenosynovitis	G. inflammation of a tendon and synovial membrane

12. The following terms are related to the treatment of joint diseases. Match column A with column B.

Column A	Column B
1. ____ arthrodesis	A. removal of a vertebral cartilage
2. ____ arthroplasty	B. binding vertebrae together
	C. repair of a joint

Column A

3. ____ capsulorrhaphy
4. ____ diskectomy
5. ____ ganglionectomy
6. ____ meniscectomy
7. ____ osteoarthrotomy
8. ____phalangectomy
9. ____ range of motion exercises
10. ____ reduction
11. ____ spinal fusion
12. ____ synovectomy

Column B

D. removal of a crescent-shaped cartilage
E. fusion of a joint
F. putting a bone back in place
G. movement of joints
H. incision into a bone at a joint
I. repair of a joint capsule
J. removal of a synovial membrane
K. removal of a finger or toe
L. removal of a benign cyst

PRETEST/ POSTTEST **ANSWERS** FOR CHAPTER **8**

1. **1.** allow motion of the musculoskeletal system
2. bear weight
3. hold the skeleton together

2. **1.** the joining of bones, a joint
2. combining form meaning joint
3. capability of being bent
4. movable or fixed place where two bones come together

3. **1.** C **2.** A **3.** B **4.** C **5.** B **6.** A **7.** C **8.** A **9.** C

4. **1.** D **2.** C **3.** E **4.** A **5.** B

5. **1.** J **2.** D **3.** G **4.** L **5.** A **6.** E **7.** H **8.** B **9.** F **10.** P **11.** M **12.** O **13.** K **14.** N **15.** I **16.** C

6. **1.** shoulder; hip
2. elbow; between bones of fingers and toes (interphalangeal); knee; ankle (talocrural)
3. between first and second cervical vertebrae (atlantoaxial); the juncture of the radius and ulna at the elbow
4. temporomandibular joint; the wrist; the joints between the bones of the palm of the hand of the foot

5. the thumb
6. between the vertebrae; between the ribs and vertebrae; at the shoulder; between the wristbones; between the tibia and fibula; between the anklebones

7. saclike, lubricate
under the skin
under the fascia
under tendons

8.

1. G	3. D, K	5. L*	7. M	9. B	11. J	13. F
2. I	4. K, D	6. N*	8. A	10. E	12. H	14. C

9. 1. Only the heel touches the floor.
2. Foot is shaped like a horse's hoof.
3. Joints of the foot are turned outward.
4. Joints of the foot are turned inward.

10. 1. back bent sideways
2. hunchback, abnormal curve of the thoracic portion of the spine
3. swayback, abnormal curve of the lumbar portion of the spine

11.

1. D	2. A	3. F	4. E	5. B	6. C	7. G

12.

1. E	3. I	5. L	7. H	9. G	11. B	12. J
2. C	4. A	6. D	8. K	10. F		

* To remember varus and valgus associate the length of the terms varus, valgus and inward, outward. Inward is a shorter word, as is varus. Thus varus/inward, valgus/outward.

9 THE NERVOUS SYSTEM

OBJECTIVES

At the end of this chapter you will be able to do the following:

1 Describe the nervous system.
2 List the parts of the nervous system.
3 Describe the structures in the central nervous system.
4 Describe the peripheral nervous system.
5 Describe the autonomic nervous system.
6 Analyze terms related to diseases involving the nervous system.
7 Analyze terms related to signs and symptoms of diseases of the nervous system.
8 Analyze terms related to the diagnosis and treatment of diseases of the nervous system.
9 Analyze terms related to drugs that affect the nervous system.
10 Analyze selected terms related to anesthetic drugs.

THE NERVOUS SYSTEM

The nervous system is the most complex system in the body. The information included here on the workings of the system is very general.

The function of the nervous system is to receive impressions from the external environment, organize the information, and provide appropriate responses. In other words, the nervous system allows the body to react to outside influences (environment).

Outside information enters the nervous system through nerve endings in the skin and through nerve endings in the special sense organs. These nerve endings are referred to as *receptors.*

Nerve endings in the skin are sensitive to pain, touch, pressure, and temperature.

Special sense nerve endings are responsible for taste, smell, vision, hearing, and sense of position and movement.

Sensations from the environment are picked up by these receptors and sent to the central nervous system by way of the peripheral nervous system. The central nervous system sorts out the information and sends back a message, again by way of the peripheral nervous system.

For example, if you put your hand on a hot stove, the nerve endings in your hand will pick up sensations of heat and pain. The message travels to the brain. The brain sends back a message to the muscles of the hand to pull the hand away.

The nervous system, along with the endocrine system, also maintains the internal environment, or the balance of the many activities within the body.

PARTS OF THE NERVOUS SYSTEM

The nervous system consists of all the nerve tissue in the body. The structure of the nervous system may be divided into a *central nervous system* (CNS) and a *peripheral nervous system* (PNS).

The CNS consists of the brain and spinal cord.

The PNS consists of nerves that carry impulses between the CNS and muscles, glands, skin, and other organs that are located outside (peripheral) the CNS. A part of the PNS that has nervous control over smooth muscle, the heart muscle, and glands is called the *autonomic nervous system.*

For purposes of study, terms related to the nervous system will be presented in three groups:

the central nervous system
the peripheral nervous system
the autonomic nervous system

Central Nervous System

The central nervous system is the center (*central*) of all nervous control. It consists of the brain and spinal cord.

The brain is located in the cranial cavity, and the spinal cord extends down the center of the vertebrae (Figure 9-1).

Descriptions of structures shown in Figure 9-1 are as follows:

brainstem: the stemlike (*stem*) portion of the brain which connects the cerebrum with the spinal cord. It contains the pons and the medulla oblongata.

cerebrum: the largest portion of the brain (*cerebrum*) that controls voluntary movements and coordinates mental activity. The cerebrum is divided into right and left cerebral hemispheres. A hemisphere is made of one-half (*hemi*) of the ball (*sphere*) of the brain. The names of the lobes, or divisions, of the cerebral hemispheres correspond to the bones under which they lie. The lobes of the cerebrum are the frontal, temporal, parietal, and occipital lobes. The outer layer of the cerebrum, the cerebral cortex, is made of gray matter, which is gray nervous tissue.

diencephalon: the portion of the brain between (*di,* variation of *dia*) the front and back halves of the brain (*encephalon*). The structures in the diencephalon include the thalamus and the hypothalamus. The term *thalamus* means "inner chamber," which signifies its location in the brain. The hypothalamus is under (*hypo*) the thalamus.

midbrain: the middle (*mid*) part of the brain. Also called the *mesencephalon,* or the middle (*mes*) of the brain (*encephalon*).

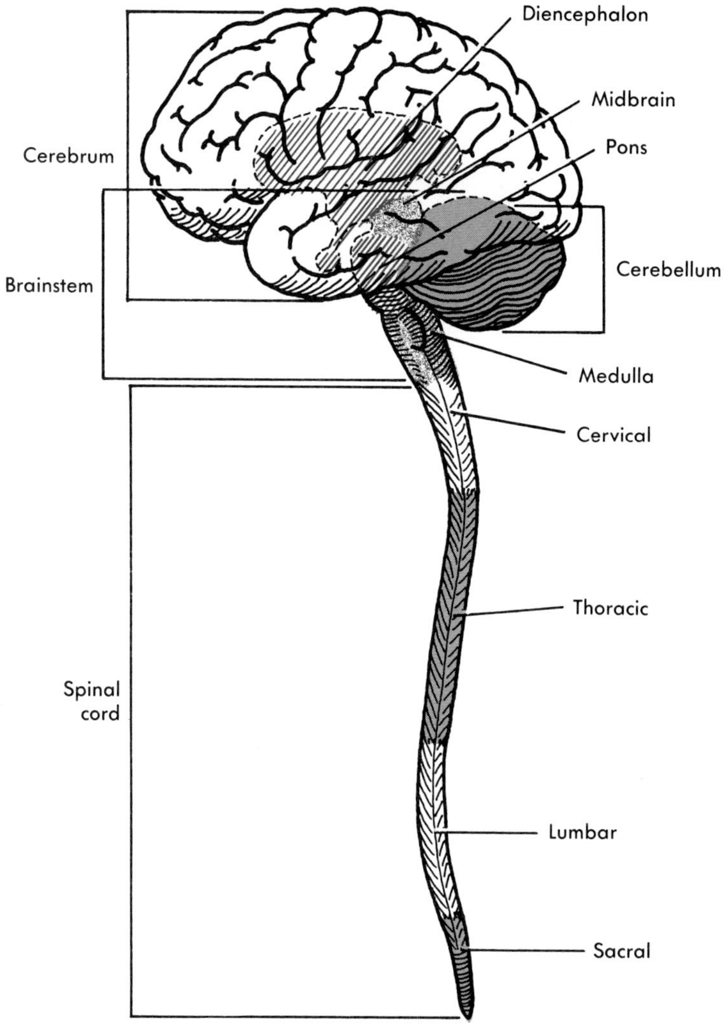

FIGURE 9-1
Lateral view of the central nervous system.

cerebellum: the small (*lum*) round mass of brain (*cerebe*) tissue located in the posterior section of the cranial cavity. It consists of three lobes: two lateral lobes and a central lobe called the flocculonodular lobe. This lobe looks like a rounded mass (*nodular*) of wool (*flocculo*).

pons: the bridgelike [bridge (pons)] structure that lies anterior to the cerebellum and between the midbrain and the medulla. This structure links, or bridges, the parts of the brain and serves as a relay station from the medulla to the higher structures in the brain.

medulla: this structure is more commonly known as the *medulla oblongata.* It is an oblong (*oblongata*) structure that is continuous with the pons and the soft tissue in the center (*medulla*) of the spinal column.

spinal cord: the spinal cord is a column of nervous tissue that extends down the center of the vertebrae. The sections of the spinal cord correspond to the various vertebrae that make up the spinal column. A root word that refers to the spinal cord is *myelo*. This term means soft, marrowlike center. *Myelo* may also refer to bone marrow.

Other structures of the CNS:

ventricles: the ventricles of the brain are little (*cle*) bellylike (*ventr*) cavities in the center of the brain that are continuous with the central cavity of the spinal cord. There are four ventricles of the brain that are all connected with each other, and through which cerebrospinal fluid circulates.

meninges: the brain and spinal cord are covered by three layers of membranes (*meninges*). The three layers from the outside in are as follows:

dura mater: the outermost layer, it is the hard (*dura*) layer. The term mater means "mother," which reflects an old custom of naming parts of the body for family members.

arachnoid layer: the cobweblike [cobweb (arachn), like (oid)] membrane that is the middle of the three meninges.

pia mater: the innermost membrane that is the soft (*pia*) layer.

meningeal spaces: There are two spaces between the meninges. The *subdural space* is the space under (*sub*) the dura (*dura*), between the dura and the arachnoid layer. The *subarachnoid space* is the space under (*sub*) the arachnoid and between it and the pia mater.

cerebrospinal fluid: the fluid that circulates in the ventricles and between the meninges is called the cerebrospinal fluid. This fluid protects the brain (*cerebro*) and spinal (*spinal*) cord by acting as a fluid protection from outside impact.

Peripheral Nervous System

The peripheral nervous system is made up of cranial and spinal nerves. The term *nerve* refers to a bundle of nerve fibers outside the spinal cord or brain.

There are basically two types of nerves; sensory neurons and motor neurons.

The nerves going to the brain are called *sensory* or *afferent* nerves. The nerves coming from the brain are called *motor* or *efferent* nerves.

Terms related to nerves:

afferent nerves: nerves that carry (*ferent*) messages to (*af,* variation of *ad*) the CNS. They are also known as sensory nerves because they pick up and transmit sensation (*sen*).

efferent nerves: nerves that carry (*ferent*) messages away (*ef,* variation of *ex*) from the CNS. They are also known as motor nerves because the messages from the brain result in motion (*motor*).

cranial nerves: the 12 pairs of nerves that arise from the brainstem in the cranium (*cranial*).

spinal nerves: the 31 pairs of nerves that come off the spinal cord.
ganglion: a mass of nerve cell bodies located outside the CNS. *Ganglia* is the plural form of ganglion.
neuro: the root word meaning "nerve."

The peripheral nervous system is composed of 12 pairs of cranial nerves and 31 pairs of spinal nerves. The cell bodies of some of these nerves form structures known as *ganglia.*

Cranial nerves

The 12 pairs of cranial nerves that arise from the brainstem in the cranial cavity are named for the function they carry out or for a physical characteristic of the nerve. See Table 9-1.

TABLE 9-1
The Cranial Nerves

Number	Name	Function
1	olfactory	the nerve of the sense of smell (olfaction)
2	optic	the nerve of the sense of vision (optic = eye)
3	oculomotor	the nerve that moves (*motor*) the eyeball (*oculo*), the eyelid, and the pupil
4	trochlear	the nerve of the muscle on top of the eye; associated with the trochlea, which is the pulleylike projection from the frontal bone
5	trigeminal	a nerve with three (*tri*) divisions; a nerve of the eye, nose, face, and mouth
6	abducens	the nerve which abducts, or moves, the eye away from the midline
7	facial	the nerve of the face and facial expression
8	acoustic or vestibulocochlear	the nerve of the ear (*acoustic*), which provides hearing and sense of equilibrium, dealing with the inner ear (*vestibul*) and the spiral organ (*cochlear*) of the ear
9	glossopharyngeal	the nerve of the tongue (*glosso*) and the pharynx (*pharyngeal*)
10	vagus	the nerve that wanders (*vagus*) in many directions; involved in the function of the pharynx, larynx, and thoracic and abdominal organs
11	spinal accessory	the nerve that controls movement of the head and shoulders and has some involvement in the pharynx and larynx; so named because although it is a cranial nerve, it has a root in the upper part of the spinal cord
12	hypoglossal	the nerve that lies under (*hypo*) the tongue (*glossal*) and allows movement of the tongue.

Spinal nerves

The 31 pairs of spinal nerves are attached to the spinal cord along almost its entire length. They are named for the region of the spinal column through which they exit. See Table 9-2.

Many of the spinal nerves are in groups of nerves called *somatic nerve plexuses.* The term *somatic* refers to the body wall. Thus these nerve plexuses contain nerves that are involved with the wall of the body as opposed to the organs within the body. A *plexus* is a network of intertwined (plexus) nerves.

The major plexuses of spinal nerves:

cervical plexus: the first plexus coming off the cervical portion of the spinal cord, which contains the major nerve of the diaphragm, the phrenic nerve
brachial plexus: the plexus that provides the entire nerve supply to the arm (*brachium*)
lumbar plexus: the plexus located near the lumbar vertebrae
sacral plexus: the network of nerves from which the sciatic nerve originates; arises from the sacrum

The roots of spinal nerves arising from the lower end of the spinal cord proceed downward and merge to form a structure called the *cauda equina.* This collection of spinal nerves resembles the hairs in a horse's (*equina*) tail (*cauda*).

Autonomic nervous system

The autonomic nervous system is the part of the peripheral nervous system that is an automatic or self-governing [self (auto), governing (nomic)] system. It is also called the *involuntary system* because the effects of this system are not (*in*) under voluntary control.

This is a system of efferent nerves and ganglia. The efferent nerves carry impulses away from the nervous system to the viscera, or internal organs of the body. This system does not pick up sensations from the organs. Each nerve that leaves the spinal cord passes into a *ganglion* that is located either near the vertebral column or on the organ that is involved.

TABLE 9-2
The Spinal Nerves

Number of Pairs	Region of the Spinal Cord
8	cervical
12	thoracic
5	lumbar
5	sacral
1	coccygeal

There are three types of ganglia:

vertebral ganglia: the ganglia that run along the vertebral column. These are sometimes called the *paravertebral ganglia,* or the ganglia near (*para*) the vertebral column (*vertebral*).
prevertebral ganglia: the ganglia lying in front of (*pre*) the vertebral column.
terminal ganglia: the ganglia in the walls of the organs where the nerves terminate (*terminal*).

There are two divisions of the autonomic nervous system: the *sympathetic division* and the *parasympathetic division.*

The sympathetic division controls the body's response to feelings (*sympath*). The nerves in this division come off the thoracic and lumbar segments of the spinal cord; therefore this division is sometimes referred to as the *thoracolumbar division.* The action resulting from these nerves includes the fight-or-flight response to fear. The reaction of some organs include an increase in the rate of the heart, dilation of the pupils, and increase in adrenalin secretion. A person may sometimes exhibit great strength as a result of a sympathetic response.

The nerves in the parasympathetic division come off the cranial nerves and sacral segments of the spinal cord; thus, it is sometimes called the *craniosacral division.*

The parasympathetic division in general causes effects opposite (*para*) to those caused by the sympathetic system. The effects include the constriction of the pupils, the return of the heart rate to normal, and the stimulation of the lacrimal glands to produce tears.

There are also plexuses of the autonomic nervous system. These intertwined nerves (*plexus*) are called the *autonomic plexuses.* Some examples of these plexuses are the cardiac plexus, or the intertwined nerves of the heart (*cardia*) and the celiac plexus, or the intertwined nerves of the organs of the abdomen (*celiac*). This last plexus is sometimes called the *solar plexus* because of the sun ray (*solar*) fashion in which the nerves come out of the plexus.

It is important to note that although divisions of the nervous system may be treated independently, they do not function independently.

DISEASE AND THE NERVOUS SYSTEM

Disease of the nervous system has an effect on almost every other system of the body.

The system most affected is the muscular system. Disorders involving movement or muscular control are very often caused by disorders of the nervous system.

Disease Conditions of the Nervous System

Analysis of selected terms related to diseases involving the nervous system:

amyotrophic lateral sclerosis: a progressive wasting away or atrophy of muscles (*myo*) resulting from a disease condition (*osis*) characterized by hardening (*scler*) of nerve tissue.
cerebral aneurysm: a sac (*aneurysm*) formed by the localized dilation of a blood vessel in the cerebrum (*cerebral*).

cerebral palsy: a form of paralysis (*palsy*) caused by a cerebral (*cerebral*) defect characterized by involuntary motions and difficulty in the control of voluntary muscles.

cerebral vascular accident: a sudden interference (*accident*) in brain function (*cerebral*) resulting from an interruption in the blood flow through the blood vessels (*vascular*) in the brain. Also known as a *stroke* or *CVA*.

encephalitis: inflammation (*itis*) of the brain (*encephal*).

encephalopathy: general term meaning a disease (*pathy*) in the brain (*encephalo*).

epilepsy: a disorder characterized by seizures (*epilepsy*), convulsions, or temporary loss of consciousness without convulsions.

seizure: a sudden attack or recurrence of a disease.

convulsion: violent spasmodic contractions of muscles.

grand mal seizure: a form of epilepsy in which there is a sudden loss of consciousness followed immediately by generalized convulsions. It was considered the great (*grand*) illness (*mal*). This form of epilepsy may be preceded by an aura. An *aura* is the sensation that something is going to happen. The term means "a breeze," which describes the sensation that some persons describe.

jacksonian seizure: form of epilepsy that involves only one-half of the body. Named for J. H. Jackson, a physician who first described the condition.

petit mal seizure: a form of epileptic seizure in which there is a momentary loss of consciousness with only minor muscle movement. It is the little (*petit*) illness (*mal*).

hydrocephalus: an increase in the accumulation of cerebrospinal fluid (hydro) within the ventricles of the head (*cephalus*).

infratentorial tumors: description of the location of tumors of the CNS that are below (*infra*) the tentlike (*tentorial*) membrane over the cerebellum. Thus, an infratentorial tumor is below the line between the cerebrum and cerebellum. A *supratentorial tumor* is above (*supra*) the line between the cerebrum and cerebellum.

meningioma: a tumor (*oma*) of the meninges (*meningi).*

meningitis: inflammation of the meninges.

meningocele: a protrusion (*cele*) of the meninges (*meningo*) through an opening in the skull or spinal column.

microcephalus: a condition in which the head (*cephalus*) is small (*micro*).

migraine headache: a pain or aching in the head (*headache*) that may be confined to one side (*mi,* variation of *hemi*) of the head (*graine,* variation of *crania*). Also known as *hemicrania,* or a headache of one-half (*hemi*) of the head (*crania*).

multiple sclerosis: condition (*osis*) caused by hardening (*scler*) of many (*multiple*) tissue patches in the brain and spinal cord.

myotonic dystrophy: a condition characterized by increased muscle (*myo*) tension (*tonic*). The muscles cannot relax.

narcolepsy: a condition characterized by frequent and uncontrollable need for sleep. The person is seized (*lepsy*) by sleep (*narco*).

neurofibroma: a tumor (*oma*) of the connective tissue (*fibr*) of a nerve (*nero*).

paralysis agitans: disease that produces rigid shaking tremors (*agitans*) that may lead to paralysis. Commonly known as Parkinson's disease.

poliomyelitis: inflammation (*itis*) of the gray (*polio*) matter of the spinal cord (*myel*) resulting in paralysis and muscle atrophy.
polyneuropathy: disease (*pathy*) that involves many (*poly*) nerves (*neuro*).
sciatica: severe pain in the leg along the course of the sciatic (*sciatic*) nerve.
spina bifida: a split (*bifida*) in the walls of the spinal canal (*spina*) through which a part of the spinal cord protrudes.
subarachnoid hemorrhage: an abnormal flow of blood (*hemorrhage*) into the subarachnoid space.
subdural hematoma: the presence of a localized collection of blood (*hematoma*) in the subdural space.
transection of the cord: a traumatic injury in which there is a cut (*section*) across (*trans*) the entire spinal cord.
transient ischemic attacks: the sudden (*attack*) occurrences in which there is a decreased blood supply (*ischemic*) to the brain. This attack only lasts a short time (*transient*).

Signs and Symptoms of Nervous System Disease

Analysis of selected terms related to signs and symptoms of diseases involving the nervous system:

adiadochokinesis: condition (*sis*) in which a person is unable (*a*) to perform a motion (*kine*) in which there is a rapid succession (*diadocho*) of movements. An example would be touching a surface first with the palm of the hand and then with the back of the hand, repeating the movements rapidly.
agnosia: an inability (*a*) to recognize objects or have knowledge (*gnosia*) of objects through the senses; for example, an inability to recognize different coins by feeling them. Stereognosis is the ability to have knowledge (*gnosia*) of the solidness (*stereo*) of an object; the ability to tell the different thickness of objects.
anesthesia: a partial or complete lack (*an*) of sensation (*esthesia*) or feeling.
apoplexy: a sudden loss of consciousness in which a person appears to be struck down (*apoplexy*). Commonly called a *stroke.*
apraxia: the inability (*a*) to perform certain actions (*praxia*).
athetosis: condition (*osis*) in which the hands or other parts of the body do not (*a*) remain in a fixed (*thet*) position. An example is ceaseless wringing movement, especially of the hands.
bruxism: the habitual purposeless grinding of teeth (*bruxism*), especially occurring during sleep.
chorea: ceaseless, rapid, jerky movements that may appear to be well coordinated, like dancing (*chorea*).
coma: a state of unconsciousness from which a person cannot be aroused. The person is called *comatose.*
concussion: a violent shaking (*concussion*) of the brain.
confusion: state of mind in which several facts are blended (*fuse*) with (*con*) each other, and a person is unable to distinguish one fact from another.
dyskinesia: difficulty (*dys*) in performing voluntary muscular movements (*kinesia*).

gait: a manner of walking.

festination: gait marked by an involuntary *(in)* hurrying (*festina*) walk.

scissors gait: manner of walking in which the knees are crossed over in scissor fashion.

spastic hemiparesis gait: stiff, awkward (*spastic*) movements from muscle weakness (*paresis*) on one side (*hemi*) of the body.

steppage gait: a manner of walking (*gait*) in which a person places the feet as if going up steps (*steppage*).

neuralgia: pain (*algia*) along the course of a nerve (*neur*).

neuritis: inflammation (*itis*) of a nerve (*neur*).

ophthalmoplegia: paralysis (*plegia*) of the eye (*ophthalmo*).

opisthotonos: condition in which there is severe muscle spasm or tension (*tonos*) resulting in a backward (*opistho*) curving of the body.

paralysis: loss of muscle function caused by injuries or disease of the nerves, brain, or spinal cord. The muscles appear to be loosened or cut (*lysis*) on one side (*para);* thus, they cease to function.

paresis: slight or incomplete paralysis; muscle weakness. The muscles appear to be in a state of relaxation.

paresthesia: an abnormal sensation (*esthesia*) such as numbness or tingling, around (*par,* variation of *para*) a part.

sensory ataxia: loss (*a*) of muscle coordination (*taxia*) because of a loss of feeling (*sensory),* especially the sensation of position and movement.

speech disorders: conditions of the nervous system in which a person is unable to speak normally.

aphasia: the loss (*a*) of the ability to speak (*phasia*).

aphonia: the loss (*a*) of the voice (*phonia*). Example: aphonia paralytica is loss of the voice resulting from a paralysis of the laryngeal nerves.

dysphonia: difficulty (*dys*) in speaking (*phonia*).

dysarthria: imperfect (*dys*) articulation (*arthria*) of speech.

dysphasia: impairment (*dys*) of speech (*phasia*).

singultus: a hiccup.

stupor: partial or nearly complete state of unconsciousness.

syncope: fainting, sometimes caused by the cutting short (*syncope*) of the blood supply to the brain.

tic douloureux: a sudden spasmodic involuntary muscle contraction (*tic*) that is accompanied by pain (*douloureux*).

tremor: an involuntary shaking (*tremor*).

resting tremor: shaking that occurs when a person is resting.

intention tremor: shaking that occurs when a person attempts to do something (*intent*).

Surgical and Diagnostic Procedures

Analysis of selected terms related to the surgical and diagnostic procedures done for disorders of the nervous system:

CAT scan (computerized *a*xial *t*omography *s*can): a two-dimensional picture (*scan*) that has been taken at various levels of tissue (*tomography*) by an x-ray apparatus that circles around the part on an axis (*axial*). The interpretation of the x-rays into a picture is done by computers.
cordotomy: cutting into (*otomy*) the spinal cord (*cord*); usually done to relieve pain.
craniectomy: the removal (*ectomy*) of a portion of the skull bone (*crani*).
craniotomy: an incision (*otomy*) into the cranium (*crani*) to open the skull.
cryoneurosurgery: the technique of exposing the nerve (*neuro*) tissue to extreme cold (*cryo*) in order to destroy specific areas of diseased tissue.
electroencephalogram (*EEG*): the measurement and recording (*gram*) of the electrical (*electro*) activity of the brain (*encephalo*).
laminectomy: the excision (*ectomy*) of a thin, flat plate (*lamina*) of bone of one or more vertebrae.
lobotomy: the cutting into (*otomy*) a lobe of the brain, usually the frontal lobe, to alter brain function.
lumbar puncture: also known as *spinal tap,* is the procedure done by inserting a long needle between two lumbar vertebrae to take a sample of cerebrospinal fluid, to measure cerebrospinal pressure or to anesthetize the lower part of the body.
neurectomy: removal (*ectomy*) of a part of a nerve (*neur*).
neurolysis: cutting (*lysis*) of nerve tissue.
neurotripsy: surgical crushing (*tripsy*) of a nerve.
reflex testing: a nerve is stimulated to see if the part being tested bends (*flex*) back (*re*) automatically. This is done to evaluate the nervous control of the part. Examples of reflexes that may be tested:
- *ankle:* the striking of the Achilles tendon results in plantar flexion of the ankle.
- *brachioradialis tendon* (also called *supinator reflex*): striking this tendon in the forearm causes flexion and supination, or turning, of the forearm.
- *cremasteric:* stroking of the inside of the thigh results in a pulling up of the testis by the cremaster muscle of the abdomen on the side being tested.
- *plantar response:* when the sole (plantar) of the foot is stroked, dorsiflexion of the great toe, or pointing of the toe toward the head, may indicate a disease. Also known as the *Babinski response*.

sympathectomy: excision (*ectomy*) of part of a sympathetic (*sympath*) nerve.
trephination: a process of cutting out a circular piece of bone from the skull using an instrument called a trephine.
vagotomy: the cutting into (*otomy*) a branch of the vagus nerve.
ventricular shunting: a procedure done to divert (*shunt*) cerebrospinal fluid to another part of the body to release some of the fluid that collects in the ventricles (*ventricular*) that causes hydrocephalus.

EFFECT OF DRUGS ON THE NERVOUS SYSTEM

Analysis of selected terms related to drugs that affect the nervous system:

analeptic: a drug that acts as a stimulant or restorative, such as caffeine, amphetamines, etc. It restores (*analeptic*) wakefulness.

analgesic: a drug that takes away (*an*) pain (*alges*).
narcotic analgesic: analgesic capable of causing stupor (*narco*).
nonnarcotic analgesic: analgesic not capable (*non*) of causing stupor (*narco*).
anticonvulsant: drug that works against (*anti*) or controls convulsions.
antiepileptic: drug that works against (*anti*) or controls epilepsy.
antiparkinsonism drug: drug that works against (*anti*) or to control Parkinson's disease.
antipyretic analgesic: drug that not only takes away (*an*) pain (*alges*) but also works against or controls (*anti*) fever (*pyretic*).
narcotic: preparation capable of producing stupor (*narco*) or a decrease in mental awareness.
narcotic antagonist: drug that works (*agonist*) against (*ant*) or reverses the effects of a narcotic.
parasympatholytic: drug that produces effects similar to those that would occur if the parasympathetic nerves (*parasympatho*) were cut (*lytic*).
parasympathomimetic: drug that produces effects that imitate (*mimetic,* variation of *mimic*) the action of the parasympathetic (*parasympatho*) nervous system.
sympatholytic: drug that produces effects similar to those that would occur if the sympathetic nerves were cut (*lytic*).
sympathomimetic: drug that produces effects that imitate the action of the sympathetic nervous system.

Anesthetic Drugs

Analysis of selected terms related to anesthetic drugs:

anesthetic drug: a preparation that is capable of taking away (*an*) sensation (*esthet*), especially the sensation of pain.
epidural anesthesia: the injection of an anesthetic agent into the space on top (*epi*) of the dura mater (*dura*). This type of anesthesia anesthetizes the nerves of the cauda equina area. This type of anesthesia is sometimes called a *caudal block*.
field block: the anesthetic agent is injected into the area around (*field*) the area to be operated on.
general anesthetic: a drug that is capable of producing loss of consciousness and total loss of sensation.
infiltration: a procedure in which the anesthetic agent is injected into the area to be numbed, and the drug filters through the tissue.
local anesthetic: a drug that causes anesthesia only in a particular area.
nerve block: an anesthetic agent is injected near a nerve supplying the area to be treated. The drug blocks the nerve impulses so that pain cannot be felt.
saddle block: an anesthetic agent is injected into the spinal canal in such a way as to cause anesthesia of a localized area. The area of the perineum anesthetized is the area that would come into contact with a saddle.
spinal anesthesia: an anesthetic agent is injected into the subarachnoid space to block the nerves below the level of the agent. The lower portion of the body is numbed.
topical anesthetic: an anesthetic agent that is applied on the surface (*top*) of a

structure, especially structures covered with mucous membranes. The agent is absorbed through the membrane.

PRETEST/ POSTTEST FOR CHAPTER 9

1. Write out the meaning of the following abbreviations:

1. CNS ______________

2. PNS ______________

2. The following structures are found in the central nervous system. Match column A with column B.

Column A	Column B
1. ____ brainstem	A. small, round mass located in the posterior section of the cranium
2. ____ cerebrum	B. largest portion of the brain
3. ____ diencephalon	C. column of nervous tissue down the center of the vertebrae
4. ____ midbrain	D. bridgelike structure
5. ____ cerebellum	E. portion of the brain containing the pons and medulla
6. ____ pons	F. structure that is continuous with the pons and spinal cord
7. ____ medulla	G. portion of the brain containing the thalamus and hypothalamus
8. ____ spinal cord	H. the mesencephalon

3. The following terms are related to structures in the CNS. Select the correct answer.

1. The ventricles are:
A. cavities in the brain.
B. the spaces around the spinal cord.
C. both of the above.

2. There are three meninges. The sequence of the layers from the outermost to the innermost is:
A. the dura mater, the arachnoid, and the pia mater.
B. the pia mater, the arachnoid, and the dura mater.
C. neither of the above.

3. The spaces between the meninges are:
   A. the subdural and the submeningeal.
   B. the subarachnoid and the subdural.
   C. both of the above.
4. The cerebrospinal fluid:
   A. circulates around the brain and spinal cord.
   B. circulates in the ventricles and between the meninges.
   C. both of the above.

4. The following terms are related to the peripheral nervous system. Select the best answer.

1. An afferent nerve:
   A. carries messages to the brain.
   B. is also known as a motor nerve.
   C. both of the above.
2. An efferent nerve:
   A. carries messages from the brain.
   B. is also known as a sensory nerve.
   C. both of the above.
3. The cranial nerves:
   A. arise from the brainstem.
   B. are also called ganglia.
   C. both of the above.
4. The spinal nerves:
   A. may be involved in a ganglion.
   B. arise from the spinal cord.
   C. both of the above.
5. A ganglion:
   A. is another name for an efferent nerve.
   B. is a structure made from nerve cell bodies.
   C. both of the above.
6. The root word for nerve is:
   A. neuro.
   B. neuron.
   C. both of the above.

5. The following terms are related to the names of the cranial nerves. Match column A with column B.

Column A	Column B
1. _____ olfactory	A. nerve of facial expression
2. _____ optic	B. nerve that moves the eye
3. _____ oculomotor	C. nerve of the ear
4. _____ trochlear	D. nerve of the sense of smell
	E. nerve with three parts; nerve of the eye, nose, face, and mouth

Column A	Column B
5. ____ trigeminal	F. nerve that wanders in many directions, including toward the pharynx and abdominal organs
6. ____ abducens	G. nerve of the sense of vision
7. ____ facial	H. nerve of the muscle on top of the eye
8. ____ acoustic	I. nerve which has a root in the upper part of the spinal cord
9. ____ glossopharyngeal	J. nerve under the tongue
10. ____ vagus	K. nerve of the tongue and pharynx
11. ____ spinal accessory	L. nerve which abducts the eye
12. ____ hypoglossal	

6. The following terms are related to the spinal nerves.

Set 1
List the regions of the spinal cord from top to bottom.

1. ____________________
2. ____________________
3. ____________________
4. ____________________
5. ____________________

Set 2
Describe the following structures:

1. cervical plexus ____________________
2. brachial plexus ____________________
3. lumbar plexus ____________________
4. sacral plexus ____________________
5. cauda equina ____________________

7. The following statements relate to the autonomic nervous system. Mark each statement true, *T*, or false, *F*.

1. ____ The autonomic system is under voluntary control.
2. ____ There are afferent and efferent nerves in this system.
3. ____ Each nerve leaves the spinal cord and passes into the ganglia.
4. ____ The sympathetic division is also known as the thoracolumbar division.
5. ____ A reaction caused by sympathetic nervous reaction might be the flow of tears.

6. _____ The parasympathetic division is also called the craniosacral division.
7. _____ A response of the parasympathetic division might be the increase in the heart rate.
8. _____ The celiac plexus is also known as the solar plexus.
9. _____ The autonomic nervous system, the CNS, and the PNS all work independently of each other.

8. The following terms are related to epilepsy. Using the list of terms, complete the following statements:

seizure	aura
convulsion	jacksonian
grand mal	petit mal

1. A sudden attack or recurrence of a disease is called a(n) _________.
2. The sensation that something is going to happen is called a(n) _________.
3. A form of seizure in which there is a momentary loss of consciousness is called a(n) _________ seizure.
4. A(n) _________ is a violent spasmodic contraction of muscles.
5. A form of seizure in which only one side of the body is involved is called a(n) _________ seizure.
6. A sudden loss of consciousness followed by generalized convulsions is characteristic of a(n) _________ seizure.

9. The following three sets of terms are related to diseases involving the nervous system. Separate directions will be given with each set.

Set 1
Using the list of terms complete the following statements. Choose the best answer.

cerebral vascular accident	multiple sclerosis
amyotrophic lateral sclerosis	paralysis agitans
cerebral aneurysm	transient ischemic attack
cerebral palsy	

1. An occurrence that lasts a short time in which blood supply to the brain is decreased is called a(n) _________________________.
2. Another name for a stroke is _________________________.
3. A form of paralysis in which there is involuntary motion and difficulty controlling voluntary motions is called _________________________.
4. Another name for Parkinson's disease is _________________________.

5. A progressive wasting away of muscles from hardening of nerve tissue is called

____.

6. A disease characterized by many hardening patches of nerve tissue is called

____.

7. A sac formed by localized dilation of blood vessels in the cerebrum is called a(n) ____.

Set 2

Match column A with column B.

Column A	Column B
1. ____ encephalitis	A. inflammation of the gray matter of the spinal cord
2. ____ encephalopathy	B. a small head
3. ____ infratentorial tumor	C. a tumor of the connective tissue of a nerve
4. ____ supratentorial tumor	D. inflammation of the brain
5. ____ meningioma	E. the term meaning "a disease involving many nerves"
6. ____ meningitis	F. general term for disease involving the brain
7. ____ narcolepsy	G. severe pain down the leg along the course of a nerve
8. ____ microcephalus	H. a tumor in or below the cerebellum
9. ____ neurofibroma	I. inflammation of the meninges
10. ____ poliomyelitis	J. attacks of irresistible sleepiness
11. ____ polyneuropathy	K. tumor of the meninges
12. ____ sciatica	L. tumor above the cerebellum

Set 3

Select the correct answer.

1. A migraine headache
   A. involves one-half of the head.
   B. is also known as hemicrania.
   C. both of the above.

2. A __________ is an abnormal flow of blood into the space between the arachnoid and pia mater meninges.
   A. subarachnoid hemorrhage
   B. arachnoid hemorrhage
   C. both of the above

3. A split in the walls of the spinal canal through which a part of the spinal cord protrudes is called
   A. spina bifida.
   B. neurofibroma.
   C. both of the above.

4. A ________ is an abnormal collection of blood under the dura mater.
   A. meningioma
   B. subdural hematoma
   C. both of the above

5. In transection of the cord, the spinal cord is
   A. cut across by trauma.
   B. bulging out through the vertebrae.
   C. both of the above.

6. In hydrocephalus there is an increase in the accumulation of ________ in the ventricles of the brain.
   A. cerebrospinal fluid
   B. blood
   C. both of the above

7. In meningocele there is a ________ of the meninges.
   A. protrusion
   B. rupture
   C. both of the above

10. The following five sets of terms are related to signs and symptoms of diseases involving the nervous system. In each set match column A with column B. Choose the one best answer.

Set 1

Column A	Column B
1. ____ adiadochokinesis	A. sudden loss of consciousness
2. ____ agnosia	B. inability to perform certain actions
3. ____ anesthesia	C. ceaseless, rapid, dancelike body movement
4. ____ apoplexy	D. inability to recognize objects
5. ____ apraxia	E. purposeless grinding of teeth
6. ____ athetosis	F. loss of sensation or feeling
7. ____ bruxism	G. inability to distinguish one fact from another
8. ____ chorea	H. state of unconsciousness
9. ____ coma	I. inability to perform motions in rapid succession
10. ____ concussion	J. violent shaking-up of the brain
11. ____ confusion	K. ceaseless wringing movement of the hands

Set 2

Terms related to gait or manner of walking.

Column A	Column B
1. ____ festination	A. knees crossing over
2. ____ scissors gait	B. appearing to be going up steps
3. ____ spastic hemiparesis	C. one-sided weakness
4. ____ steppage	D. hurrying gait

Set 3

Column A	Column B
1. ____ neuralgia	A. paralysis of the muscles of the eye
2. ____ neuritis	B. backward curving of the body
3. ____ ophthalmoplegia	C. inflammation of a nerve
4. ____ opisthotonos	D. pain along a nerve
5. ____ paralysis	E. abnormal sensations, such as tingling
6. ____ paresis	F. loss of muscular function
7. ____ paresthesia	G. muscle weakness; muscles appearing to be in a state of relaxation

Set 4

Terms related to speech. Select the best answer.

1. The loss of the ability to speak is called:
   A. aphasia.
   B. dysphasia.
   C. both of the above.

2. The impairment of speech is called:
   A. dysphasia.
   B. dysphagia.
   C. both of the above.

3. Difficulty in speaking is called:
   A. dysphonia.
   B. dysphasia.
   C. both of the above.

4. Dysarthria is a difficulty:
   A. in articulation or the forming of words.
   B. also called aphonia.
   C. both of the above.

Set 5

Mark the statements true, *T*, or false, *F*.

1. ____ Singultus is difficulty in singing.

2. _____ The complete loss of consciousness is called stupor.
3. _____ Syncope is a word for fainting.
4. _____ A resting tremor occurs when a person needs rest.
5. _____ An intention tremor occurs when a person attempts to do something.

11. The following terms are related to diagnostic procedures and treatment of diseases involving the nervous system. Match column A with column B.

Set 1

Column A	Column B
1. _____ CAT scan	A. measurement and recording of electrical activity of the brain
2. _____ cordotomy	B. two-dimensional picture at various depths of tissue
3. _____ craniectomy	C. removal of a piece of skull
4. _____ craniotomy	D. cutting into a lobe of the brain
5. _____ cryoneurosurgery	E. cutting into the spinal cord
6. _____ electroencephalogram	F. insertion of a needle between the vertebrae
7. _____ laminectomy	G. using extreme cold to destroy diseased tissue
8. _____ lobotomy	H. cutting into the skull
9. _____ lumbar puncture	I. excision of a thin, flat plate of bone from the vertebrae

Set 2

Column A	Column B
1. _____ neurectomy	A. removal of a piece of a sympathetic nerve
2. _____ neurolysis	B. diversion of cerebrospinal fluid
3. _____ neurotripsy	C. cutting of nerve tissue
4. _____ reflex testing	D. cutting of a branch of the tenth cranial nerve
5. _____ trephination	E. removal of a part of a nerve
6. _____ sympathectomy	F. cutting out a circular piece of bone
7. _____ vagotomy	G. crushing a nerve tissue
8. _____ ventricular shunting	H. stimulation of a part of the body to evaluate nervous control

12. The following two sets of terms are related to drugs that have an effect on the nervous system. In each set match column A with column B. Choose the one best answer.

Set 1

Column A	Column B
1. _____ analeptic	A. drug that controls convulsions
2. _____ analgesic	B. drug that controls Parkinson's disease
3. _____ anticonvulsant	C. drug that controls fever
4. _____ antiepileptic	D. drug that restores wakefulness
5. _____ antiparkinsonian	E. drug that takes away pain
6. _____ antipyretic	F. drug that controls epilepsy

Set 2

Column A	Column B
1. _____ narcotic	A. drug that has action similar to the cutting of a parasympathetic nerve
2. _____ narcotic anatagonist	B. drug that has action similar to the cutting of a sympathetic nerve
3. _____ parasympatholytic	C. drug capable of producing stupor
4. _____ parasympathomimetic	D. drug that imitates the action of a sympathetic nerve
5. _____ sympatholytic	E. drug that reverses the action of a narcotic
6. _____ sympathomimetic	F. drug that has action similar to the action of the parasympathetic nerves

13. The following terms are related to anesthetic drugs. Match column A with column B.

Column A	Column B
1. _____ general	A. drug injected near a nerve to block all sensations
2. _____ topical	B. drug capable of producing loss of consciousness
3. _____ infiltration	C. drug injected to numb the area that comes in contact with a saddle
4. _____ nerve block	D. drug injected so that it can filter through the area to be operated on
5. _____ spinal	E. drug put on the surface
6. _____ saddle block	F. drug injected into the subarachnoid space
7. _____ epidural	G. also known as a caudal anesthesia

PRETEST/ POSTTEST **ANSWERS** FOR CHAPTER **9**

1. **1.** central nervous system
   2. peripheral nervous system

2. **1.** E **2.** B **3.** G **4.** H **5.** A **6.** D **7.** F **8.** C

3. **1.** A **2.** A **3.** B **4.** C

4. **1.** A **2.** A **3.** A **4.** C **5.** B **6.** C

5. **1.** D **2.** G **3.** G **4.** H **5.** E **6.** L **7.** A **8.** C **9.** K **10.** F **11.** I **12.** J

6. **Set 1**

   1. cervical
   2. thoracic
   3. lumbar
   4. sacral
   5. coccygeal

   Set 2

   1. intertwined group of nerves that comes off the cervical portion of the spinal cord
   2. intertwined group of nerves that provides the nerves of the arm
   3. intertwined group of nerves near the lumbar vertebrae
   4. intertwined group of nerves near the sacral vertebrae
   5. collection of nerves at the end of the spinal cord that resembles a horse's tail

7. **1.** F **2.** F **3.** T **4.** T* **5.** F **6.** T* **7.** F **8.** T **9.** F

8. **1.** seizure
   2. aura
   3. petit mal
   4. convulsion
   5. jacksonian
   6. grand mal

9. **Set 1**

   1. transient ischemic attack
   2. cerebral vascular accident
   3. cerebral palsy
   4. paralysis agitans
   5. amyotrophic lateral sclerosis
   6. multiple sclerosis
   7. cerebral aneurysm

   Set 2

   1. D **2.** F **3.** H **4.** L **5.** K **6.** I **7.** J **8.** B **9.** C **10.** A **11.** E **12.** G

   Set 3

   1. C **2.** A **3.** A **4.** B **5.** A **6.** A **7.** A

---

* To avoid confusing these, think of the feeling of sympathy that comes from the heart. The heart is located in the thoracic cavity.

10. Set 1

1. I	**3.** F	**5.** B	**7.** E	**9.** H	**10.** J	**11.** G
2. D	**4.** A	**6.** K	**8.** C			

Set 2

1. D **2.** A **3.** C **4.** B

Set 3

1. D **2.** C **3.** A **4.** B **5.** F **6.** G **7.** E

Set 4

1. A **2.** A* **3.** C **4.** A

Set 5

1. F **2.** F **3.** T **4.** F **5.** T

11. Set 1

1. B	**3.** C	**5.** G	**6.** A	**7.** I	**8.** D	**9.** F
2. E	**4.** H					

Set 2

1. E	**3.** G	**4.** H	**5.** F	**6.** A	**7.** D	**8.** B
2. C						

12. Set 1

1. D **2.** E **3.** A **4.** F **5.** B **6.** C

Set 2

1. C **2.** E **3.** A **4.** F **5.** B **6.** D

13. **1.** B **2.** E **3.** D **4.** A **5.** F **6.** C **7.** G

---

* To avoid confusing dysphasia and dysphagia, associate the *phag* in dysphagia with eating.

10 THE CARDIOVASCULAR SYSTEM

OBJECTIVES

At the end of this chapter you will be able to do the following:

1 Describe the cardiovascular system, and name its parts.
2 Identify the structures and chambers of the heart.
3 Identify the blood vessels entering the heart and the valves controlling the flow of blood through the heart.
4 Describe a heartbeat and terms related to it.
5 Define terms related to the vascular system.
6 Name the major arteries of the body.
7 Name the major veins of the body.
8 Trace circulation through the heart.
9 Describe various circulations within the cardiovascular system.
10 Analyze selected diagnostic terms related to the cardiovascular system.
11 Analyze selected terms related to diseases of the cardiovascular system.
12 Analyze terms related to the treatment of cardiovascular diseases.
13 Analyze terms related to cardiac drugs.

THE CARDIOVASCULAR SYSTEM

The cardiovascular system has two parts:

1 the heart
2 the blood vessels

The heart is a hollow organ that is located in the thoracic cavity, to the left of the midline of the body, between the lungs, in a space called the mediastinum.

Blood vessels attached to the heart are linked to every cell of the body, either directly or indirectly, through a network of veins, arteries, and capillaries.

Blood is pumped through the heart and blood vessels. For the purpose of study, however, blood is covered separately, in Chapter 11.

Terms related to the cardiovascular system:

cardio-: combining form meaning "heart."
cardiovascular: the system made up of the heart (*cardio*) and blood vessels (*vascular*).

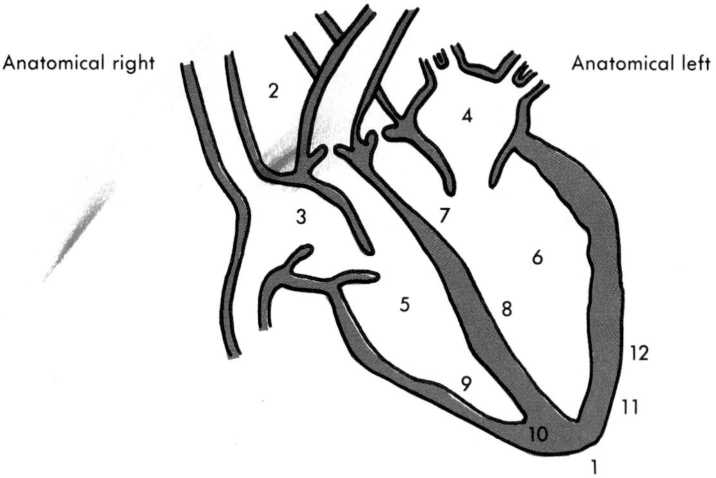

FIGURE 10-1
The structure and chambers of the heart: (1) apex, (2) base, (3) right atrium, (4) left atrium, (5) right ventricle, (6) left ventricle, (7) interatrial septum, (8) interventricular septum, (9) endocardium, (10) myocardium, (11) epicardium, and (12) pericardium.

In Figure 10-1 the structure and chambers of the heart are identified.

Flow of Blood in the Heart

The heart is the pumping station for the circulation of the body.

Blood enters the heart through the superior and inferior vena cavae and pulmonary veins, goes through a system of valves, and leaves the heart through the pulmonary artery and the aorta.

In Figure 10-2 the blood vessels entering the heart and the valves of the heart are identified.

The Heartbeat

The heartbeat is an automatic, rhythmic, and repetitive contraction of the heart muscle that produces the pumping action of the heart. This pumping action of the heart circulates blood throughout the body.

The heartbeat includes a contraction phase and relaxation phase. The contraction phase is called *systole,* and the relaxation phase is called *diastole.*

The normal heartbeat is triggered by an electrical impulse originating in the sinoatrial node in the heart. The electrical impulse travels through the heart muscle causing the contraction. This action is called *conduction.*

Terms related to the heartbeat:

conduction: action in which the electrical impulses for the contraction of the heart muscle are transferred (*conduct*) through the heart.

TABLE 10-1
Terms Related to the Anatomy of the Heart Listed in the Order Shown in Figure 10-1

1. apex: the tip (*apex*) of the heart. The pointed aspect of the heart, which is in a downward position.
2. base: the part of the heart nearest its points of attachment to the blood vessels. It is the flat part of the heart.
3. right atrium: the upper chamber where blood enters the heart, the entrance chamber (*atrium*) of the heart from the vena cavae.
4. left atrium: the entrance chamber (*atrium*) from the pulmonary veins.
5. right ventricle: the lower chamber of the heart that receives blood from the upper chamber for pumping to the lungs. The bellylike (*ventri*) area of the heart.
6. left ventricle: the lower chamber of the heart that receives blood from the upper chamber for pumping into the aorta for distribution to all parts of the body.
7. interatrial septum: the wall (*septum*) between (*inter*) the atria (*atria*).
8. interventricular septum: the wall (*septum*) between (*inter*) the ventricles (*ventricular*).
9. endocardium: the membrane lining the inside (*endo*) of the heart (*cardium*).
10. myocardium: the heart (*cardium*) muscle (*myo*).
11. epicardium: the membrane on (*epi*) the outside of the heart.
12. pericardium: the sac that is around (*peri*) the heart (*cardium*).

contraction: thickening and shortening of the heart muscle that causes it to draw the walls together (*contract*), making the space inside the heart smaller, causing blood to be forced out of the space. This is also called the *systolic phase*.

diastole: indicates that the walls of the heart are placed (*stole*) further apart (*dia*). The relaxation phase.

heartbeat: pulsation of the heart including a contraction and relaxation phase.

heart sounds: sounds that are caused by the vibration of the heart valves and walls of the heart as well as by the blood rushing through the great vessels.

pulse: impact of the ejection of blood from the left ventricle into the aorta that is felt at points throughout the body where arteries come close to the surface.

relaxation: return of the heart muscle to a resting state, increasing the space in the heart and allowing blood to flow into the heart. This is also called the *diastolic phase*.

sinoatrial node: small mass of tissue (*node*) located in a depressed (*sino*) area of the atrium (*atrial*). This tissue gives rise to the electrical impulse that triggers the heartbeat.

sinus rhythm: the normal heart rate (*rhythm*), which begins at the sinoatrial (*sinus*) node.

systole: indicates that the walls of the heart are placed (*stole*) more closely together (*sy*, variation of *syn*). The contraction phase.

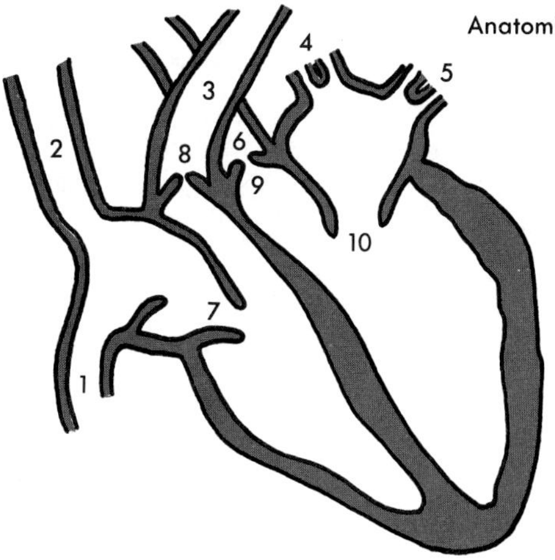

FIGURE 10-2
Blood vessels and valves of the heart: (1) inferior vena cava, (2) superior vena cava, (3) pulmonary artery, (4) right pulmonary vein, (5) left pulmonary vein, (6) aorta, (7) tricuspid valve, (8) pulmonary valve, (9) aortic valve, (10) bicuspid valve, also called the mitral valve.

THE VASCULAR SYSTEM

The vascular system is made of blood vessels that carry blood to and from the heart. The term *vascular* means "small (*cular,* variation of *cule*) vessel (*vas*)."

Terms related to parts of the vascular system:

angio-: combining form meaning "vessel," but not always blood vessel.
artery: blood vessel leading away from the heart.
arteriole: small (*iole*) artery (*arter*).
capillary: small, hair-thin (*capill*) blood vessel between the ends of arteries and beginnings of veins.
phleb-: combining form meaning "vein."
vein: blood vessel carrying blood toward the heart. Veins drain a part or organ and carry blood back to the heart. The term *vein* means "to come to"; thus, the blood comes to the heart by way of veins.
venule: small (*ule*) vein (*ven*).

Names of Arteries and Veins

Most names of arteries and veins are derived from the anatomical structures they supply or are close to, or from the root word denoting the area of the body they supply.

A review of Chapter 5 will help you associate the names of the blood vessels with the parts of the body they supply.

Most often the names of an artery supplying fresh blood to a part and a vein carrying the blood back to the heart correspond. For example, there is an axillary artery and an axillary vein.

TABLE 10-2
Terms Related to the Blood Vessels and Valves of the Heart Listed in the Order Shown in Figure 10-2

1. inferior vena cava: the vein (*vena*) carrying blood from the lower (*inferior*) part of the body. *Cava* means "hollow." This vein was so named because it was found to be empty or hollow (*cava*) after death.
2. superior vena cava: the vein (*vena*) carrying blood from the upper (*superior*) part of the heart. Also hollow (*cava*) after death.
3. pulmonary artery: the duct or blood vessel (*artery*) carrying blood to the lungs (*pulmonary*).
4. right pulmonary veins: the veins returning blood to the heart from the right lung (*pulmonary*).
5. left pulmonary veins: the veins returning blood to the heart from the left lung (*pulmonary*).
6. aorta: the main artery carrying blood from the heart to all parts of the body except the lungs.
7. tricuspid valve: the flap of tissue that controls the flow of blood between the right atrium and right ventricle. There are three (*tri*) pointed or triangular flaps (*cusps*) in this valve.
8. pulmonary valve: a semilunar valve controlling the flow of blood into the pulmonary artery from the right ventricles. The term *semilunar* refers to the three half moon-shaped [half (semi), moon (lunar)] flaps that make up this valve.
9. aortic valve: the semilunar valve controlling the flow of blood into the aorta from the left ventricle. Also has three semilunar flaps (cusps).
10. bicuspid valve: the valve with two (*bi*) triangular folds controlling the flow of blood between the left atrium and left ventricle. This valve is also called the *mitral valve* because it resembles the headdress of a bishop called the miter.

In some cases there are different names for arteries to a part and veins from a part. For example, there is a carotid artery to the head and a jugular vein from the head.

In many cases there are right and left corresponding blood vessels. For example, there is a right femoral vein and a left femoral vein.

In some cases there is only a main blood vessel. For examples, there is only one inferior vena cava. There is also only one hepatic vein.

Following are illustrations showing the principal arteries (Figure 10-3) and the principal veins (Figure 10-4).

Sections of Systemic Circulation

There are sections of the systemic circulation that have different names.

Terms denoting various sections of the circulatory system:

coronary circulation: circulation that supplies blood to the heart muscle itself. The path of the blood vessels encircles the heart in a crownlike (*coronary*) fashion (Figure 10-5).

peripheral vascular circulation: refers to the circulation of blood through blood vessels on the periphery or around the outside of the body, away from the heart. It includes circulation in the extremities.

portal or hepatic circulation: circulation that transports (*portal*) blood and absorbed food products from the intestine to the liver (*hepatic*).

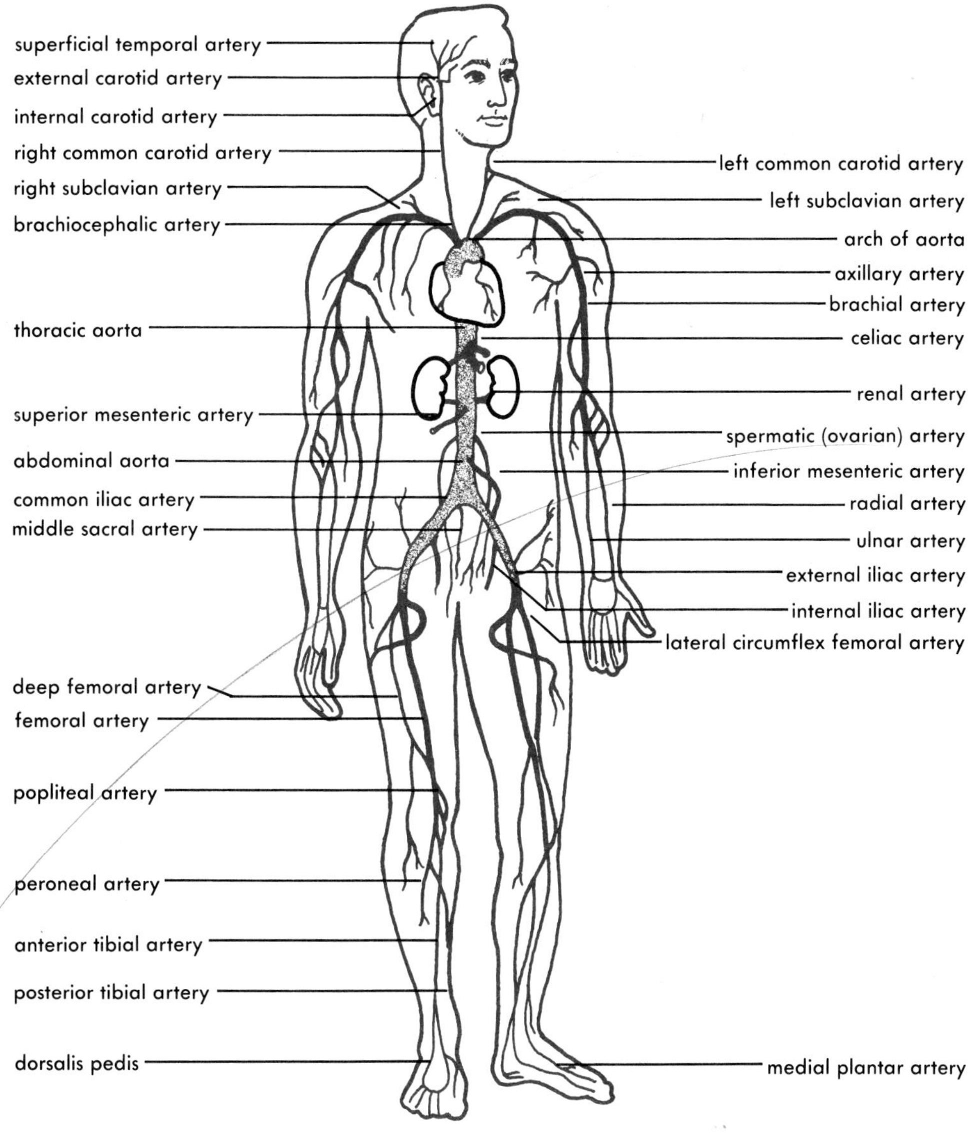

FIGURE 10-3
The principal arteries of the body.

DISEASES OF THE CARDIOVASCULAR SYSTEM

There are many diseases of the cardiovascular system.

Diseases of the heart may be the result of infection; for example, subacute bacterial endocarditis; of an interruption of the normal heartbeat, for example, heart block; or of a mechanical problem involving the pumping action, for example, valvular stenosis.

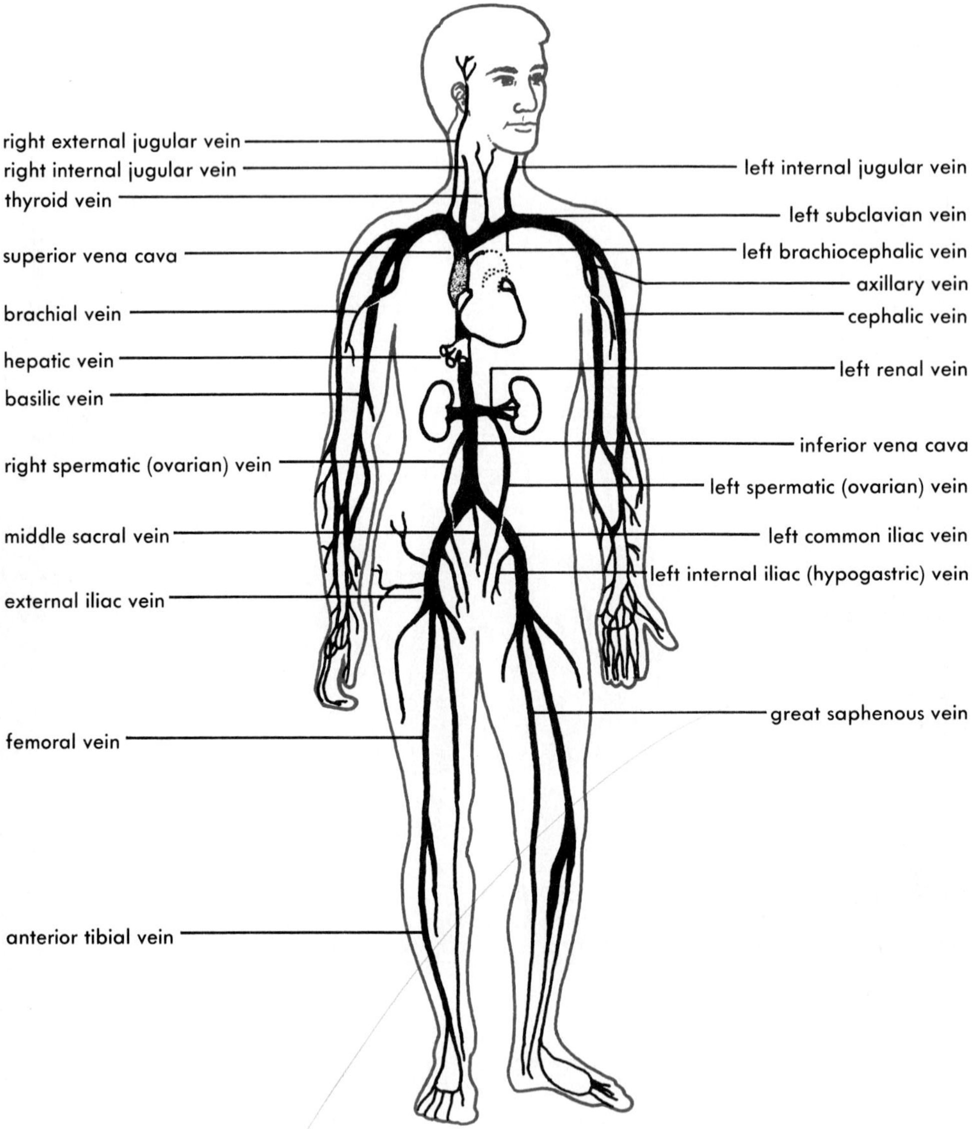

FIGURE 10-4
The pricipal veins of the body.

Disease of the blood vessels may be the result of infection, for example, phlebitis; or of a mechanical obstruction, for example, embolus.

The treatment of cardiovascular diseases includes the use of cardiac drugs that have specific actions. A separate listing of terms related to these drugs is included later in this chapter.

TABLE 10-3
An Analysis of Names of Arteries Shown in Figure 10-3 Listed in Descending Order

Right Anatomical Side

superficial temporal artery: artery close to the surface (*superficial*) over the temporal bone.

external carotid: outermost (*external*) artery to the head. It was so named because compressing the artery reduces blood flow to the brain, and the person afflicted may become stuporous (*carotid*).

internal carotid: innermost (*internal*) artery to the head.

right common carotid: artery on the right that leads to both (*common*) the external and internal carotid arteries.

right subclavian: artery on the right that goes under (*sub*) the collarbone (*clavicle*).

brachiocephalic: artery branching from the aorta that supplies the arms (*brachio*) and the head (*cephalic*).

thoracic aorta: portion of the aorta in the thoracic cavity.

superior mesenteric: artery that supplies the upper portion of the mesentery.

abdominal aorta: portion of the aorta in the abdominal cavity.

common iliac: artery that leads to all (*common*) of the branches that go through or are near the ilium (*iliac*).

middle sacral: artery that goes through the middle of the sacrum.

deep femoral: artery near the femur (*femoral*) that is deeply situated.

femoral: artery near the femur.

popliteal: artery that goes in back of the knee (*popliteal*).

peroneal: artery near the fibula (*peroneal*).

anterior tibial: artery in front of (*anterior*) the tibia (*tibial*).

posterior tibial: artery in back of (*posterior*) the tibia (*tibial*).

dorsalis pedis: artery on the top front aspect of the foot (*pedis*). The term *dorsum* means "back." In this case the top of the foot is called the dorsum. It corresponds to the dorsum, or back, of the hand.

Left Anatomical Side

left common carotid: artery on the left corresponding to the right common carotid artery.

left subclavian: artery on the left corresponding to the right subclavian artery.

arch of aorta: curved portion of the large main (*aorta*) vessel that carries blood from the heart.

axillary: artery located at the armpit (*axilla*).

brachial: artery of the upper arm (*brachia*).

celiac: artery leading to the organs in the abdomen (*celiac*).

renal: artery leading to the kidney (*renal*).

spermatic (ovarian): artery leading to the organs that produce sperm in the male and ova in the female. The artery to the reproductive organs.

inferior mesenteric: artery that supplies the lower (*inferior*) part of the mesentery.

radial: artery that goes along and crosses over the radius (*radial*) in the forearm.

ulnar: artery that lies near the ulna (*ulnar*) in the forearm.

(*Continued.*)

TABLE 10-3
An Analysis of Names of Arteries Shown in Figure 10-3 Listed in Descending Order *(continued)*

Left Anatomical Side

external iliac: artery that goes through the ilium, (*iliac*) to supply organs outside (*external*) the pelvis.

internal iliac: artery that supplies organs inside (*internal*) the ilium, (*iliac*).

lateral circumflex femoral: artery that bends (*flex*) around (*circum*) the femur (*femoral*) toward the side (*lateral*).

medial plantar: artery along the sole of the foot (*plantar*) toward the midline (*medial*).

TABLE 10-4
An Analysis of Names of Veins Shown in Figure 10-4 Listed in Descending Order

Right Anatomical Side

right external jugular: outermost (*external*) vein of the throat (*jugular*).

right internal jugular: innermost (*internal*) vein of the throat (*jugular*).

thyroid: vein from the thyroid gland.

superior vena cava: vein (*vena*) draining the top part (*superior*) of the body. The term *cava* means "empty," and the name comes from the fact that this blood vessel is empty after death.

brachial: vein of the upper arm (*brachia*).

hepatic: vein from the liver (*hepatic*).

basilic: prominent (*basilic*) vein of the arm.

right spermatic (ovarian): vein on the right draining the male or female reproductive organs.

middle sacral: vein at the middle of the sacrum.

external iliac: vein draining the organs outside (*external*) the ilium (*iliac*).

femoral: vein that lies near the femur (*femoral*).

anterior tibial: vein in front of (*anterior*) the tibia (*tibial*).

Left Anatomical Side

left internal jugular: vein on the left corresponding to the right internal jugular vein.

left subclavian: vein on the left corresponding to the right subclavian vein.

left brachiocephalic: vein on the left draining the arm (*brachio*) and the head (*cephalic*).

axillary: vein at the armpit.

cephalic: outer vein of the arm that drains the blood from the arm toward the heart in the direction of the head (*cephalic*).

left renal: vein that drains the left kidney.

inferior vena cava: vein that drains the lower part (*inferior*) of the body. See superior vena cava earlier in Table 10-4.

left spermatic (ovarian): vein on the left corresponding to the right spermatic or ovarian vein.

(*Continued.*)

TABLE 10-4
An Analysis of Names of Veins Shown in Figure 10-4 Listed in Descending Order *(continued)*

Left Anatomical Side

left common iliac: vein on the left that drains all (*common*) branches of the iliac vein.

left internal iliac (hypogastric): vein on the left that drains the organs inside (*internal*) the ilium (*iliac*), also called the hypogastric vein because it is below (*hypo*) the stomach (*gastric*).

great saphenous: longest (*great*) vein of the body. This vein in the leg is a superficial vein. The name means "standing," apparently so applied because the vein may become visible when a person is standing.

DISEASES OF THE CARDIOVASCULAR SYSTEM

Diagnostic Terms, Including Signs and Symptoms

Analysis of selected diagnostic terms including signs and symptoms related to the cardiovascular system:

acrocyanosis: bluish tinge (*cyano*) to the tips (*acro*) of the extremities.

angina pectoris: strangling (*angina*) pain in the chest area (*pectus*).

angiogram: x-ray procedure done to blood vessels (*angio*) involving the injection of a radiopaque substance into the selected blood vessel.

apical rate: pulse rate at the apex (*apical,* variation of apex) of the heart.

arrhythmia: condition (*ia*) in which the normal rhythm (*rhythm*) of the heart is absent (*a*).

arteriography: x-ray films (*graphy*) taken of the arteries (*arterio*).

atrial flutter: rapid contraction (*flutter*) of the atria of the heart.

auscultation: process of listening (*auscul*) for heart sounds.

blood pressure (BP): pressure of the blood against the inner walls of the blood vessels. The blood pressure is recorded in two numbers, one over the other. The top number indicates the pressure during contraction of the heart, or systole; the bottom number indicates the pressure during relaxation, or diastole. Example: 120/80, 120 systolic over 80 diastolic. Remember the *d* number for *d*iastolic is *down* under the line.

bradycardia: condition in which the heart rate (*cardia*) is slower (*brady*) than normal.

bruise: discoloration of the skin that results from the breaking (*bruise*) of superficial blood vessels with the release of blood into the tissue.

bruit: abnormal heart sound heard by listening with a stethoscope.

cardiac catheterization: passage of a catheter, which is a tube for injecting or removing fluid, into the heart for the purpose of obtaining blood samples directly from the heart and taking pressure readings in the heart. This is done to determine abnormalities in cardiac circulation.

cardiac output: amount of blood pumped (*output*) by the heart (*cardiac*) each minute.

cardiomegaly: condition in which the heart (*cardio*) is enlarged (*megaly*).

claudication: lameness or limping (*claudication*) that results from a decrease in the blood supply to the legs.

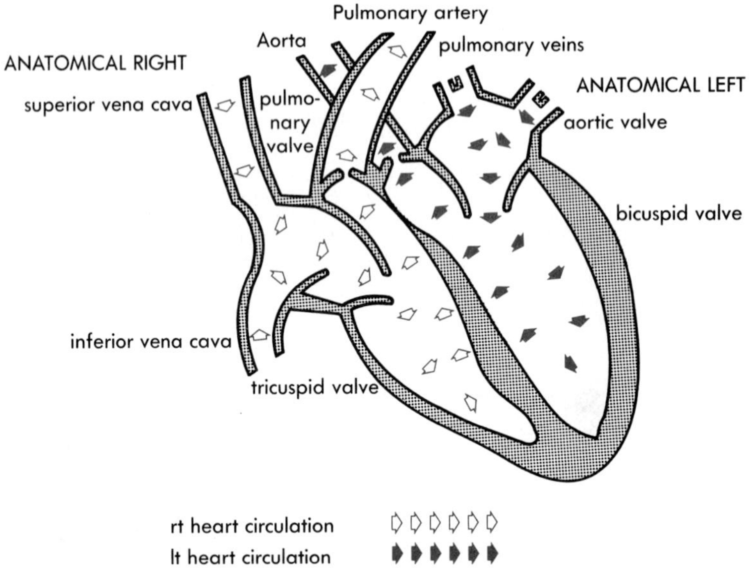

FIGURE 10-5
Circulation of blood through the heart. *Right heart circulation:* Unoxygenated blood enters the right atrium through the superior and inferior vena cavae. It goes through the tricuspid valve into the right ventricle. It is pumped through the pulmonary valve into the pulmonary artery to the lungs where it is oxygenated. (This is the only artery that carries unoxygenated blood.) *Left heart circulation:* Oxygenated blood returns to the left atrium by way of the pulmonary veins. (These are the only veins that carry oxygenated blood.) From the left atrium, blood goes through the bicuspid (mitral) valve into the left ventricle. It is pumped through the aortic valve into the aorta and into general circulation.

ecchymosis: condition (*osis*) in which there is an outpouring (*ec*, variation of *ex*) of fluid (*chym*) that is blood under the skin resulting in a purple spot.

echocardiogram: use of sound to produce a picture (*gram*) of the sound waves (*echo*) from different parts of the heart (*cardio).*

electrocardiogram (EKG or ECG): record (*gram*) of the electrical (*electro*) activity of the heart (*cardio*).

edema: condition in which there is swelling (*edema*) of parts of the body from an accumulation of fluid outside the blood vessels.

extrasystole: the heart contracts (*systole*) more often (*extra*) than it should: the heart does not get an opportunity to relax before the next contraction starts. Sometimes referred to as premature contraction of the heart.

fibrillation: action of (*tion*) uncontrolled twitching of the fibers (*fibrill*) of the heart muscle. May be *atrial fibrillation,* in which the atria twitch, or *ventricular fibrillation,* in which the ventricles twitch.

murmur: sound heard through a stethoscope produced by abnormal opening and closing of the valves in the heart or by abnormal flow of blood through the heart. Murmurs are not always considered to be abnormal.

palpitation: awareness of an abnormally strong or abnormally rapid beating of the heart.

plethysmography: test done to measure and record (*graphy*) variations in size (*plethysmo*) of blood vessels or extremities because of variations in the amount of blood passing through a blood vessel or contained in a part.

pulse pressure: pressure resulting from subtracting the diastolic pressure from the systolic pressure. Example: systolic pressure of 120 minus diastolic pressure of 80 indicates a pulse pressure of 40.

radial rate: pulse rate at the wrist that can be felt near the end of the radius (*radial*).

sphygmomanometer: instrument for measuring the pressure (*manometer*) of the blood by measuring the force of the pulse (*sphygmo*). The device is used for a measurement of blood pressure. Also known as a blood pressure cuff.

stethoscope: instrument used to "view" (*scope*), or hear, the sounds produced in the chest (*stetho*).

tachycardia: condition in which the heart (*cardia*) beats faster (*tachy*) than normal.

thrill: fine vibration felt by the hand on the chest surface, resulting from a loud murmur.

vasoconstriction: constriction or narrowing of the diameter of the blood vessels (*vaso*).

vasodilation: dilation, or widening, of diameter of blood vessels (*vaso*).

ventricular hypertrophy: increase (*hyper*) in size (*trophy*) of the ventricle or the ventricles of the heart.

Disease Conditions of the Cardiovascular System

Analysis of selected terms related to disease conditions of the cardiovascular system:

aneurysm: dilation or widening (*eury*) of (*an*, variation of *ana*) a blood vessel caused by a weakness in the wall of the blood vessel. Abdominal aortic aneurysm (AAA): a weakening in the walls of the abdominal aorta.

arteriosclerosis: disease (*osis*) characterized by hardening (*scler*) of the walls of arteries (*arterio*). Arteriosclerotic heart disease (ASHD): disease state of the heart in which the arteries (*arterio*) have become hardened (*sclerotic*).

arteritis: inflammation (*itis*) of an artery (arter).

atherosclerosis: form of arteriosclerosis in which fatty substances (*athero*) deposit in and between the layers of the lining of the arteries.

avascular necrosis: condition in which there is death of tissue (*necrosis*) because of the lack (*a*) of blood supply through the blood vessels (*vascular*).

bacterial endocarditis: inflammation (*itis*) of the inside (*endo*) lining of the heart (*card*) caused by bacteria.

cardiomyopathy: disease (*pathy*) of the heart (*cardio*) muscle (*myo*).

circulatory collapse: sudden failure (*collapse*) of the circulatory system and respiratory system resulting in a profound degree of shock.

congenital heart defect: heart defect that a child is born (*genital*) with (*con*).

congestive heart failure: condition in which the heart fails to pump blood adequately and there is resultant congestion or backup of blood.

cor pulmonale: form of heart (*cor*) disease resulting from disease in the lungs (*pulmonale*).

coronary artery disease (CAD): disease of the arteries involved in coronary circulation, which supplies blood to the heart itself.

coronary occlusion: obstruction (*occlusion*) in the circulation to the heart.

embolus: ball (*bolus*) of clotted blood and possibly other substances that is carried within (*em*) the bloodstream.

heart attack: sudden seizure (*attack*) of pain and inability of the heart to function because an interference in the coronary circulation.

heart block: normal path of the electrical conduction through the heart is blocked, preventing a normal contraction of the heart.

hemangioma: tumor (*oma*) consisting of blood (*hem*) vessels (*angi*). Also called an *angioma.*

hematoma: tumor (*oma*) or swelling that contains blood (*hemat*).

hemorrhoid: dilated vein filled with blood (*hemo*) in the area of the anal sphincter.

hypertension: elevation (*hyper*) of the blood pressure (*tension*) above normal limits. High blood pressure.

hypotension: condition of low (*hypo*) blood pressure (*tension*).

myocardial infarction: necrosis or death (*infarct*) of a portion of the heart (*cardial*) muscle (*myo*).

myocardial insufficiency: action of the muscle (*myo*) of the heart (*cardial*) is not (*in*) adequate (*sufficient*).

myocardial ischemia: decrease (*isch*) in the blood (*hemia*) supply to the muscle (*myo*) of the heart (*cardial*).

phlebitis: inflammation (*itis*) of a vein (*phleb*).

pulmonary stenosis: condition (*osis*) in which there is constriction or narrowing (*sten*) of the main blood vessel to the lungs (*pulmonary*).

rheumatic heart disease: damage to the heart and scarring of the heart valves resulting from rheumatic fever.

shock: collapse of circulatory function.

- *anaphylactic shock:* reaction from a severe allergy. The shock occurs because the person is not (*ana*) protected (*phylactic*) from a particular protein substance.
- *cardiogenic shock:* shock that is produced (*genic*) from failure of the heart (*cardio*).
- *neurogenic shock:* shock that is produced (*genic*) from a failure of the nervous system.
- *hypovolemic shock:* shock caused from a decrease (*hypo*) in the volume (*vol*) of circulating blood (*emic*).

subacute bacterial endocarditis (SBE): a bacterial inflammation (*itis*) of the inside (*endo*) of the heart (*card*). It is below (*sub*), the acute stage.

tamponade, cardiac: condition in which fluid accumulates in the pericardial sac around the heart muscle. The accumulated fluid builds to a point where the heartbeat is impaired; thus, the flow of blood is blocked (*tampon*). Also called *hemopericardium.* Hemopericardium means that there is blood (*hemo*) in the sac around the heart (*pericardium*).

thromboangiitis obliterans: inflammation (*itis*) of a blood vessel (*angi*) that results in the formation of a blood clot (*thrombo*) that obstructs (*obliterans*) the flow of blood through the vessel.

thrombophlebitis: inflammation (*itis*) of a vein (*phleb*) that results in the formation of a blood clot (*thrombo*).

thrombus: blood clot (*thrombus*) attached to the wall inside a blood vessel.

valvular disease: disease of the valves of the heart can be of three types:

valvular insufficiency: valve does not work efficiently.

valvular regurgitation: valve does not close completely, allowing some blood to flow (*gurgita*) back (*re*).

valvular stenosis: condition (*osis*) in which there is a narrowing (*sten*) of the opening of a valve.

varicose veins: enlarged, twisted veins, particularly in the lower extremities.

Treatment of Cardiovascular Disease

Analysis of terms related to the treatment of disease of the cardiovascular system:

angioplasty: procedure in which a small catheter with a balloon end is insered into a blood vessel (*angio*) to reshape (*plasty*) the inside of the vessel.

bypass surgery: surgery done on blood vessels for the purpose of installing a graft that will bypass an occluded blood vessel. A graft carries the blood supply around the point of occlusion in a blocked vessel, thereby passing the occlusion.

cardiopulmonary resuscitation (CPR): act of restoring consciousness (*resuscitate*) by forcing air into the lungs (*pulmonary*) and forcing blood from the heart (*cardio*).

defibrillation: stopping (*de*) the uncontrolled twitching (*fibrillation*) of the heart through the use of medications or electric shock.

embolectomy: surgical removal (*ectomy*) of a blood clot (*embol*).

endarterectomy: surgical removal (*ectomy*) of a thrombus and the abnormally thickened inside (*end,* combining form of *ando*) lining of an artery (*arter*).

heart transplant: procedure in which the heart of one person is put into the body of another person (see Glossary of Terms related to Transplantation).

intravenous therapy: injection into (*intra*) a vein (*venous*) of essential nutrients or drugs for the treatment (*therapy*) of disease.

mitral commissurotomy: surgical cutting (*otomy*) of the seam (*commissure*) of the two flaps of the mitral valve. An operation for mitral stenosis.

open-heart surgery: surgical procedure done during which the heart is opened.

phlebotomy: opening (*otomy*) into a vein (*phleb*) for the purpose of removing blood.

pacemaker implant: implanting of an artificial device that keeps (*maker*) the rate (*pace*) of the heart in a desirable range.

portacaval shunt: procedure done in which a branch of the portal vein (*porta*) is sewn to the vena cava (*caval*). The portal blood is thus diverted (*shunt*) around the liver.

valve replacement: surgical procedure in which the heart is opened and a valve that is defective is replaced with a new valve.

venipuncture: puncture of a vein (*veni*) with a needle, or the insertion of a catheter for a diagnostic procedure.

Use of Drugs in Treatment

Analysis of selected terms related to the treatment of cardiovascular diseases by the use of drugs:

anticoagulant drugs: drugs that work against (*anti*) the clotting (*coagulant*) of blood, commonly called "blood thinners."

antiangina drugs: drugs that work against (*anti*) the strangling (*angina*) pain in the chest.

antiarrhythmic drugs: class of medicines that work against (*anti*) the lack of (*a*) rhythm (*rrhythm*) of the heart. These drugs restore the normal rhythm of the heart.

cardiotonic drugs: class of medicines that invigorate and strengthen (*tonic*) the heart (*cardio*).

chronotropic drug action: action of a drug that changes (*tropic*) the timing (*chrono*) of the heart rate. A positive chronotropic action increases the heart rate, and a negative chronotropic effect decreases the heart rate.

dromotropic drug action: action of a drug that changes (*tropic*) the rate at which the conduction of the electrical impulse runs (*dromo*), or courses (*dromo),* through the heart. A positive dromotropic action speeds the conduction rate, and a negative dromotropic action decreases the conduction rate.

inotropic drug action: action of a drug that changes (*tropic*) the action of the heart muscle fibers (*ino).* A positive inotropic action increases the ability of the muscle to contract, and a negative inotropic effect decreases the ability of the heart muscle to contract.

vasoconstrictors: drugs that act to narrow or constrict (*constrictor*) the blood vessels (*vaso*).

vasodilators: drugs which act to widen or dilate (*dilator*) the blood vessels (*vaso).*

PRETEST/ POSTTEST FOR CHAPTER 10

1. Label the diagram (Figure 10-6) that shows the structures and chambers of the heart.

2. The following terms are related to the blood vessels and valves of the heart. Match column A with column B. Choose the one best correct answer.

Column A	Column B
1. _____ inferior vena cava	A. the main artery of the body
	B. the valve leading from the left ventricle
2. _____ superior vena cava	C. returns blood from the left lung

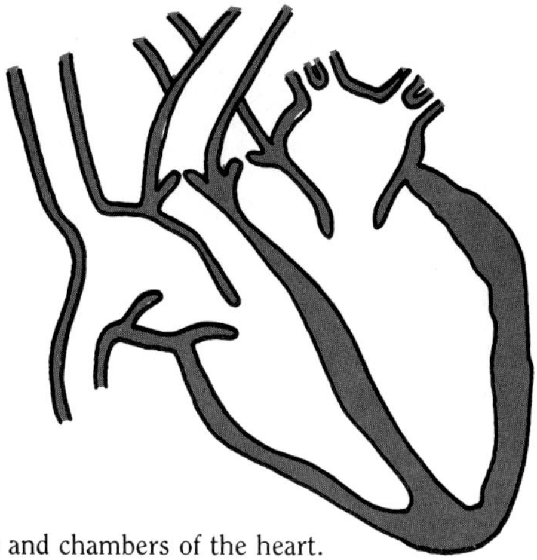

FIGURE 10-6
The structures and chambers of the heart.

Column A	Column B
3. _____ pulmonary artery	D. blood vessel carrying blood to the lungs
4. _____ right pulmonary vein	E. valve leading from the right ventricle
5. _____ left pulmonary vein	F. valve on the right side of the heart between the atrium and ventricle
6. _____ aorta	G. drains blood from the lower parts of the body
7. _____ tricuspid valve	H. valve on the left side of the heart between the atrium and ventricle
8. _____ pulmonary valve	I. drains blood from the upper part of the body
9. _____ aortic valve	J. returns blood from the right lung
10. _____ bicuspid or mitral valve	

3. The following terms are related to the heartbeat. Choose the correct phrase.

1. The heartbeat:
- A. includes a contraction phase and a relaxation phase.
- B. includes a systolic phase and a contraction phase.

2. Conduction refers to the action in which there is a transfer of _________ through the heart.
- A. electrical impulses
- B. heart sounds

3. The thickening and shortening of the heart muscle occurs during:
- A. contraction.
- B. relaxation.

4. In relaxation the heart is said to be in the ________ phase.
   A. systolic
   B. diastolic

5. The sinoatrial node is located:
   A. in the atrium.
   B. in the ventricle.

6. Heart sounds are caused by:
   A. the contraction of the heart muscle.
   B. blood rushing through the heart.

7. A pulse is felt as a result of:
   A. the impact of blood on the artery walls.
   B. the relaxation of the left ventricle.

8. The normal rate and rhythm of the heart is called:
   A. arrhythmia.
   B. sinus rhythm.

4. The following terms are related to blood vessels. Match column A with column B. Choose the one best answer.

Column A	Column B
1. ____ angio-	A. small artery
2. ____ artery	B. hair-thin blood vessel
3. ____ arteriole	C. root word meaning vein
4. ____ capillary	D. leading toward the heart
5. ____ phleb-	E. vessel
6. ____ vein	F. small vein
7. ____ venule	G. leading away from the heart

5. The following listed arteries are illustrated in Figure 10-3. Briefly describe the artery. The terms are selected from Table 10-3.

Artery	Description
1. superficial temporal	________________
2. external carotid	________________
3. subclavian	________________
4. brachiocephalic	________________

5. thoracic aorta ____________________
6. superior mesenteric ____________________
7. common iliac ____________________
8. middle sacral ____________________
9. femoral ____________________
10. popliteal ____________________
11. peroneal ____________________
12. posterior tibial ____________________
13. dorsalis pedis ____________________
14. axillary ____________________
15. brachial ____________________
16. celiac ____________________
17. renal ____________________
18. spermatic or ovarian ____________________
19. radial ____________________
20. ulnar ____________________
21. lateral circumflex femoral ____________________
22. medial plantar ____________________

6. The following veins are illustrated in Figure 10-4. Briefly describe the vein. The terms are selected from Table 10-4.

Vein	Description
1. external jugular	____________________
2. thyroid	____________________
3. superior vena cava	____________________
4. brachial	____________________
5. hepatic	____________________
6. basilic	____________________
7. right spermatic or ovarian	____________________
8. external iliac	____________________
9. femoral	____________________
10. anterior tibial	____________________

Vein	Description
11. left subclavian	______________________
12. axillary	______________________
13. cephalic	______________________
14. left renal	______________________
15. inferior vena cava	______________________
16. left common iliac	______________________
17. left internal iliac	______________________
18. great saphenous	______________________

7. The following terms are related to circulation. Circle the letter indicating the correct statement.

1. In pulmonary circulation the blood:
A. is pumped from the right ventricle to the lungs and returns to the right atrium.
B. is pumped from the left ventricle to the lungs and returns to the left atrium.
C. is pumped from the right ventricle to the lungs and returns to the left atrium.
D. is pumped from the left ventricle to the lungs and returns to the right atrium.

2. In systemic circulation the blood:
A. is pumped from the right ventricle to all parts of the body and returns to the right atrium.
B. is pumped from the left ventricle to all parts of the body and returns to the left atrium.
C. is pumped from the right ventricle to all parts of the body and returns to the left atrium.
D. is pumped from the left ventricle to all parts of the body and returns to the right atrium.

3. Coronary circulation:
A. involves the circulation in the coronal plane.
B. is the circulation that supplies blood to the heart muscle.

4. Peripheral vascular circulation:
A. involves the circulation of blood around the outside of the heart.
B. involves blood vessels around the outside of the body away from the heart.

5. Portal circulation:
A. transports blood and absorbed food products to the liver.
B. transports blood from the liver to the intestine.
C. transports blood and food products to the heart.
D. transports blood from the heart to the liver.

8. The following sets of diagnostic terms are related to the cardiovascular system. Match column A with column B. Choose the one best answer.

Set 1

Column A	Column B
1. _____ angina pectoris	A. pulse rate at apex of the heart
2. _____ angiogram	B. pressure against inner walls of blood vessels
3. _____ apical rate	C. pain in the chest
4. _____ arrhythmia	D. slow heart rate
5. _____ arteriography	E. x-ray of blood vessels including both arteries and veins
6. _____ auscultation	F. x-ray of arteries
7. _____ atrial flutter	G. listening for heart sounds
8. _____ blood pressure	H. normal rhythm of the heart is absent
9. _____ bradycardia	I. discoloration of skin
10. _____ bruise	J. rapid contraction of the atria

Set 2

Column A	Column B
1. _____ cardiac catheterization	A. test to determine abnormalities in cardiac circulation
2. _____ cardiac output	B. record of the electrical activity of the heart
3. _____ cardiomegaly	C. use of sound waves to produce a picture of the heart
4. _____ claudication	D. amount of blood pumped by the heart each minute
5. _____ ecchymosis	E. limping caused by decreased circulation
6. _____ echocardiogram	F. purple spot under the skin
7. _____ electrocardiogram	G. swelling of parts of the body
8. _____ edema	H. enlarged heart
9. _____ extrasystole	I. uncontrolled twitching of parts of the heart
10. _____ fibrillation	J. premature contraction of the heart

Set 3

Column A	Column B
1. _____ murmur	A. fast heart rate
2. _____ palpitation	B. increase in the size of the ventricle or ventricles

Column A	Column B
3. _____ plethysmography	C. sound produced by blood pumping through the heart
4. _____ pulse pressure	D. awareness of abnormally strong or rapid heartbeat
5. _____ radial rate	E. pulse rate at the wrist
6. _____ sphygmomanometer	F. test to record changes in size of a part caused by the differences in blood volume passing through a part
7. _____ stethoscope	G. difference between systolic and diastolic pressure
8. _____ tachycardia	H. widening of the diameter of blood vessels
9. _____ thrill	I. instrument used to measure blood pressure
10. _____ vasoconstriction	J. instrument used to hear sounds produced in the chest
11. _____ vasodilation	K. narrowing of the diameter of blood vessels
12. _____ventricular hypertrophy	L. fine vibration felt on chest wall from a loud murmur

9. The following sets of terms are related to disease conditions of the cardiovascular system. Match column A with column B. Choose the one best answer. Be specific.

Set 1

Column A	Column B
1. _____ aneurysm	A. death of tissue because of destruction of blood vessels to that tissue
2. _____ arteriosclerosis	B. general term for disease of heart muscle
3. _____ arteritis	C. condition a child is born with
4. _____ atherosclerosis	D. failure of heart as a pump, which results in congestion
5. _____ avascular necrosis	E. widening or weakening of a blood vessel
6. _____ bacterial endocarditis	F. inflammation of an artery
7. _____ cardiomyopathy	G. hardening of the arteries
8. _____ circulatory collapse	H. inflammation inside the heart
9. _____ congenital heart defect	I. general phrase referring to diseases involving blood vessels in the heart
10. _____ congestive heart failure	J. obstruction in circulation to the heart
11. _____ cor pulmonale	
12. _____ coronary artery disease	

Column A	Column B
13. ____ coronary occlusion	K. fatty deposits in blood vessel causing hardening of arteries
	L. heart disease resulting from lung disease
	M. sudden failure of the circulatory system

Set 2

Column A	Column B
1. ____ embolus	A. normal path of conduction through the heart blocked
2. ____ heart attack	B. action of heart muscle inadequate
3. ____ heart block	C. common term referring to sudden seizure of pain and inability of heart to function
4. ____ hemangioma	D. necrosis or death of heart muscle
5. ____ hematoma	E. dilated vein containing blood in the anal area
6. ____ hemorrhoid	F. low blood pressure
7. ____ hypertension	G. swelling containing blood
8. ____ hypotension	H. high blood pressure
9. ____ myocardial infarction	I. ball of blood or other substances in the bloodstream
10. ____ myocardial insufficiency	J. tumor consisting of blood vessels
11. ____ myocardial ischemia	K. decrease in the blood supply to the heart

Set 3

Column A	Column B
1. ____ phlebitis	A. inflammation of blood vessel with clot that obstructs flow of blood
2. ____ pulmonary stenosis	B. constriction or narrowing of blood vessels to the lungs
3. ____ rheumatic heart disease	C. blood accumulates around the heart
4. ____ shock	D. inflammation of a vein that results in the formation of a clot
5. ____ subacute bacterial endocarditis	E. less than acute inflammation of the inside of the heart
6. ____ cardiac tamponade	F. enlarged twisted veins, especially in lower extremity
7. ____ thromboangiitis obliterans	G. damage to the heart and scarring of the heart valves
8. ____ thrombophlebitis	
9. ____ thrombus	

Column A	Column B
10. ____ valvular disease	H. disease of the valves of the heart
11. ____ varicose veins	I. inflammation of a vein
	J. collapse of circulatory function
	K. blood clot that is obstructing a blood vessel

10. The following terms are related to the treatment of cardiac diseases. Match column A with column B.

Column A	Column B
1. ____ bypass surgery	A. surgical removal of a clot
2. ____ cardiopulmonary resuscitation	B. use of artificial device to control heart rate
3. ____ defibrillation	C. stopping uncontrolled twitching of the heart
4. ____ embolectomy	D. puncture of vein with a needle
5. ____ intravenous therapy	E. surgery done to go around an occluded blood vessel
6. ____ open-heart surgery	F. surgical procedure for defective heart valve
7. ____ phlebotomy	G. act of restoring breathing
8. ____ pacemaker implant	H. group of surgical procedures in which the heart is opened
9. ____ valve replacement	I. injection of substance into vein for treatment of disease
10. ____ venipuncture	J. removal of blood
11. ____ angioplasty	K. reshaping the inside of a blood vessel

11. The following terms are related to drugs used in the treatment of cardiovascular diseases. Match column A with column B.

Column A	Column B
1. ____ anticoagulant	A. changes timing of the heart rate
2. ____ antianginal	B. changes rate of conduction through the heart
3. ____ antiarrhythmic	C. blood thinner
4. ____ cardiotonic	D. drug that narrows blood vessels
5. ____ chronotropic	E. drug that widens blood vessels
6. ____ dromotropic	F. used for pain in chest
7. ____ inotropic	G. restores normal rhythm of heart
8. ____ vasoconstrictor	H. changes action of heart muscle fibers
9. ____ vasodilator	I. invigorates and strengthens the heart

PRETEST/ POSTTEST **ANSWERS** FOR CHAPTER **10**

1. See Figure 10-1.

2. **1.** G **2.** I **3.** D **4.** J **5.** C **6.** A **7.** F* **8.** E **9.** B **10.** H*

3. **1.** A **2.** A **3.** A **4.** B **5.** A **6.** B **7.** A **8.** B

4. **1.** E **2.** G **3.** A **4.** B **5.** C **6.** D **7.** F

5.
1. artery close to the surface over the temporal bone
2. outermost artery to the head
3. artery under the collarbone
4. artery supplying the arm and head
5. portion of the aorta in the thoracic cavity
6. artery supplying upper mesentery
7. artery that leads to all branches of artery going through the ilium
8. artery that goes through the middle of the sacrum
9. artery near the femur
10. artery that goes in back of knee
11. artery near the fibula
12. artery in back of the tibia
13. artery at the top of the foot
14. artery at the armpit
15. artery of the upper arm
16. artery to the organs in abdomen
17. artery to the kidney
18. artery to reproductive organs
19. artery at the wrist
20. artery near ulna
21. artery that circles the femur toward the side
22. artery along the sole of the foot toward the midline

6.
1. outermost vein of the throat
2. vein from thyroid gland
3. vein draining upper part of body
4. vein in the upper arm
5. vein from the liver
6. prominent vein in the arm
7. vein from reproductive organs

* To remember the location of the tricuspid and bicuspid valves, think of the number 32. There are 3 lobes of the right lung and 2 lobes of the left lung. There are 3 cusps on the right valve and 2 cusps on the left valve. Remember this refers to anatomical right and left.

8. vein draining organs outside ilium
9. vein near the femur
10. vein in front of tibia
11. vein under collarbone
12. vein in the armpit
13. vein in arm that carries blood back to heart in direction of the head
14. vein from left kidney
15. vein draining blood from lower part of the body
16. vein on left that drains all branches of the iliac vein
17. vein on left that drains organs inside ilium (also called hypogastric)
18. largest vein of the body located in the leg

7. 1. C 2. D 3. B 4. B 5. A

8. Set 1
1. C 2. E 3. A 4. H 5. F 6. G 7. J 8. B 9. D 10. I

Set 2
1. A 2. D 3. H 4. E 5. F 6. C 7. B 8. G 9. J 10. I

Set 3
1. C 2. D 3. F 4. G 5. E 6. I 7. J 8. A 9. L 10. K 11. H 12. B

9. Set 1
1. E 2. G 3. F 4. K 5. A 6. H 7. B 8. M 9. C 10. D 11. L 12. I 13. J

Set 2
1. I 2. C 3. A 4. J 5. G 6. E 7. H 8. F 9. D 10. B 11. K

Set 3
1. I 2. B 3. G 4. J 5. E 6. C 7. A 8. D 9. K 10. H 11. F

10. 1. E 2. G 3. C 4. A 5. I 6. H 7. J 8. B 9. F 10. D 11. K

11. 1. C 2. F 3. G 4. I 5. A 6. B 7. H 8. D 9. E

11 THE HEMATOLOGICAL SYSTEM

OBJECTIVES

At the end of this chapter you will be able to do the following:

1 List the body functions in which blood is involved.
2 Name the components of whole blood.
3 List the ways red blood cells are evaluated.
4 Define terms related to red blood cells.
5 Define the various types of white blood cells.
6 Define *platelet.*
7 List the major proteins in plasma.
8 Describe hemostasis.
9 Describe the ABO system of blood typing.
10 Describe classifications of blood diseases.
11. Analyze selected terms related to diseases of blood, including changes in blood resulting from other diseases.
12 Analyze selected terms related to the treatment of diseases of the blood.

FUNCTIONS OF BLOOD

Blood is one of the connective tissues of the body. It connects the outside of the body to the inside of the body and connects each section, organ, and system of the body to all other sections, organs, and systems.

Blood is involved in the following functions:

1 *nutrition:* the products of digestion are absorbed into the bloodstream and carried to the various cells.
2 *excretion:* waste products of cells are carried to the kidneys, sweat glands, and lungs for removal from the body.
3 *internal respiration:* the blood circulates through the lung tissue, where it picks up oxygen and releases carbon dioxide.
4 *fluid balance:* fluid moves back and forth between the cells of tissue and the blood.
5 *chemical balance:* the blood contains certain elements that help control the chemical balance in the body.

don't NEED to know All

TABLE 11-1
Components of Blood

Erythrocytes (Red Blood Cells)	Leukocytes (White Blood Cells)	Thrombocytes	Plasma
reticulocytes	granulocytes: neutrophils, eosinophils, basophils nongranulocytes: lymphocytes, monocytes	platelets	water globulin albumin fibrinogen prothrombin

6 *protection:* the blood contains many cells and chemicals that serve a protective function, e.g., in phagocytosis.
7 *temperature regulation:* the blood serves as a heating and/or cooling fluid.
8 *endocrine function:* blood carries and distributes the hormones from the endocrine glands.

Terms related to blood:

corpuscle: an old term for a blood cell. It means small (*cle*) rounded body (*corpus*).
-emia, hemia-, hemo-, hemato-, sangui-: forms meaning "blood."

COMPOSITION OF BLOOD

Blood consists of formed elements suspended in a fluid. The site for most of the development of formed blood elements is the bone marrow. The formation of blood cells is called *hematopoiesis.*

The fluid in which these elements are suspended is called *plasma.* See Table 11-1.

Erythrocytes

Erythrocytes are red blood cells containing hemoglobin that gives blood its red color.

Hemoglobin functions to transport oxygen and carbon dioxide to and from the cells and lungs.

Red blood cells are described in health and disease in three ways:

1 according to the shape of the cell. This is called *morphology* or the study (*ology*) of shapes (*morph*).
2 according to the quantity of blood cells, or the *cell count.* Example: anemia means a lack (*an*) of blood (*emia*). The amount of blood is low.
3 according to the color and size of blood cells. Examples: normochromic red blood cells have a normal (*normo*) color (*chronic*); therefore the cells contain a normal amount of hemoglobin. Microcytic red blood cells are cells (*cytic*) that are smaller (*micro*) than normal.

Terms describing red blood cells:

Red blood cells are produced in bone marrow.

Cells in bone marrow called *hematocytoblasts* function to produce blood cells.

The production of the various cells of blood is very complicated. A hormone from the kidney called *erythropoietin* is involved in the production of red blood cells.

Terms related to red blood cells:

erythrocytes: red (*erythro*) blood cells (*cytes*)
erythropoietin: hormone (*in*) that regulates the production (*poiet*) of red (*erythro*) blood cells
hemoglobin: protein (*globin*) substance in red blood (*hemo*) cells that is capable of attaching to oxygen
reticulocytes: young red blood cells (*cytes*) containing a network (*reticulo*) of dark-staining material

Leukocytes

Leukocytes are white (*leuko*) blood cells (*cytes*) that function in the body's defense against infections and foreign substances.

There are two basic types of leukocytes: granulocytes and nongranulocytes.

Granulocytes

A *granulocyte* is a white blood cell that contains small, beadlike granules. There are three types of granulocytes that are named according to their reaction to chemical stains or dyes. The three types of granulocytes are neutrophils, eosinophils, and basophils.

Terms related to granulocytes:

basophil: white blood cell that stains, or loves (*phil*) basic (*baso*) dyes.
eosinophil: white blood cell that stains, or loves (*phil*), a rose-colored (*eosin*) dye.
neutrophil: white blood cell that stains, or loves (*phil*), neutral (*neutro*) dye.
polymorphonuclear leukocyte: another name for neutrophil that means a white (*leuko*) blood cell (*cyte*) with a nucleus (*nuclear*) having many (*poly*) shapes (*morpho*).

Some granulocytes carry on the function of phagocytosis. *Phagocytosis* is a process in which the white blood cell (*cyt*) ingests, or eats (*phago*), a foreign harmful substance. This is a protective mechanism.

Nongranulocytes

A nongranulocyte is a white blood cell (*cyte*) that does not (*non*) contain granules (*granulo*). These cells are also called *agranular leukocytes,* or white (*leuko*) blood cells (*cytes*) without (*a*) granules (*granular*).

Types of nongranulocytes:

lymphocyte: a white blood cell (*cyte*) that is found in large numbers in lymphoid (*lymph*) tissue.
monocyte: a white blood cell (*cyte*) that has one (*mono*) nucleus. These cells are sometimes called *large mononuclear leukocytes.*

Thrombocytes

Platelets are blood cells that function in the clotting of blood. They are known as platelets because of their small (*let*) platelike (*plate*) appearance. They are also called *thrombocytes*. A thrombocyte is a cell (*cyte*) that functions in the clotting (*thrombo*) of blood.

This cell is only one part functioning in the complicated mechanism of blood clotting. See the discussion of hemostasis later in this chapter.

Plasma

Plasma is the straw-colored fluid in which the formed elements of blood are suspended.

Plasma is composed of water and plasma proteins.

Plasma proteins

The four major proteins are albumin, globulin, fibrinogen, and prothrombin. Albumin is the most abundant, and prothrombin is the least abundant.

albumin: a protein that coagulates like egg white (albumen) when heated.
globulin: a protein that in solution tends to assume a spherical or globelike (*globul*) shape.
fibrinogen: a protein substance that produces (*gen*) fibers (*fibren*) during the clotting of blood.
prothrombin: the protein that exists before (*pro*) thrombin. This protein is changed to thrombin, which causes the blood to clot (*thromb*).

HEMOSTASIS

Blood clotting or coagulation is also known as *hemostasis*. Hemostasis is another protective mechanism of blood. The term means stopping (*stasis*) of blood (*hemo*). It prevents the loss of large amounts of blood when a blood vessel is opened.

Hemostasis may be divided into three phases:

1 *vascular phase:* in which the cut blood vessel constricts, thus somewhat mechanically squeezing the open end of the cut blood vessel.
2 *platelet phase:* in which platelets stick to the injured blood vessel wall and to each other and form a temporary clot.
3 *coagulation phase:* in which the liquid blood is changed into a jellylike or curdled (*coagula*) mass, and a more permanent fibrin clot is formed. The formation of the fibrin clot involves a complicated mechanism in which the plasma proteins thrombin and fibrinogen and other elements in the blood called *factors* interact.

Other selected terms related to blood clotting:

factor VIII, or the antihemophilic factor: an element in blood that works against (*anti*) bleeding (*hemophilic*).
heparin: natural substance in the body that prevents the clotting of blood. Also used as a medication to prevent blood clotting.
prothrombin: one of the factors in the blood plasma that is believed to come before (*pro*) thrombin, which is needed to clot blood.
serum: clear, pale-yellow liquid that remains after a clot is formed.

BLOOD TYPING

Blood grouping is a process in which types of blood are grouped to enable the transfusion of blood from one person to another.

ABO System

All human blood can be grouped into four major blood types. This is called the *ABO system*.

The four groups are as follows:

A B AB O

In the use of blood transfusion as a life-saving treatment, grouping or typing of blood is essential. Blood is a protein substance and thus is capable of causing a severe allergic reaction if given to a person who has a different blood type than that which is transfused.

In the ABO system of grouping, blood donors and blood recipients are matched so that an allergic reaction will not occur.

Blood type AB is called the *universal recipient,* because it will not react to any of the other blood groups.

Blood type O is called the *universal donor,* because it can be given to any other person. Persons with O blood can give blood to any other person, but can only be given O-type blood.

TABLE 11-2
Donor and Recipient Matching in Blood Transfusion

Recipient Type	Donor Type
A	A and O
B	B and O
AB	A, B, AB, and O
O	O

Rh Factor

Another difference noted when blood transfusions are necessary is the Rh factor. If your blood contains the Rh factor, you are considered Rh-positive. If your blood does not contain the Rh factor, you are considered Rh-negative.

Persons with Rh-positive blood may receive blood that is Rh-positive and Rh-negative.

Persons with Rh-negative blood may receive only Rh-negative blood because they will have an allergic reaction to Rh-positive blood.

If your blood type and Rh factor matches the blood type and Rh factor of another person, your blood is said to be *compatible* with that person's blood.

There are many factors that must be tested for blood compatibility. The Rh factor is only one example.

CLASSIFICATION OF BLOOD DISEASES

Diseases of blood may occur from lack of blood (*anemias*). This lack may be from inadequate production of blood cells (aplastic), excessive destruction or breakdown of blood cells (hemolysis), or loss of blood through bleeding (hemorrhage).

Blood diseases may also occur from the overproduction or underproduction of various elements of blood (leukemia), or the production of abnormal blood cells (hypochromic microcytic anemia).

A delicate balance of numbers and amounts of blood elements is essential to life. A slight variation in the proportions of blood elements signals disease. For example, the normal white blood cell count is 5000 to 10,000. If a white cell count is 4000 or 12,000, there may be disease.

Blood is involved in almost every disease known. A blood test is done for almost all diseases.

The diseases listed here are selected because they are diseases of the blood or blood-forming organs, or are diseases whose signs are evident in blood.

Terms Related to Diseases Evident in Blood

Analysis of terms related to diseases of the blood including changes in blood from other diseases:

agranulocytosis: condition (*osis*), in which there is a lack (*a*) of granulocytes.

anemia: ~~condition in which there is a lack (*an*) of blood (*emia*)~~.

There are many causes and variations of this condition:

- *aplastic anemia:* anemia characterized by the lack (*a*) of blood cell formation (*plastic*).
- *hemolytic anemia:* anemia resulting from the breakdown (*lytic*) of blood (*hemo*) cells.
- *hypochromic microcytic anemia:* anemia characterized by a decrease (*hypo*) in the normal color (*chromic*) of blood cells (*cytic*), and which are smaller (*micro*) than normal.
- *iron-deficiency anemia:* anemia caused by the lack of (deficiency) sufficient iron to produce normal red blood cells.

macrocytic anemia: anemia characterized by the appearance of large (*macro*) red blood cells (*cytic*).

pernicious anemia: anemia that may lead to (*per*) death (*nici,* variation of *necro*).

sickle-cell anemia: anemia characterized by presence of crescent, or sickle-shaped, red blood cells.

thalassemia: type of blood (*emia*) disease so named because it is found mostly in persons from the Mediterranean Sea (*thalass*) region. It is a hemolytic-type disease.

anisocytosis: condition (*osis*) in which the sizes of red blood cells (*cyt*) are unequal or dissimilar (*aniso*).

anoxia: deficiency (*an*) of oxygen (*oxia*) in the blood.

acidosis: condition (*osis*) in which the blood is more acid than normal.

alkalosis: condition (*osis*) in which the blood is more alkaline (*alkal*) than normal.

dyscrasia: general term for disorders that may be used for a blood condition (*ia*) and that then refers to defective or abnormal (*dys*) mixture (*cras*) of formed blood elements.

embolus: clump, usually of blood products, which acts as a stopper (*bolus*) inside (*em*) a blood vessel. This clump travels through the blood vessels until it reaches a blood vessel too small for it to pass through.

erythrocytosis: condition (*osis*) in which there is an excess of red blood cells (*erythrocyt*).

erythropenia: deficiency (*penia*) of red blood cells (*erythro*).

exsanguination: occurrence in which all of the blood (*sanguin*) is let out (*ex*) of the body.

extravasation: condition resulting from (*tion*) blood outside (*extra*) a blood vessel (*vasa*).

granulocytopenia: condition in which there is a decrease (*penia*) in the number of granulocytes.

hemolysis: breaking down (*lysis*) of red blood (*hemo*) cells.

hemophilia: hereditary blood disease in which the time it takes for the blood to coagulate is prolonged, as though there were a love (*philia*) of blood (*hemo*). A hemophiliac is commonly called a "bleeder."

hemorrhage: event in which there is a break in a blood vessel causing the release or bursting forth (*rrhage*) of blood (*hemo*).

hemostasis: stopping or stagnation (*stasis*) of blood (*hemo*) resulting from poor circulation.

hyperglycemia: condition in which there is an excessive (*hyper*) amount of glucose (*glyc*) or sugar in the blood (*emia*).

hypoglycemia: condition in which there is a decrease (*hypo*) in the amount of glucose (*glyc*) or sugar in the blood (*emia*).

hypoxia: condition (*ia*) in which there is a decrease (*hyp*) in the amount of oxygen (*ox*) in the blood.

leukemia: condition (*ia*) characterized by the presence of abnormally high numbers of white blood cells (*leuk*) in the blood (*em*).

leukopenia: abnormal decrease (*penia*) in the number of white blood cells (*leuko*).

myelocytic leukemia: increase in the large cells (*cytic*) in bone marrow (*myelo*) from which leukocytes are derived. See leukemia.

pancytopenia: reduction (*penia*) in all (*pan*) cellular (*cyto*) elements of the blood.

poikilocytosis: condition (*osis*) in which red blood cells (*cytes*) have varied or irregular (*poikilo*) shapes.

polycythemia: condition in which there is an excess (*poly*) of blood (*hemia*) cells (*cyt*).

septicemia: condition in which there is invasion of disease-causing (*septic*) substances into the blood (*emia*); an infection in the blood commonly called "blood poisoning."

thrombocythemia: condition in which there is an increase in the numbers of platelets (*thrombocyt*) in the blood (*hemia*).

thrombocytopenia: condition in which there is a decrease (*penia*) in the number of platelets (*thrombocytes*). One type is called ITP, *idiopathic thrombocytopenic purpura:* the cause of the disease (*pathic*) is peculiar (*idio*) to that person. The cause is unknown. The results of the disease are purple (*purpura*) areas from bleeding under the skin.

thrombosis: condition (*osis*) in which there is a clotting (*thromb*) of blood in a blood vessel.

TREATMENT OF DISEASES OF THE BLOOD

Analysis of selected terms related to the treatment of diseases of the blood*:

chemotherapy: treatment (*therapy*) of disease by the use of drugs or chemical (*chemo*) agents.

heparinization: action taken to prevent blood clotting by the administration of the drug *heparin*.

irradiation therapy: treatment (*therapy*) of blood diseases by radiation of blood-forming organs to slow down the abnormal production of blood cells.

phlebotomy: cutting into (*otomy*) a vein (*phleb*) for the drawing off of blood. Also called *venesection*.

transfusion: intermingling (*transfusion*) of the blood of one person with the blood of another compatible person. A transfusion may include the injection of whole blood or of one of the parts of whole blood. Packed cells, platelets, or plasma may be given. The choice of the element transfused depends on the reason for the needed transfusion. If the problem is hemorrhage, whole blood may be given. If the problem is thrombocytopenia, platelets alone may be given.

* Note: terms related to treatment of blood diseases that directly affect blood vessels are covered in Chapter 10.

PRETEST/ POSTTEST FOR CHAPTER 11

1. List five combining forms meaning blood:

1. ________ 4. ________

2. ________ 5. ________

3. ________

2. The following terms relate to the components of blood. Match column A with column B.

Column A	Column B
1. ____ erythrocytes	A. thrombocytes
2. ____ leukocytes	B. fluid of blood
3. ____ platelets	C. red blood cells
4. ____ plasma	D. white blood cells
5. ____ hemoglobin	E. hormone regulating the production of red blood cells
6. ____ erythropoietin	F. red coloring in red blood cells
7. ____ reticulocytes	G. young red blood cells

3. The following terms are related to white blood cells and platelets. Select the best answer.

1. A granulocyte is a(n) ____.
   A. erythrocyte
   B. leukocyte
   C. both of the above
2. There are three types of granulocytes. Choose three terms.
   A. thrombocyte
   B. basophil
   C. eosinophil
   D. monocyte
   E. neutrophil
   F. platelet
3. The nucleus in a polymorphonuclear leukocyte is
   A. a nucleus with many shapes.
   B. a nucleus that picks up many stains.
4. A ________ does not contain granules.
   A. nongranulocyte

B. eosinophil
C. both of the above

5. ________ are found in large numbers in lymphoid tissue.
A. Granulocytes
B. Lymphocytes
C. both of the above

6. A ________ has one nucleus.
A. monocyte
B. polymorphonuclear leukocyte
C. both of the above

7. Phagocytosis is a process in which the white cell ________ a foreign harmful substance.
A. coagulates
B. ingests
C. both of the above

8. A platelet is also known as a ________.
A. blood cell that looks like a plate
B. thrombocyte
C. both of the above

4. The following terms are related to plasma. Match column A with column B.

Column A	Column B
1. ____ albumin	A. protein substance that becomes spherical in solution
2. ____ globulin	B. protein which produces fibers
3. ____ fibrinogen	C. protein substance that coagulates like an egg white when heated
4. ____ prothrombin	D. protein which is involved in blood clot production

5. Choose the best answer.

Plasma is the ________ liquid in which the formed elements of blood are suspended.
A. straw-colored
B. red-colored

6. The following terms are related to blood clotting. Circle the letter indicating the correct statement.

1. Hemostasis involves three phases. The order of these phases is as follows:
A. vascular, platelet, and coagulation
B. coagulation, platelet, and vascular
2. The antihemophilic factor

A. causes bleeding.
B. works against bleeding.

3. Heparin
   A. is a drug used to clot blood.
   B. is a substance that prevents the clotting of blood.
4. Prothrombin
   A. is a drug used to prevent the clotting of blood.
   B. is a substance that is needed to clot blood.
5. Serum
   A. is the fluid remaining after a clot is formed.
   B. is another name for blood.

7. Fill in the blanks.

1. The process of blood grouping involves the __________ system.
2. The four major blood types are _____, _____, _____, and _____.
3. Blood type _____ is called the universal recipient type.
4. Blood type _____ is called the universal donor type.
5. Another factor besides types of blood, examined for compatibility is the __________.

8. The following sets of terms are related to diseases of blood. Match column A with column B. Be specific.

Set 1

Column A	Column B
1. _____ agranulocytosis	A. unequal or dissimilar red blood cells
2. _____ anemia	B. blood more acid than normal
3. _____ anisocytosis	C. blood more alkaline than normal
4. _____ anoxia	D. deficiency of oxygen in the blood
5. _____ acidosis	E. lack of blood
6. _____ alkalosis	F. abnormal mixture of blood elements
7. _____ dyscrasia	G. lack of granulocytes

Set 2

Column A	Column B
1. _____ aplastic	A. anemia resulting from the breakdown of blood cells
2. _____ hemolytic	B. anemia found mostly in persons who live near the Mediterranean Sea
3. _____ hypochromic microcytic	C. anemia with large red blood cells

Column A	Column B
4. ____ iron-deficiency	D. anemia resulting from the lack of blood cell production
5. ____ macrocytic	E. anemia with crescent-shaped blood cells
6. ____ pernicious	F. anemia with blood cells decreased in color and size
7. ____ sickle cell	G. anemia that may lead to death
8. ____ thalassemia	H. anemia caused by lack of iron
9. ____ erythrocytosis	I. decrease in red blood cells
10. ____ erythropenia	J. all blood let out of the body
11. ____ exsanguination	K. excess of red blood cells

Set 3

Column A	Column B
1. ____ granulocytopenia	A. person with this condition known as a "bleeder"
2. ____ hemolysis	B. break in a blood vessel resulting in a flow of blood
3. ____ hemophilia	C. excessive amount of glucose in the blood
4. ____ hemorrhage	D. stopping of blood
5. ____ hemostasis	E. decrease in the amount of sugar in the blood
6. ____ hyperglycemia	F. decrease in the numbers of granulocytes
7. ____ hypoglycemia	G. decrease in the amount of oxygen in the blood
8. ____ hypoxia	H. breaking down of blood cells

9. The following statements are related to blood diseases. Circle the best answer to complete the statement.

1. Leukemia is a condition characterized by
   A. an increase in the number of white blood cells.
   B. a decrease in the number of white blood cells.
   C. neither of the above.
2. Leukocytosis is a condition characterized by
   A. an increase in the number of white blood cells.
   B. a decrease in the number of white blood cells.
   C. neither of the above.
3. Leukopenia is a condition in which there is
   A. an increase in the number of white blood cells.
   B. a decrease in the number of white blood cells.
   C. neither of the above.

4. An event resulting in blood outside a blood vessel is called
   A. extravasation.
   B. hemorrhage.
   C. both of the above.

5. ________ is a condition in which there is clotting of blood in a blood vessel.
   A. Thrombosis
   B. Thrombocytosis

6. An infection in the blood is sometimes called
   A. idiopathic purpura.
   B. septicemia.

10. Using the following list of terms fill in the blanks of the statements below.

myelocytic leukemia	polycythemia
pancytopenia	thrombocythemia
poikilocytosis	thrombocytopenia

1. A condition in which red blood cells have varied or irregular shapes is called ____________________.
2. A condition in which there is an increase in the number of platelets is called ____________________.
3. A reduction of all cellular elements in the blood is called ____________________.
4. A decrease in the number of platelets is called ____________________.
5. A condition involving the increase in the large cells of bone marrow is called ____________________.
6. A condition in which there is an increase in blood cells is called ____________________.

PRETEST/ POSTTEST **ANSWERS** FOR CHAPTER **11**

1. 1. emia- 2. hemia- 3. hemo- 4. hemato- 5. sangui-

2. 1. C 2. D 3. A 4. B 5. F 6. E 7. G

3. 1. B 2. B, C, E 3. A 4. A 5. B 6. A 7. B 8. C

4. 1. C 2. A 3. B 4. D

5. A

6. **1.** A **2.** B **3.** B **4.** B **5.** A

7. **1.** ABO
2. A, B, AB, O
3. AB*
4. O*
5. Rh factor

8. **Set 1**
1. G **2.** E **3.** A **4.** D **5.** B **6.** C **7.** F

Set 2
1. D **2.** A **3.** F **4.** H **5.** C **6.** G **7.** E **8.** B **9.** K **10.** I **11.** J

Set 3
1. F **2.** H **3.** A **4.** B **5.** D **6.** C **7.** E **8.** G

9. **1.** A **2.** A **3.** B **4.** C **5.** A **6.** B

10. **1.** poikilocytosis
2. thrombocythemia
3. pancytopenia
4. thrombocytopenia
5. myelocytic leukemia
6. polycythemia

---

* To remember these blood types, associate *AB* with *a*ll *b*lood. A person with this type can receive all blood. The type O person cannot receive any blood but type O.

12 THE LYMPHATIC SYSTEM AND THE IMMUNE SYSTEM

OBJECTIVES

At the end of this chapter you will be able to do the following:

1 Describe the functions of the lymphatic system.
2 Describe the structures in the lymphatic system.
3 Identify the location of the lymph ducts and lymph nodes.
4 Describe the other organs in the lymphatic system: tonsils, thymus, and spleen.
5 Analyze selected terms related to conditions of the lymphatic system.
6 Analyze selected terms related to the diagnosis and treatment of conditions of the lymphatic system.
7 Define humoral and cellular immunity.
8 Analyze selected terms related to immunology.

THE LYMPHATIC SYSTEM

The lymphatic system is responsible for several functions. The system operates in the following ways:

1 It returns vital substances, such as plasma protein, to the bloodstream from the tissues of the body.
2 It helps in the maintenance of fluid balance by draining fluid from the body tissues.
3 It helps in the body's defense against disease-producing substances.
4 It helps in the absorption of fats from the digestive system.

The lymphatic system is a network of channels and nodes in which a substance called *lymph* travels. Lymph is a clear, watery fluid (*lymph*) similar to plasma. Unlike the cardiovascular system, travel in the lymphatic system goes only in one direction.

The system collects and drains lymph from different areas of the body and carries it through the lymphatic channels back to the venous system. There it is deposited, mixed with venous blood, and recirculated.

Lymph capillaries are found close to and parallel to veins that carry blood to the heart (Figure 12-1).

The ends of the lymphatic capillaries meet to form larger lymph vessels. The lymph

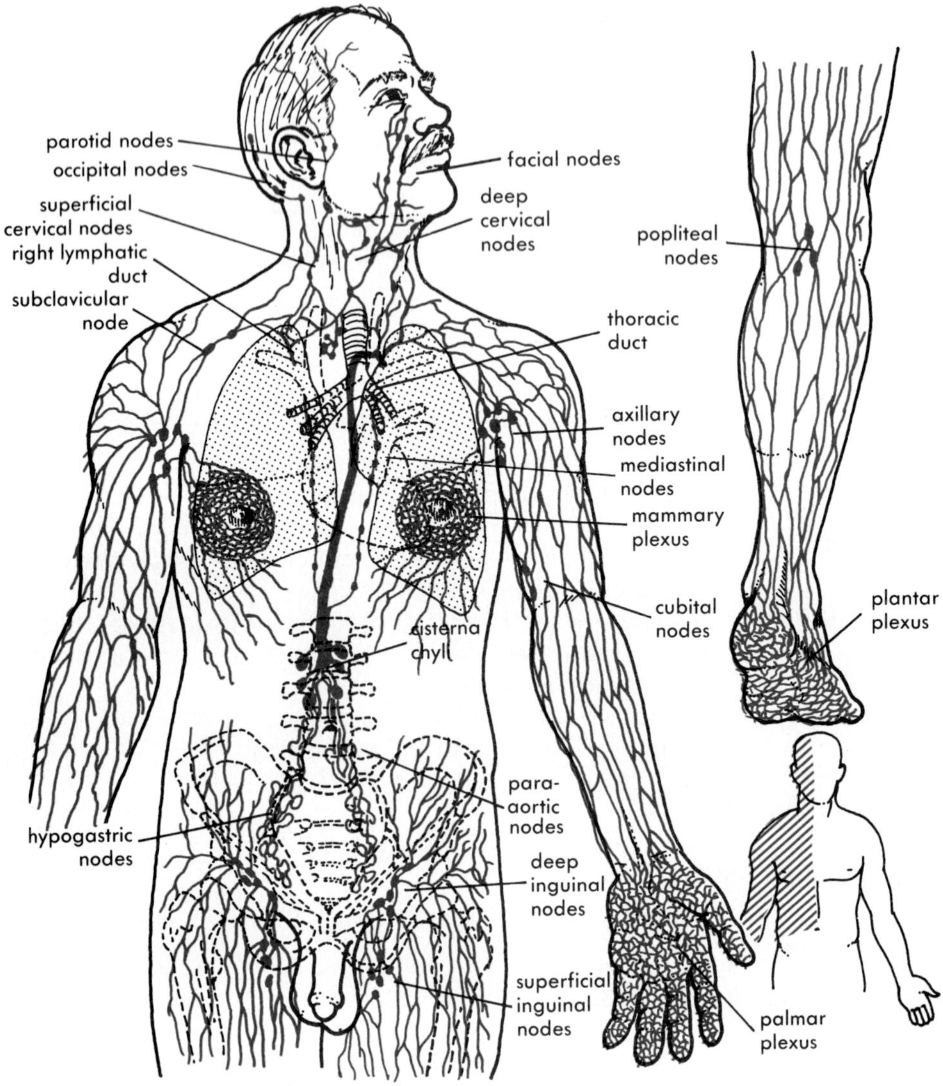

FIGURE 12-1
Principal lymph vessels and nodes.

vessels in the right chest and right arm join the right lymphatic duct (see Figure 12-1), which drains into the right subclavian vein (see Figure 12-1, lower right).

The lymph vessels from all other parts of the body join to meet the thoracic duct, which drains into the left subclavian vein.

The *cisterna chyli* is a receiving area for lymph before the lymph passes into the thoracic duct. The cisterna is a receptacle (*cistern*) for lymph that is known as *chyle.* Chyle is a milky fluid containing fat that has been digested and absorbed into the lymphatic system. The fat from the intestines travels through the lymphatic system and enters the bloodstream by this mechanism.

Throughout the lymph system are lymph nodes. Lymph nodes are small bodies present in the path of the lymph channels that act as filters for lymph before it returns to the bloodstream.

Following is a description of the lymph nodes shown in Figure 12-1. Nodes shown on the right anatomical side:

parotid nodes: the nodes around (*para*) or in front of the ear (*otid*)
occipital nodes: the nodes over the occipital bone at the back of the head
superficial cervical nodes: the nodes close to the surface (*superficial*) of the neck (*cervic*)
subclavicular nodes: the nodes under (*sub*) the collarbone (*clavicular*)
hypogastric nodes: the nodes in the area beneath (*hypo*) the stomach (*gastric*)

Nodes on the left anatomical side:

facial nodes: the nodes draining the tissue in the face
deep cervical nodes: deeply situated (*deep*) nodes in the neck (*cervic*)
axillary nodes: nodes in the armpit (*axilla*)
mediastinal nodes: nodes in the mediastinal section of the thoracic cavity
cubital nodes: nodes of the elbow (*cubit*)
paraaortic nodes: nodes around (*para*) the aorta (*aortic*)
deep inguinal nodes: deeply situated (*deep*) nodes in the groin (*inguin*)
superficial inguinal nodes: the nodes in the groin (*inguin*) close to the surface (*superficial*)
popliteal nodes: nodes in back of the knee (*popliteal*)

There are plexuses of lymph channels throughout the body. These intertwined channels are found in the following areas (see Figure 12-1):

mammary plexus: lymphatic vessels around the breasts
palmar plexus: lymphatic vessels in the palm (*palmar*) of the hands
plantar plexus: lymphatic vessels in the sole (*plantar*) of the feet

Other Organs in the Lymphatic System

The spleen, tonsils, adenoids, and thymus gland are organs that are related to the lymphatic system.

Spleen

The spleen is a soft, oval organ located in the left upper quadrant beneath the diaphragm and behind the lower ribs. The spleen is composed of a spongelike network of cells and blood channels called *sinusoids.*

Among the functions of the spleen are the following:

1 The destruction of worn-out red blood cells to make room for new red blood cells.
2 The filtering out of harmful organisms from the blood.

Tonsils and adenoids

The tonsils and adenoids are collections of lymphoid tissue near the back of the throat.

These collections of lymphatic tissue guard the entrance of the digestive and respiratory system from bacteria.

The tonsils are oval masses of lymphoid tissue attached to the side walls of the back of the mouth.

The adenoids are glandlike [gland (*aden),* like (oid)] masses of lymphoid tissue located against the back wall of the nasopharynx.

Thymus

The thymus gland is located in the upper part of the chest behind the sternum. This gland is one of the central controllers of the body's immune system. It also has an endocrine function (see Chapter 16). It is relatively large in the fetus and very young child but begins to atrophy after adolescence.

DISEASE OF THE LYMPHATIC SYSTEM

Analysis of selected terms related to disease of the lymphatic system including terms related to signs and symptoms of disease:

chylothorax: condition in which the milky lymphatic fluid (*chyle*) drains into the thoracic (*thorax*) cavity.

dependent edema: swelling (*edema*), usually in the lower legs, that occurs as a result of the hanging down (*dependent*) of the legs. The lymph does not drain; thus, there is an accumulation of fluid (edema).

elephantiasis: disease (*iasis*) condition in which lymph collects in the limb causing the limb to swell to a point where it resembles an elephant's leg. May also occur in the external genitals.

infectious mononucleosis: a lymph disease (*osis*) that is spread from person to person (*infectious).* This disease is characterized by the development of white blood cells that are mononuclear (*mononucle).* Sometimes called *glandular fever.*

lymphadenitis: inflammation (*itis*) of lymph (*lymph*) glands (*aden).*

lymphadenopathy: general term meaning disease (*pathy*) of the lymph (*lymph*) glands (*adeno*).

lymphatic metastasis: condition in which disease moves from one place (*stasis*) to another (*meta*) by way of the lymph system.

lymphoma: tumor of the lymph (*lymph*) nodes. One type is called *Hodgkin's disease.* Also known as a neoplasm of lymphatic tissue.

lymphosarcoma: malignant (*sarc*) tumor (*oma*) of the lymph (*lympho*) nodes.

splenomegaly: condition in which the spleen (*spleno*) is enlarged (*megaly).*

tonsillitis: inflammation (*itis*) of the tonsil (*tonsil).*

Diagnosis and Treatment

Analysis of selected terms related to the diagnosis and treatment of conditions related to the lymphatic system:

node biopsy: the excision of a segment of lymph node tissue (biopsy) for microscopic examination.

splenectomy: removal (*ectomy*) of the spleen (*splen).*

staging procedure: surgical procedure done to determine the extent or stage of lymphatic disease. The abdomen may be opened, and lymph nodes are biopsied. If only one area contains diseased lymph nodes, the disease is said to be in stage I. If many are involved in both the abdomen and thorax, the disease is said to be in stage IV.

T & A: an abbreviation of the following two terms:
tonsillectomy: the removal (*ectomy*) of the tonsils.
adenoidectomy: the removal (*ectomy*) of the adenoids.

THE IMMUNE SYSTEM

The human body has the ability to resist organisms or toxins that tend to damage the tissues and organs that make up the body.

This ability is called immunity.

There are basically two types of immunity in the body: humoral immunity and cellular immunity. Each type has specific characteristics (Table 12-1).
Analysis of selected terms related to immunology:

acquired immunity: resistance (*immunity*) to a particular disease developed by people who have had (*acquired*) the disease.

acquired immune deficiency syndrome (*AIDS*): group of symptoms (syndrome) caused by the transmission (acquired) of a virus that causes a breakdown (deficiency) of the immune system. (See Glossary of Terms Related to AIDS)

active immunity: resistance (*immunity*) in which the antibodies that have been produced by a person currently exist.

TABLE 12-1
Humoral and Cellular Immunity

Humoral Immunity	Cellular Immunity
This system is dependent on the body's ability to develop circulating antibodies, which attack the invading agent.	This system is dependent on the body's ability to develop lymphocytes, which attach to the invading agent and destroy it.
The antibodies circulate in the fluids of the body; thus, the name humoral (fluid) immunity.	The lymphocytes are specialized white blood cells; thus, the name cellular immunity.
This type of immunity is under the influence of tissues that are similar to tissue in birds known as the *bursa of Fabricius.* Because of the *b* in birds and *b* in bursa, this form of immunity is also known as *B-cell immunity.*	This type of immunity is under the influence of the thymus gland; thus, it is sometimes referred to as *T-cell immunity.*
This immunity protects the body against some bacteria and some viral infections.	This immunity protects the body against viruses, fungi, some bacteria, and cancers, and it works against organs that have been transplanted.

allergy: state of hypersensitivity to a particular substance. The immune system overreacts [over, (*hyper*), reacts (*sensitive*)], to foreign substances and physical changes occur.

antigen: substance that stimulates the immune response.

antihistamines: class of drugs whose action is directed against (*anti*) the histamine that is released by cells in an allergic reaction.

antitoxin: special kind of antibody that fights against (*anti*) the poisonous (*toxin*) substances given off by some disease-producing germs.

autoimmunity: condition in which an individual produces antibodies (*immunity*) that are directed against that person's own (*auto*) tissue.

booster dose: dose of an immunizing substance given to maintain or renew (*boost*) the level of resistance to a particular disease.

desensitization: type of therapy given to reduce (*de*) the sensitivity (*sensitiza*) of a person to a particular substance.

immunization: action (*tion*) taken that results in a person's having resistance (*immunity*) to a particular disease. For example, babies are immunized against diseases such as diphtheria, pertussis (whooping cough), and tetanus. They are given "baby shots" to be immune to these diseases.

immunosuppressant: preparation (*ant*) used to stop or decrease (*suppress*) the immune (*immuno*) response that leads to tissue injury or transplant rejection.

natural immunity: type of resistance (*immunity*) a newborn child has received from its mother. This may also refer to the type of immunity one has following an exposure to or an episode of a disease.

passive immunity: type of immunity in which persons do not form (*passive*) their own antibodies but rather are given antibodies against a particular disease from another source.

susceptible: said of a person who is capable (*ible*) of acquiring (*suscept*) a particular disease.

toxoid: preparation used in immunization, which resembles (*oid*) the disease-causing (*tox*) substance but is not strong enough to cause the disease itself.

vaccination: action of (*ion*) immunizing against smallpox in which a form of a germ-causing cow (*vacca*) pox is used.

vaccine: general term used to describe a preparation used against particular diseases in the immunization process.

PRETEST/ POSTTEST FOR CHAPTER 12

1. The following terms are related to the major ducts of the lymphatic system. Select the best answer.
   1. The right lymphatic duct drains:
      A. the right arm and leg.
      B. the right arm and chest.
      C. both of the above.
   2. The thoracic duct drains:
      A. the lower extremities and the left chest.
      B. the left chest and arm.
      C. both of the above.
   3. The cisterna chyli:
      A. carries a milky form of lymph.
      B. drains into the thoracic duct.
      C. both of the above.
   4. The major ducts of the lymphatic system:
      A. drain toward the heart.
      B. drain away from the heart.
      C. both of the above.

2. The following are groups of lymph nodes. Write in the location of these lymph nodes.
   1. parotid ______________________________
   2. occipital ______________________________
   3. facial ______________________________
   4. cervical ______________________________
   5. subclavicular ______________________________
   6. axillary ______________________________
   7. mediastinal ______________________________
   8. cubital ______________________________
   9. paraaortic ______________________________
   10. hypogastric ______________________________
   11. inguinal ______________________________
   12. popliteal ______________________________

3. The following are lymphatic plexuses. Write in the location of these plexuses.

   1. mammary ____________________
   2. palmar ____________________
   3. plantar ____________________

4. Describe the location of the spleen. ____________________

   ____

5. Describe the location of the tonsils. ____________________

   ____

6. Describe the location of the adenoids. ____________________

   ____

7. Describe the location of the thymus gland. ____________________

   ____

8. The following terms are related to diseases of the lymphatic system. Match column A with column B. Choose the one best answer.

Column A	Column B
1. _____ chylothorax	A. general term meaning disease of the lymph glands
2. _____ dependent edema	B. sometimes called glandular fever
3. _____ elephantiasis	C. a neoplasm of the lymphatic tissues
4. _____ infectious mononucleosis	D. milky lymph in the chest cavity
5. _____ lymphadenitis	E. inflammation of lymph glands
6. _____ lympadenopathy	F. inflammation of the tonsils
7. _____ lymphatic metastasis	G. swelling of the legs from being held in a hanging position
8. _____ lymphoma	H. malignant tumor of the lymph glands
9. _____ lymphosarcoma	I. disease in which a limb has swollen to a very large size
10. _____ splenomegaly	J. enlargement of the spleen
11. _____ tonsillitis	K. the spread of disease through the lymphatic system

9. The following terms are related to the diagnosis and treatment of conditions affecting the lymphatic system. Match column A with column B.

Column A	Column B
1. _____ node biopsy	A. surgical procedure to evaluate the extent of lymphomas
2. _____ splenectomy	B. removal of the adenoids

Column A	Column B
3. ____ staging procedure	C. removal of the tonsils
4. ____ tonsillectomy	D. removal of the spleen
5. ____ adenoidectomy	E. microscopic examination of lymph tissue

10. The following terms are related to types of immunity. Select the best answer.

1. Humoral immunity:
 A. is based on the body's ability to develop lymphocytes.
 B. is based on the body's ability to develop antibodies.

2. Humoral immunity is also known as:
 A. B-cell immunity.
 B. T-cell immunity.

3. Cellular immunity:
 A. is under the influence of the thymus gland.
 B. is based on the body's ability to form specialized white blood cells.

11. The following three sets of terms are related to immunology. Separate directions will be given for each set.

Set 1

Using the list of terms complete the following statements.

acquired immunity	natural immunity
autoimmunity	passive immunity

1. A condition in which there are antibodies directed against one's own tissue is called ________________.

2. The type of immunity a child has received from its mother is called ________________.

3. The type of immunity one has after actually having had a disease is referred to as ________________ or ________________.

4. A type of immunity in which a person does not form his or her own antibodies, but rather receives them from another source is called ________________.

Set 2

Match column A with column B. Choose the one best answer.

Column A	Column B
1. ____ active immunity	A. hypersensitivity to a particular substance
2. ____ allergy	B. drug that works against the substance released during an allergic reaction
3. ____ antigen	C. state of being currently resistant to a particular disease
4. ____ antihistamine	D. given to renew the level of resistance to a particular disease
5. ____ antitoxin	

Column A	Column B
6. _____ booster dose	E. substance that stimulates the immune response
	F. special kind of antibody that fights poisonous substances

Set 3
Match column A with column B.

Column A	Column B
1. _____ desensitization	A. preparation used to stop the immune response
2. _____ immunization	B. preparation used to immunize a person against particular diseases
3. _____ immunosuppressant	C. type of therapy given to reduce sensitivity
4. _____ susceptible	D. preparation used that resembles the disease-causing substance
5. _____ toxoid	E. action taken to reduce a person's susceptibility to particular diseases
6. _____ vaccination	F. the act of immunizing a person against smallpox
7. _____ vaccine	G. being able to acquire a particular disease

PRETEST/ POSTTEST **ANSWERS** FOR CHAPTER **12**

1. **1.** B **2.** C **3.** C **4.** A

2. **1.** in front of or near the ear
   2. over the bone in back of the head
   3. in the face
   4. at the neck
   5. under the collarbone
   6. in the armpit
   7. in the mediastinum or center of the thoracic cavity
   8. near the elbow
   9. around the aorta
   10. beneath the stomach
   11. in the groin

12. in back of the knee

3. 1. the breast
   2. the palm of the hand
   3. the sole of the foot

4. The spleen is beneath the diaphragm, behind the ribs, in the left upper quadrant.

5. The tonsils are attached to the side walls at the back of the mouth.

6. The adenoids are located against the back wall of the nasopharynx.

7. The thymus is located in the upper part of the chest cavity behind the sternum.

8. 1. D 2. G 3. I 4. B 5. E 6. A 7. K 8. C or H 9. C or H 10. J 11. F

9. 1. E 2. D 3. A 4. C 5. B

10. 1. B 2. A 3. B

11. **Set 1**
   1. autoimmunity
   2. natural immunity
   3. acquired immunity or natural immunity
   4. passive immunity

   Set 2
   1. C 2. A 3. E 4. B 5. F 6. D

   Set 3
   1. C 2. E 3. A 4. G 5. D 6. F 7. B

13 THE RESPIRATORY SYSTEM

OBJECTIVES

At the end of this chapter you will be able to do the following:

1 Describe the functions of the respiratory system.
2 List the structures involved in respiration.
3 Define terms related to the nose, the nasal cavity, and the paranasal sinuses.
4 Define terms related to the anatomy of the larynx and the production of sound.
5 Define terms related to the trachea, bronchi, and alveoli.
6 Describe the lungs and identify terms related to the anatomy of the lungs.
7 Define *respiration* and related terms.
8 Analyze terms related to pathological conditions of the respiratory system.
9 Analyze terms related to diagnostic and surgical procedures done on the respiratory system.

THE RESPIRATORY SYSTEM

The respiratory system functions to supply oxygen and remove carbon dioxide from the cells of the body. There are two phases of respiration: external and internal. External respiration involves the absorption of oxygen from the air by the lungs and the transport of carbon dioxide from the lungs back into the air. Internal respiration involves the exchanges of oxygen and carbon dioxide in the cells of the body.

The terms discussed in this chapter will deal with the external respiration process.

The respiratory system comprises both an upper respiratory tract and the lungs (see Figure 13-1).

Nose, Nasal Cavity, and Paranasal Sinuses

The nose is composed of bone and cartilage. As a part of the respiratory system, the nasal cavity consists of passageways, spaces, walls, and protective membranes.

The function of the nasal cavity is the filtering, cooling or warming, and moistening of air. It is also necessary for the sense of smell.

There are paranasal sinuses around the nasal cavity. The paranasal sinuses come in

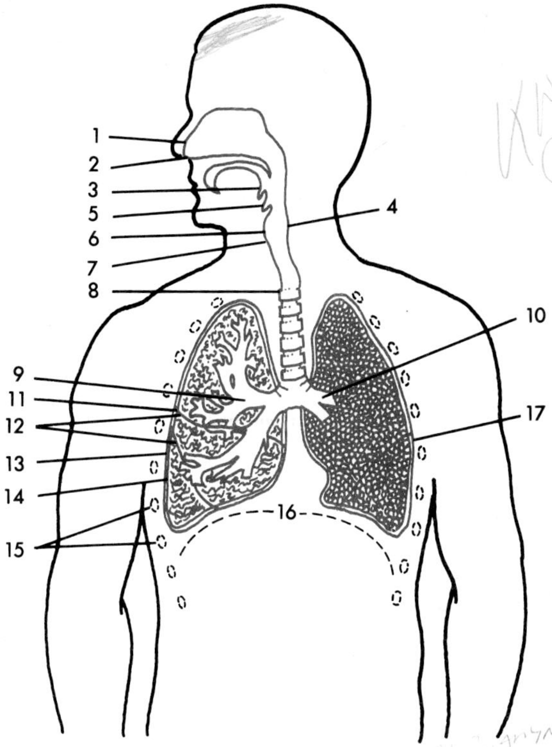

FIGURE 13-1
The respiratory system: (1) nasal cavity, (2) nasopharynx, (3) pharynx, (4) esophagus, (5) epiglottis, (6) vocal cords, (7) larynx, (8) trachea, (9) right main-stem bronchus, (10) left main-stem bronchus, (11) right lung (lobar and segmental bronchi are exposed), (12) lobe divisions, (13) parietal pleura, (14) visceral pleura, (15) ribs, (16) diaphragm, and (17) left lung.

pairs, one on each side, and are named according to the bone they are in. Thus, there are frontal, ethmoid, sphenoid, and maxillary sinuses. The main function of the sinuses is to make the skull bone lighter. The spaces also function in the production of sound. The air in them vibrates, giving the voice a pleasant, resonant sound.

Terms related to the nose, nasal cavity, and paranasal sinuses:

meatus: channel (*meatus*) with an opening in the sides of the nasal cavity for the passage of air and mucus from the paranasal sinuses.
nares: external openings of the nose.
nasal septum: wall (*septum*) dividing the nose (*nasal cavity*) into right and left halves.
nostrils: holes (*trils*) in the nose (*nos*).
olfactory cells: cells which function in the sensation of smell (*olfaction*) located in the nose.
paranasal sinuses: airspaces (*sinuses*) which are near (*para*) the nasal (*nasal)* cavity.
rhino-: root word meaning "nose."
vibrissae: visible hairs in the nose. These hairs vibrate (*vibrissae*) on respiration.

Pharynx and Esophagus

The nasal cavity is continuous with the nasopharynx and oropharynx. The pharynx is the cavity connecting the nose and mouth with the esophagus and trachea (see Chapter 14).

The esophagus is the tube that leads to the stomach in which food passes (see Chapter 14).

Larynx

The larynx is located in the throat between the end of the pharynx and the beginning of the trachea. The larynx is shaped like a triangular box and is composed of nine cartilages. The most prominent of these cartilages is the thyroid cartilage. It is covered by a special cartilaginous flap called the *epiglottis,* which prevents food from entering the larynx. The opening into the larynx is the *glottis.*

The larynx is also known as the "voice box" because it contains the vocal cords and its chief function is phonation, the production of the sound that constitutes the human voice.

Terms related to the larynx:

epiglottis: lidlike cartilage over (*epi*) the opening of the larynx (*glottis*).
glottis: opening at the upper part of the larynx.
phonation: action (*tion*) of passing air through the vocal cords, which vibrate and produce the sound (*phon*) of the voice (*phon*).
thyroid cartilage: largest cartilage in the larynx. In the male this cartilage increases in size at puberty, during which time the voice changes. This enlarged cartilage is also known as the Adam's apple, as if the first man, Adam, in taking a bite of the forbidden fruit was unable to swallow, and a piece of it became lodged in his throat.
vocal cords: folds (*cords*) of tissue in the larynx responsible for the production of the voice (*vocal).*
voice box: boxlike structure in the throat containing the vocal cords, which produce the voice. Also called the *larynx.*

Trachea and Bronchi

The trachea extends from the larynx to the main-stem bronchus. It functions as a passageway for air to reach the lungs.

The term *trachea* means "rough," which may relate to its physical appearance. Its popular meaning is "windpipe" although it is only one part of a series of pipes that permit the passage of air.

The *main-stem bronchus* is the first division of the windpipe. The *bronchi* (plural of *bronchus*) extend from the trachea in a branchlike fashion. Each bronchus continues to decrease in diameter as it enters the lung, where the smaller branches are called *bronchioles.*

The bronchioles terminate at the *alveolar ducts.* The alveolar ducts lead into the *alveoli,* which are the small saclike cavities where the exchange of oxygen and carbon dioxide takes place.

Terms related to the trachea and bronchi are listed here from the largest structure to the smallest:

trachea: the windpipe.
main-stem bronchus: main branch of the trachea, which leads (*stem*) to the lung. The bronchus is a continuation of the windpipe.
bronchiole: smaller (*iole*) section of the windpipe (*bronch*).
alveolar ducts: tubes at the end of the bronchioles that lead to the alveoli.
alveoli: saclike (*alveoli*) structures arranged in clusters in which the exchange of oxygen and carbon dioxide takes place.

Lungs

The lungs are cone-shaped organs that are made up of a network of pulmonary arteries, veins, bronchi, alveoli, and connective tissue. Since the alveoli are air sacs, the lungs are lightweight organs.

The lungs fill the spaces in the thoracic cavity called the *pleural spaces.* The other space in the thoracic cavity is called the *mediastinum.* It contains the heart, great vessels, trachea, and esophagus.

Lungs are held in an inflated state by the negative pressure, or suction, which exists between the outside surface of the lung, called the *visceral pleura,* and the inside wall of the chest, called the *parietal pleura.*

The lungs are divided into lobes. The right lung has three lobes: superior lobe, middle lobe, and inferior lobe. The left lung has two lobes: superior lobe and inferior lobe. The heart is located in the space where the middle lobe of the left lung would be.

Each lung may be further divided into bronchopulmonary segments. The bronchi of each lung supply air to segments of that lung, so that each branch or bronchus has a particular lung space to which it is connected.

Terms related to the lungs and pleura:

lungs: two lightweight (*lung*) organs of respiration.
lobes: major divisions of the lungs. There are three lobes on the right and two on the left.
bronchopulmonary segments: each lobe is further divided into lung (*pulmon*) sections (*segments),* each of which is attached to a stem of the bronchus (*broncho).*
pleura: general term meaning "side." The pleura is a membrane that covers the surfaces of the lungs and lines the inside wall of the thoracic cavity.
parietal pleura: the membrane lining the wall (*parietal*) of the thoracic cavity.
visceral pleura: the covering of the lungs, which are the organs (*viscera*) of respiration.
pleural space: area between the two layers of pleura.
pneumo-: root word meaning "lung," or "air" or "breath."
pulmon-: root word meaning "lungs."
mediastinum: space that stands (*stinum*) in the middle (*media*) between the two lungs.

TABLE 13-1
Structures Involved in Respiration

Upper Respiratory Tract*
nose and nasal cavity
nasopharynx
trachea
main-stem bronchus to the right and left lungs
Lungs†
lobes and segmental divisions
bronchioles
alveolar ducts
alveoli
Adjacent Structures‡
parietal pleura
visceral pleura
ribs
diaphragm

*See Figure 13-1, numbers 1 to 10.
†See Figure 13-1, numbers 11, 12, and 17.
‡See Figure 13-1, numbers 13 to 16.

RESPIRATION

The maintenance of the process of respiration is an automatic mechanical action. In the healthy individual, breathing is an involuntary activity.

The muscles involved in breathing are the diaphragm and the intercostal muscles. These muscles may also be controlled voluntarily.

As the diaphragm contracts, it pulls downward and increases the space in the thorax. The intercostal muscles contract, lifting the ribs up and out, which also increases the space. The greatly increased space is filled by the outside air. These muscles relax, space decreases, and air is forced out.

Terms related to the anatomy and physiology of breathing:

aer-: root word meaning "air."
airway: another name for the upper respiratory tract.
breath: air inhaled and exhaled during respiration.
breathe: to take air in and expel air out. To inhale and exhale.
breath sounds: noise heard from air moving in and out of the lungs.
diaphragm: muscular wall (*phragm*) across (*dia*) the trunk between the thoracic and abdominal cavities.

exhale: to force (*hale*) air out (*ex*).
inhale: to pull (*hale*) air in (*in*).
phrenic: relating to the diaphragm. There are two meanings for this word, diaphragm and mind, the result of an old belief that the diaphragm may be associated with the mind.
-pnea: word ending that means "breathing."
respiration: to breathe (*spiration*) again (*re*).
spiro-: root word meaning "to breathe."
stertor: heavy snoring (*stertor*) sound.
ventilate: to provide new air through a blowing (*vent*) force.

DISEASE CONDITIONS OF THE RESPIRATORY SYSTEM

Analysis of terms related to disease conditions of the respiratory system including terms related to signs and symptoms:

apnea: situation in which there is an absence (*a*) of breathing (*pnea*).
atelectasis: incomplete (*atel*) dilation (*ectasis*) of lung tissue, collapse of lung tissue.
bronchiectasis: excessive dilation (*ectasis*) of the bronchi (*bronchi*) characterized by the accumulation of mucus in the dilated space.
bronchitis: inflammation (*itis*) of the bronchi (*bronch*).
chronic obstructive pulmonary disease (COPD): long-term (*chronic*) disease in which there is an obstruction (*obstructive*) in the lungs (*pulmonary*) causing respiratory difficulty.
cough: sudden noise signaling expulsion of air from the lungs.
dyspnea: difficult (*dys*) or labored breathing (*pnea*).
emphysema: condition (*ma*) in which the alveoli of the lungs have been blown (*physe*) in (*em*); the lungs have been permanently overinflated.
epistaxis: nosebleed during which blood drips (*staxis*) upon (*epi*) a surface.
hemoptysis: spitting (*ptysis*) of blood (*hemo*) from the respiratory tract.
hemothorax: condition in which there is blood (*hemo*) in the thoracic cavity (*thorax*) between the two pleura.
hyperventilation: excessive (*hyper*) breathing (*ventilation*).
laryngitis: inflammation (*itis*) of the larynx.
laryngospasm: sudden contraction (*spasm*) of the larynx (*laryngo*).
laryngotracheobronchitis: inflammation (*itis*) of the larynx, trachea, and bronchi.
nasal polyp: projecting growth (*polyp*) arising from the mucous membrane of the nose (*nasal*).
orthopnea: condition in which breathing (*pnea*) is easier when a person is in an upright, or straight (*ortho*), position.
pleural effusion: flowing of fluid (*effusion*) into the pleural space.
pleurisy: inflammation (*isy,* variation of *itis*) of the pleura (*pleur*).
pneumonia: disease condition (*ia*) of the lungs (*pneumon*), usually an inflammation of the lungs.
pneumoconiosis: lung (*pneumo*) condition (*osis*) caused by inhalation of various types of dust particles (*coni*).

pneumothorax: condition in which there is air (*pneumo*) in the thoracic cavity (*thorax*) outside the lungs between the two pleura.

pulmonary edema: condition in which there is excessive fluid (*edema*) in the lungs (*pulmonary*).

pyothorax: condition in which there is pus (*pyo*) in the thoracic cavity (*thorax*) between the two pleura.

sinusitis: inflammation (*itis*) of the paranasal sinuses.

tachypnea: abnormally fast (*tachy*) breathing.

tracheoesophageal fistula: abnormal opening (*fistula*) between the trachea and esophagus.

tuberculosis: condition (*osis*) usually of the lung in which small nodes (*tubercles*) develop as part of the disease process.

Diagnostic and Therapeutic Procedures

Analysis of selected terms related to diagnostic and therapeutic procedures done for diseases of the respiratory system:

adventitious breath sounds: abnormal (*adventitious*) or unusual noises heard in the lungs through a stethoscope.

- *pleural friction rub:* sound heard as inflamed pleura rub against (*friction*) each other.
- *rales:* abnormal rattling (*rale*) or crackling sound.
- *rhonchi:* coarse snoring (*rhonchi*) sound.
- *wheeze:* high-pitched continuous blowing (*wheeze*) sound.

bronchogram: x-ray picture (*ogram*) of the bronchi (*bronch*) taken following the injection of a radiopaque substance.

bronchophony: abnormal increase in the intensity of the voice sounds (*phony*) heard while listening to the lungs (*broncho*).

bronchoscope: a viewing device (*scope*) used to visualize the bronchi (*broncho*).

egophony: sounds (*phony*) heard through a stethoscope that resemble the high-pitched bleating of a goat (*ego,* variation of aigo).

lavage of sinuses: washing (*lavage*) of the sinuses, usually to remove infectious material.

laryngectomy: removal (ectomy) of the voice box (*larynx*).

lobectomy: removal (*ectomy*) of one of the lobes of the lungs.

pectoriloquy: sound of the whispered word (*loquy*) is unusually loud when listened to through the chest (*pectori*) wall.

pneumonectomy: removal (*ectomy*) of one of the lungs (*pneumo*).

spirometry: test used to measure (*metry*) the efficiency of breathing (*spiro*).

thoracentesis: surgical puncture (*centesis*) into the thoracic (thora) cavity for the removal of fluid. Also called *pleurocentesis,* or puncture of the pleura.

thoracotomy: making an opening (*otomy*) into the thorax to carry out a surgical procedure.

tracheostomy: surgical procedure done to make a somewhat permanent opening (*ostomy*) into the trachea.

tracheotomy: surgical procedure done to cut into (*otomy*) the trachea.
vital capacity: term used to indicate the largest amount of air that can be exchanged during respiration. The term means "the volume (*capacity*) of life (*vital*)."

Drugs Used in Treatment

Analysis of selected terms related to drugs used to treat diseases of the respiratory system:

antitussive: drug that works against (*anti*), or controls, coughing (*tussive*).
bronchodilator: drug that causes the dilation (*dilator*) of the bronchi (*broncho*).
expectorant: drug used to help expel (*ex*) mucus from the chest (*pect*).

PRETEST/ POSTTEST FOR CHAPTER 13

1. The following terms are related to the nose and nasal cavity. Select the best answer.

1. A root word meaning nose is _____.
A. rhino
B. -pnea

2. The terms that mean the external opening of the nose are _____.
A. nares and nostril
B. nostril and meatus

3. The wall dividing the nasal cavity is called the _____.
A. paranasal septum
B. nasal septum

4. An opening from a nasal sinus into the back of the nasal cavity is called a _____.
A. meatus
B. glottis

5. The hairs in the nose are called _____.
A. vibrisae
B. vibrissae

6. The cells that function in the sensation of smell are called _____.
A. olfactory cells
B. paranasal cells

7. The airspaces near the nasal cavity are called the ____.
   A. paranasal sinuses
   B. olfactory sinuses

2. The following terms are related to the larynx. Match column A with column B.

Column A	Column B
1. ____ epiglottis	A. vibration of air as it passes through the vocal cords
2. ____ glottis	B. lidlike cover over the opening to the larynx
3. ____ phonation	C. Adam's apple
4. ____ thyroid cartilage	D. the larynx
5. ____ vocal cords	E. opening to the larynx
6. ____ voice box	F. folds of tissue in the larynx

3. The following terms are related to the trachea and bronchi. Match column A with column B.

Column A	Column B
1. ____ trachea	A. small bronchus
2. ____ main-stem bronchus	B. large branchlike structure from the trachea
3. ____ bronchiole	C. saclike structure in which oxygen and carbon dioxide are exchanged
4. ____ alveolar duct	D. windpipe
5. ____ alveolus	E. tube at the end of a bronchiole

4. The following terms are related to the lungs and pleura. Match column A with column B.

Column A	Column B
1. ____ left lung	A. membrane on the walls of the chest cavity
2. ____ right lung	B. has two lobes
3. ____ parietal pleura	C. area between the lungs and the walls of the chest
4. ____ visceral pleura	D. has three lobes
5. ____ pleural space	E. root word meaning lungs, air, or breath
6. ____ pneumo	F. space between the two lungs
7. ____ pulmon	G. membrane covering the lungs
8. ____ mediastinum	H. root word meaning lungs

5. The following terms are related to the process of breathing. Choose the best answer.

1. The common term for the upper respiratory tract is:
   A. airway.
   B. windpipe.
   C. both of the above.
2. The term meaning to take in and to expel air is:
   A. to breathe.
   B. stertor.
   C. both of the above.
3. Breath sounds are noises heard:
   A. with movement of air past the vocal cords.
   B. with movement of air in the lungs.
   C. both of the above.
4. The _____ is a muscular wall across the abdomen.
   A. diaphragm
   B. abdominoseptum
   C. both of the above
5. To pull in and force out air is called:
   A. respiration.
   B. inhalation and exhalation.
   C. both of the above.
6. The term that means snoring is:
   A. stertor.
   B. ventilate.
   C. both of the above.
7. A root word meaning diaphragm is:
   A. septo.
   B. phrenic.
   C. both of the above.
8. The term ventilate means:
   A. to provide new air through blowing force.
   B. a noise made by the movement of air in the lungs.
   C. both of the above.
9. Terms meaning breathing are:
   A. aer- and spiro.
   B. spiro and -pnea.
   C. both of the above.
10. The term meaning air is:
    A. aer.
    B. spiro.
    C. -pnea.

6. The following sets of terms are related to diseases of the respiratory tract. In all sets match column A with column B. Be specific.

Set 1

Column A	Column B
1. _____ apnea	A. sudden noisy expulsion of air from the lungs
2. _____ atelectasis	B. excessive dilation of lung tissue with an accumulation of mucus
3. _____ bronchiectasis	C. inflammation of the bronchi
4. _____ bronchitis	D. nosebleed
5. _____ chronic obstructive pulmonary disease	E. absence of breathing
6. _____ cough	F. incomplete dilation of lung tissue
7. _____ dyspnea	G. alveoli permanently blown in
8. _____ emphysema	H. difficulty in breathing
9. _____ epistaxis	I. long-term lung disease in which there is an obstruction in the lungs

Set 2

Column A	Column B
1. _____ hemoptysis	A. sudden contraction of the larynx
2. _____ hemothorax	B. projecting growth inside the nose
3. _____ hyperventilation	C. excessive breathing
4. _____ laryngitis	D. condition in which breathing is easier in an upright position
5. _____ laryngospasm	E. spitting of blood from the respiratory tract
6. _____ laryngotracheo-bronchitis	F. inflammation of the pleura
7. _____ nasal polyp	G. inflammation of the larynx, trachea, and bronchi
8. _____ orthopnea	H. fluid in the pleural space
9. _____ pleural effusion	I. blood in the thoracic cavity between the pleura
10. _____ pleurisy	J. inflammation of the larynx

Set 3

Column A	Column B
1. _____ pneumonia	A. air in the thoracic cavity outside the lungs between the two pleura
2. _____ pneumoconiosis	B. fast rate of breathing
3. _____ pneumothorax	C. pus in the thoracic cavity between the two pleura

Column A	Column B
4. _____ pulmonary edema	D. disease condition of the lungs, usually inflammation
5. _____ pyothorax	E. lung condition caused by inhalation of dust particles
6. _____ sinusitis	F. abnormal opening between the trachea and esophagus
7. _____ tachypnea	G. excessive fluid in the lungs
8. _____ tracheoesophageal fistula	H. condition in which small nodes develop usually in the lungs
9. _____ tuberculosis	I. inflammation of the paranasal sinuses

7. The following terms are related to diagnostic therapeutic procedures performed for diseases of the respiratory system. Match column A with column B. Be specific.

Column A	Column B
1. _____ adventitious breath sounds	A. removal of the voice box
2. _____ artificial ventilation	B. abnormal noises in the lungs
3. _____ bronchogram	C. x-ray of the bronchi
4. _____ bronchoscopy	D. washing of the sinuses
5. _____ lavage of sinuses	E. removal of a lobe of the lung
6. _____ laryngectomy	F. puncture into thoracic cavity
7. _____ lobectomy	G. forced respiration by use of machines
8. _____ pneumonectomy	H. making a somewhat permanent opening in the trachea
9. _____ thoracentesis	I. removal of a lung
10. _____ thoracotomy	J. passing of a viewing device inside the bronchi
11. _____ tracheostomy	K. cutting into the trachea
12. _____ tracheotomy	L. measurement of breathing efficiency
13. _____ spirometry	M. largest amount of air that is exchanged during breathing
14. _____ vital capacity	N. cutting into the thoracic cavity

8. The following terms are related to drugs used to treat diseases of the respiratory system. Describe each type of drug.

1. antitussives ______________________________

2. bronchodilators ______________________________

3. expectorants ______________________________

PRETEST/ POSTTEST **ANSWERS** FOR CHAPTER **13**

1. **1.** A **2.** A **3.** B **4.** A **5.** B **6.** A **7.** A

2. **1.** B **2.** E **3.** A **4.** C **5.** F **6.** D

3. **1.** D **2.** B **3.** A **4.** E **5.** C

4. **1.** B* **2.** D* **3.** A **4.** G **5.** C **6.** E **7.** H **8.** F

5. **1.** A **2.** A **3.** B **4.** A **5.** C **6.** A **7.** B **8.** A **9.** B **10.** A

6. **Set 1**
1. E **2.** F **3.** B **4.** C **5.** I **6.** A **7.** **H** **8.** G **9.** D

Set 2
1. E **2.** I **3.** C **4.** J **5.** A **6.** G **7.** B **8.** D **9.** H **10.** F

Set 3
1. D **2.** E **3.** A **4.** G **5.** C **6.** I **7.** B **8.** F **9.** H

7. **1.** B **2.** G **3.** C **4.** J **5.** D **6.** A **7.** E **8.** I **9.** F **10.** N **11.** H **12.** K **13.** **L** **14.** **M**

8. **1.** drugs used to control coughing
2. drugs used to dilate the bronchi
3. drugs used to help expel mucus from chest

* To remember the numbers of lobes in each lung, think again of the number 32. There are three lobes of the lung on the anatomical right and two lobes of the lung on the anatomical left. Recall that there are three cusps in the valve on the right side of the heart and two cusps in the valve on the left.

14 THE DIGESTIVE SYSTEM

OBJECTIVES

At the end of this chapter you will be able to do the following:

1 List the functions of the digestive system.
2 List the sequence of organs in the digestive system, and name the accessory organs.
3 Define terms related to the oral cavity, including the lips, cheeks, tongue, teeth, and salivary glands.
4 Define terms related to the oral pharynx, esophagus, stomach, small intestine, large intestine, and rectum.
5 Define terms related to the accessory organs, including the liver.
6 Analyze selected terms related to pathological conditions of the digestive system, including terms related to signs and symptoms of disease.
7 Analyze selected terms related to the diagnostic and surgical procedures done for diseases of the digestive system.
8 Analyze selected terms related to drugs used in the treatment of diseases of the digestive system.

THE DIGESTIVE SYSTEM

The digestive system has three major functions:

1 the digestion of food
2 the absorption of nutrients into the bloodstream and lymphatic system
3 the elimination of solid waste products

Specific terms related to the digestive process are not covered in this chapter. Selected terms related to disease processes are included.

The digestive system is known by other names. It is also called the gastrointestinal system, GI system, and the alimentary tract.

Terms related to the digestive system:

alimentary tract: the tract through which food (aliment) passes.
bowel: the intestine, the organs that look like little sausages (*bowel*).
celiac: term pertaining to (*iac*) the contents of the belly (*celi*).

digestion: process by which food is broken up physically and more or less dissolved (*digest*) and changed into a substance suitable for absorption and use by the body.
entero: root word meaning "intestine."
gastro: root word meaning "stomach."
gastrointestinal system: the system that includes the stomach (*gastro*) and intestines (*intestinal*).

The anatomy of the system can be compared to that of a long muscular tube that travels a path through the body. The organs of the digestive system transport food through the muscular tube. There are other organs called accessory organs. These accessory organs carry on functions directly related to digestion and are connected to the system by way of ducts.

Figure 14-1 shows the digestive system from the anterior view. There are several organs shown in the illustration only to demonstrate their locations relative to the digestive system. They are not considered part of the system; these structures are, from the top of the illustration to the bottom, the nasopharynx, trachea, lungs, and spleen.

Table 14-1 lists the organs in the digestive system and the accessory organs.

Oral Cavity

Digestion begins in the oral cavity. Both a mechanical and a chemical effect occur here. The teeth tear, grind, and chew food to make it easier to swallow. The salivary glands secrete a digestive juice that begins the chemical breakdown of food.

Terms related to the oral cavity will be listed in the following sets:

1 the mouth: lips, cheeks, and tongue
2 the teeth
3 the salivary glands

Terms related to the mouth:

bucca: inside of the cheek (*bucca*) that makes up the wall of the mouth.
cheil: root word meaning "lip."
fauces: opening at the back of the mouth that is the passage (*fauces*) to the throat.
frenulum: small (*ulum*) fold of membrane that holds, or bridles (*fren*), the tongue to the floor of the mouth.
glossa: root word meaning "tongue."
labia: lips. The term comes from the word *to take*. Food is taken into the mouth by the action of the lips and tongue.
lingua: root word meaning "tongue."
malar: relating to the cheek, which consists of the bones and the flesh over the bones.
os, ora: opening into the mouth.
palate: roof (*palate*) of the mouth. The hard palate consists of the anterior portion of the roof of the mouth. It is formed by the bones of the roof of the mouth; therefore it is hard. The soft palate is the posterior of the roof of the mouth, which is composed of muscles; therefore it is soft.

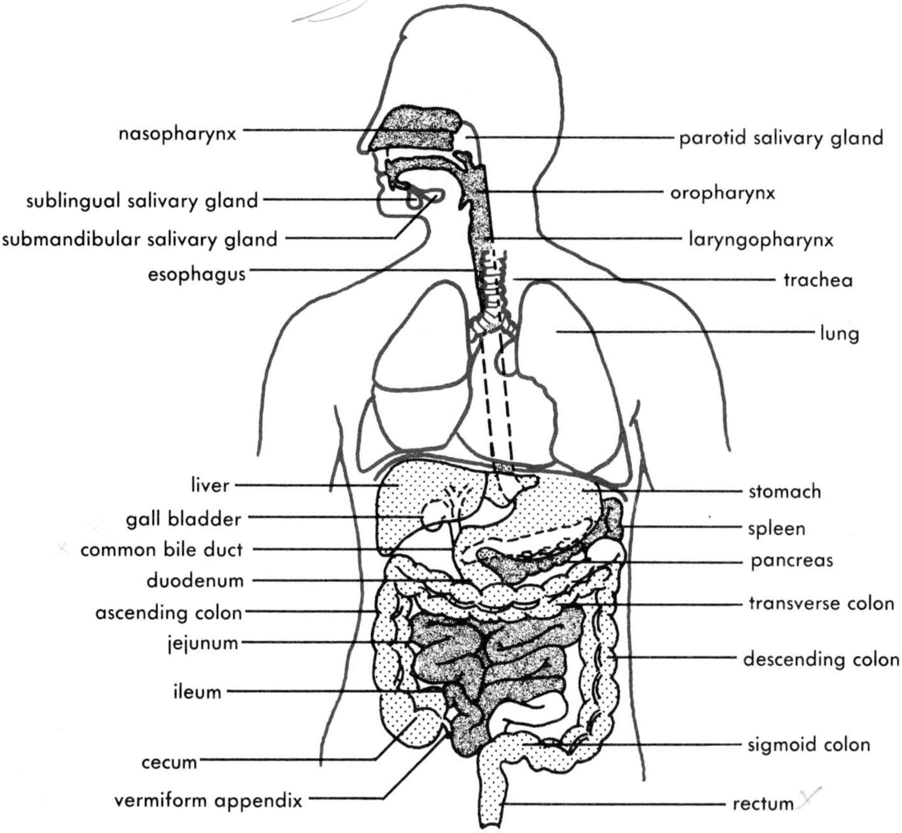

FIGURE 14-1
The digestive system.

stoma: mouth. This is also a general term for a mouthlike opening.

tongue: highly movable muscular structure that functions to mix saliva with food and aids in chewing and swallowing. Numerous taste buds are located on its surface.

tonsil: prominent oval mass of tissue on each side of the back of the mouth at the fauces.

uvula: small (*ula*) grapelike (*uv*) structure hanging down from the back edge of the soft palate. Staphyl is the combining form of uvula.

Teeth

The teeth have an important function in the digestive process: the mechanical breaking down of foodstuffs.

Each person normally has two sets of teeth. The first set of 20 teeth is commonly referred to as the *deciduous teeth* (baby teeth). The second set of 32 teeth are the

TABLE 14-1
Digestive System

Sequence of Anatomical Structures in the Digestive Tract	Relative Location of Openings for Deposit of Digestive Juices Secreted by the Accessory Organs
oral cavity	salivary glands
lips	parotid
mouth	submandibular
teeth	sublingual
tongue	
pharynx	
esophagus	
stomach	
small intestine	
duodenum	common bile duct
jejunum	liver
ileum	gallbladder
	pancreas
large intestine	
cecum	
ascending colon	
transverse colon	
descending colon	
sigmoid colon	
rectum	
anus	

permanent teeth (adult teeth). Some persons have an occasional third tooth. Some persons have a third set of manufactured teeth, referred to as *dentures* (false teeth).

Terms related to sets of teeth:

deciduous teeth: also called *milk teeth, baby teeth.* The teeth that normally fall (*ciduous*) out (*de*) and are replaced by permanent teeth.
dentures: artificial replacements of one or several teeth (partial dentures) or of all of the teeth (full dentures) of either or both jaws.
permanent teeth: any of the 32 adult teeth that replace the 20 deciduous teeth.

Terms related to parts of a tooth:

alveoli: bony socket of the maxillar or mandible in which the teeth are rooted.
cementum: tissue on the outer surface of the root of the tooth that holds the tooth firmly (*cement*) in place.
crown: part of the tooth above the gum.
dent: root word meaning "tooth."
dentin: hard section of the tooth.

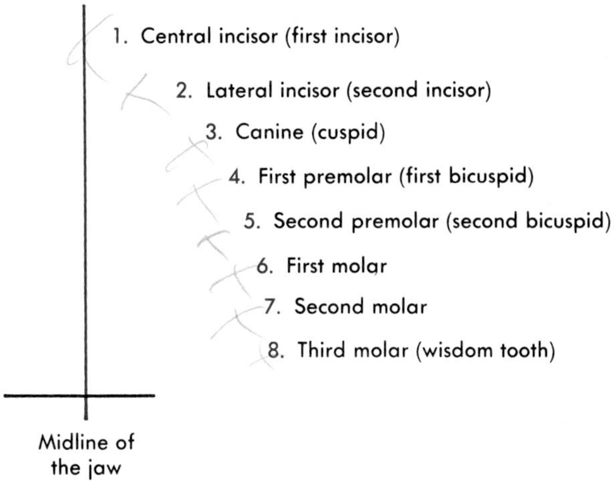

FIGURE 14-2
Names of the teeth of one quadrant of the jaw.

enamel: hard, glossy covering of the crown of a tooth.
gingiv: root word meaning "gums." The term means "beget" and is used because the teeth begin in the gums.
gum: firm, fleshy tissue covering the alveolar parts of either jaw and enveloping the necks of the teeth.
neck: region of the tooth where the crown narrows as it joins the roots.
periodontal membrane: the fibrous connective tissues around (*peri*) the tooth (*odontal*).
pulp cavity: central hollow (*cavity*) portion of the tooth that contains pulp, the inner substance of the tooth.
root: portion of the tooth embedded in the alveolus.
root canal: cavity (*canal*) in the root or roots of the teeth.

Terms related to the various surfaces of a tooth:

buccal surface: surface of a tooth that touches the cheek (*bucca*). The teeth to which this applies include premolars and molars.
distal surface: surface away from (*distal*) the midline of the jaw.
labial surface: surface of a tooth that touches the lips (*labia*). The teeth to which this applies include incisors and cuspids.
lingual surface: surface next to the tongue (*lingua*). All teeth have this surface.
mesial surface: surface of a tooth that is toward the front of the mouth or toward the medial (*mesi*), or midline, of the jaw.

There are eight types of teeth in an adult. To learn the names of the teeth divide the upper jaw in half and start at the first front tooth. Touch each tooth in sequence toward the back of the jaw. The names of the teeth are listed in Figure 14-2 using both names for a tooth where appropriate.

The names of the permanent teeth are the same in all four quadrants of the mouth.
Terms related to the names of teeth:

1 Central or first incisor: center front tooth, the first tooth next to the midline.
2 Lateral or second incisor: tooth to the side (*lateral*) of the central incisor. It is the second tooth from the midline. Incisor teeth are used in the process of (*or*) cutting (*incis*) food.
3 Canine or cuspid: tooth that is most prominent in dogs (*canine*). This tooth has a single projected point (*cusp*).
4 First premolar or first bicuspid: first of two teeth in front of (*pre*) the molars. Also the first tooth with two (*bi*) points (*cusp*).
5 Second premolar or second bicuspid: second of two teeth in front of the molar. Also the second tooth with two (*bi*) cusps.
6 First molar: first tooth that grinds (*mol,* variation of *mill*) or pulverizes food.
7 Second molar: second tooth that grinds food.
8 Third molar or wisdom tooth: third tooth that grinds food. It is the last tooth to appear and appears at the so-called age of reason (*wisdom*).

Salivary Glands

There are three pairs of salivary glands that play an important part in the digestive process. They are considered accessory organs because they aid in digestion but are located outside the so-called tube of the digestive system.

The three pairs of salivary glands are the following (see Figure 14-1):

1 parotid glands
2 submandibular glands
3 sublingual glands

Terms related to the salivary glands:

parotid: salivary glands situated around (*par*) the front of each ear (*otid*).
saliva: colorless, watery fluid secreted into the mouth by the salivary glands and containing digestive juices.
sial: root word meaning "salivary gland."
sublingual: salivary gland located under (*sub*) the tongue (*lingual*).
submandibular: salivary gland located under (*sub*) the lower jawbone (*mandibular*).

Pharynx

The pharynx is the area that serves as a passageway for both the digestive system and the respiratory system. The pharynx allows a person to breathe through the nose and mouth. It connects the oral and nasal cavities with the esophagus and trachea.

Terms related to the pharynx:

adenoids: enlarged glandlike (*adenoid*) mass of tissue in the nasopharynx.
nasopharynx: section of pharynx in the nasal (*naso*) cavity.

oropharynx: section of pharynx that connects the mouth (*ora*) with the back of the throat.

pharynx: gulflike cavity (*pharynx*) that connects the oral and nasal cavities with the esophagus and trachea.

throat: area of the body including the pharynx that is the passageway for food and drink to the stomach and for air to the lungs.

Esophagus

The esophagus extends from the pharynx to the stomach. It is located in the thoracic cavity and lies vertically between the trachea and the vertebral column. It allows a direct passage into the stomach.

The term esophagus means an inner (*eso*) tube through which food that has been eaten (*phagus*) passes into the stomach.

The common name for the esophagus is the *gullet.*

Stomach

The stomach is the most dilated portion of the digestive system. It is involved in digestion and produces, among other things the digestive juice pepsin. The stomach action mechanically breaks down foodstuff into a liquid mass called *chyme.* The chyme is stored in the stomach while it is slowly released into the small intestine.

Terms related to the anatomy of the stomach listed in sequence from the beginning of the stomach to the end:

cardiac sphincter: circular band of muscle fibers that keeps the entrance to the stomach, which is near the heart (*cardiac*), closed tightly (*sphincter*).

fundus: upper portion of the stomach toward the left.

body: middle portion of the stomach.

rugae: wrinkles or folds (*rugae*) of the stomach wall that permit the stomach to expand.

antrum: chamber (*antrum*) of the stomach that is the entranceway to the duodenum.

pylorus: opening between the stomach and intestine. The term means "gatekeeper." The action of the pylorus controls the emptying of the stomach.

pyloric sphincter: circular band of muscle that keeps the exit from the stomach closed tightly.

Small Intestine

The small intestine consists of three sections: the duodenum, the jejunum, and the ileum (see Figure 14-1).

Digestion continues in the small intestine because of the various digestive juices secreted by the intestine and also because of the digestive juices from the accessory organs.

The duodenum is the first portion of the small intestine. It extends from the stomach to the jejunum. In the duodenum is the opening from the duct system that carries digestive juices from the liver, gallbladder, and pancreas.

The ileum is the distal, or last, portion of the small intestine. It is connected to the large intestine at the cecum. The opening between the ileum and the cecum is called the ileocecal valve.

Terms related to the small intestine:

duodenum: first portion of the small intestine, which is 12 fingerbreadths long. The name comes from the words for 2 (*duo*) and 10 (*denum*), which add up to 12.

ampulla: small (*ulla*) flasklike (*amp*) dilation with an opening into the duodenum. It is called the ampulla of Vater. This ampulla is also known as the *hepaticopancreatic ampulla* (see the Accessory Organs later in this chapter).

jejunum: middle section of the small intestine so named because it has been found to be empty (*jejunum*) at death.

ileum: last section of the small intestine, so named because it is the most twisted (*ileum*) part of the intestines.

ileocecal valve: structure controlling the flow (*valve*) of intestinal contents from the ileum (*ileo*) to the cecum (*cecal*).

Large Intestine

The function of the large intestine is mainly the absorption of water. The removal of water changes the intestinal contents to a more solid consistency.

The large intestine is circled by bands that cause it to be in pouches, or to have a sausagelike appearance.

The colon is approximately 5 feet long.

Terms related to the large intestine are listed here in anatomical sequence. Follow the structures in Figure 14-1.

appendix: wormlike (*vermiform*) organ hanging (*pend*) down (*ap*) from the end of the cecum. Commonly called the appendix, though its full name is the *vermiform appendix.*

cecum: beginning part of the large intestine, which has a blind (*cecum*) pouch.

colon: large intestine.

ascending colon: section of large bowel that moves upward (*ascend*).

transverse colon: section of large intestine that goes across (*transverse*) the abdomen.

descending colon: section of large intestine that moves downward (*descend*).

sigmoid colon: part of the large intestine that is shaped like (*oid*) the Greek letter sigma.

rectum: part of the large intestine that is straight (*rect*).

anus: ringlike (*anus*) opening at the end of the alimentary tract through which solid wastes of digestion are excreted. This opening has a sphincter that allows a person to hold the anus closed tightly.

Abdominal Membranes

The contents of the abdominal cavity are held in place by various sheets of membranous tissue.

Terms related to these membranes:

mesentery: membrane attached to the intestines (*entery*) that holds them more or less in the middle (*mes*) of the abdominal cavity.
peritoneum: membrane lining the abdominal cavity enclosing the abdominal organs. It stretches (*tone*) around (*peri*) the abdominal contents.
omentum: fold of peritoneum hanging like an apron (*omentum*) from the stomach to adjacent organs in the abdominal cavity.

Activity of the Digestive System

There is much activity throughout the digestive system.

Selected terms related to the activity of the digestive system in order of occurrence:

mastication: act (*tion*) of chewing (*mastica*).
deglutition: act of (*tion*) swallowing (*gluti*) or passing food down (*de*) the throat.
peristalsis: progressive waves of contractions (*stalsis*) around (*peri*) the walls of the digestive organs that move contents through the digestive tract.
absorption: action (*ion*) in which the end products of digestion are taken away or sucked up (*sorb*) from the digestive system into the lymphatic system and bloodstream.
defecation: act of (*tion*) removing waste matter of the intestines (*feca,* variation of *feces*) from (*de*) the body.
bowel movement (*BM*): action resulting from the peristalsis (*movement*) of the large intestine (*bowel*) during which waste products are excreted.
excretion: act of (*tion*) eliminating waste (*cret*) from (*ex*) the body.
flatus: release or blowing (*flatus*) of accumulated air from the intestine.

Accessory Organs

The organs that are considered accessory organs to the digestive system are the liver, gallbladder, and the pancreas.

The function of the liver is very complex and varied. It is considered a part of the digestive system because it produces bile.

Terms related to the liver:

bile: bitter, yellow or greenish liquid secreted by the liver which is one of the digestive juices.
chole: root word meaning "bile."
gall: common term meaning "bile."
hepar: root word meaning "liver."
pyle: root word meaning "portal vein."

The gallbladder is a small, saclike structure located near the interior surface of the liver. Its function is to store and concentrate bile.

The term for gallbladder is *cholecyst;* sac (*cyst*) containing bile (*chole*).

The pancreas is a fleshy organ located near the duodenum. It produces and secretes digestive juices that act on all three major foodstuffs, which are carbohydrates, fats, and proteins. Special cells in the pancreas produce insulin (see Chapter 16).

Pancreas means an organ that appears to be all (*pan*) flesh (*creas*).

Accessory organ ducts

The accessory organs that excrete digestive juices into the duodenum are connected by a series of ducts.

The ducts are the hepatic, cystic, pancreatic, and common bile ducts. The ducts carry the digestive juices, including bile and pancreatic juices, into the duodenum (see Table 14-1).

Terms related to the duct system:

hepatic duct: tube (*duct*) that leads from the liver (*hepatic*).
cystic duct: tube (*duct*) that leads from the gallbladder (*cystic*).
common bile duct: duct formed by the joining of the hepatic and cystic ducts that goes on to join the pancreatic duct.
pancreatic duct: tube that carries the digestive enzymes from the pancreas to the duodenum.
hepatopancreatic ampulla: small (*ulla*), dilated portion (*amp*) of the ducts from the liver (*hepato*) and pancreas (*pancreatic*) that opens into the duodenum. The opening has a nipplelike appearance; thus, it is sometimes referred to as a *papilla.*

DISEASES OF THE DIGESTIVE SYSTEM

Diseases of the digestive system may be of an inflammatory nature, a disruption in the digestive process, or malignant tumors.

In cases of cancer of organs in the digestive system the treatment often involves the removal of the tumor. When a tumor is removed from the digestive system, the system must be reconnected in some way so that the intestinal tube can continue until it reaches the outside of the body.

The terms related to the varieties of surgical reconnections are numerous. If you have learned the root words and combining forms, you can figure out almost any of the possible reconnections. Not all possible surgical connections are listed here.

Signs and Symptoms of Disease Conditions

Analysis of selected terms related to disease conditions of the digestive system and its accessory organs including terms related to signs and symptoms of disease conditions:

anorexia: condition (*ia*) in which there is a loss of (*an*) desire for food, loss of appetite.
appendicitis: inflammation (*itis*) of the appendix.
ascites: fluid accumulation in the abdominal cavity resulting in a baglike (*asc*) appearance of the abdomen. not in the stomach
borborygmus: rumbling or gurgling sounds made by movement of gas in the intestine.

caries: decay (*caries*) of teeth. Cavities in teeth as a result of decay of the surfaces of the teeth.

cholecystitis: inflammation (*itis*) of the gallbladder (*cholecyst*).

choledocholithiasis: condition in which there are stones (*lithiasis*) in the bile (*chole*) ducts (*docho*).

cholelithiasis: condition in which there are bile (*chole*) stones (*lithiasis*). Most commonly formed and found in the gallbladder, but may also be found in the duct system.

cirrhosis: condition (*osis*) of the liver in which the organ takes on a dark yellowish (*cirrh*) color.

constipation: condition of the bowels in which the contents are packed (*stipa*) with (*con*) fecal matter because there has been no bowel movement.

dehiscence: splitting open of the walls of the abdomen.

diarrhea: condition in which the intestinal contents flow (*rrhea*) rapidly through (*dia*) the digestive system before digestion is complete.

diverticulosis: condition (*osis*) in which a small (*cul*) tubular projection turns (*verti*) or grows out from (*di,* variation of *de*) the inside surface of the intestinal tract.

duodenal ulcer: sore (*ulcer*) in the lining of the duodenum (*duodenal*).

dysentery: disease condition of the bowels. There is disease or difficulty (*dys*) in the intestines (*entery*).

dyspepsia: condition (*ia*) in which there is difficulty (*dys*) in digestion (*peps*). Also known as *"indigestion."*

dysphagia: difficulty (*dys*) in swallowing (*phagia*).

emesis: an action in which the contents of the stomach are sent forth (*eme,* variation of *emit*), or vomited.

eructation: belching forth air from the stomach. Burping.

evisceration: event following an operation or other wound in which the abdominal organs (*viscera*) come out (*e*) through the opening.

gastritis: inflammation (*itis*) of the stomach (*gastr*).

hematemesis: vomiting (*emesis*) of blood (*hemat*).

hemorrhoids: veins near the anus that have become dilated and full of blood (*hemo*).

hepatitis: inflammation (*itis*) of the liver (*hepat*).

hernia: protrusion of an organ from its usual location.

- *femoral hernia:* organ passes through the femoral ring, where the femoral artery and vein pass out from the abdominal cavity.
- *hiatal hernia:* protrusion of the stomach into the thoracic cavity through an opening (*hiatal*) in the diaphragm. Also known as a *diaphragmatic hernia.*
- *inguinal hernia:* hernia in the groin (*inguin*) area.
- *umbilical hernia:* protrusion at the navel; also called *omphalocele,* an outpouching (*cele*) at the navel (*omphal*).
- *incarcerated hernia:* protruding part of the organ is trapped (*carcer*) in the abnormal space.
- *incisional hernia:* protrusion occurs at the site of a previous incision.
- *strangulated hernia:* protruding part is squeezed in the unnatural space to the point where circulation is cut off (*strangulated*).

hyperacidity: amount of acid (*acidity*) in the digestive tract is higher (*hyper*) than normal.

indigestion: condition in which the normal process of digestion is not (*in*) occurring.

intestinal obstruction: condition in which there is a blockage (*obstruct*) somewhere along the intestinal tract.

intussusception: slipping (*susception*) of one section of the intestine within (*intus*) another section.

jaundice: condition in which the skin takes on a yellow (*jaundice*) color from an excess of bile or bilelike substances in the bloodstream. Also known as *icterus* (*yellow*).

malocclusion: condition in which the teeth of the upper and lower jaw do not (*mal*) close (*occlusion*) together when the jaws are closed.

paralytic ileus: condition in which the ileum is twisted (*ileus*) and paralyzed; therefore peristalsis is absent. The bowel contents stop moving through the digestive system.

pendulous abdomen: condition in which the muscles of the abdomen are hanging (*pendulous*) loosely.

peptic ulcer: an erosion (*ulcer*) of the lining of the stomach or duodenum that may be caused by the action of the digestive juice pepsin (*peptic*).

perforated viscus: condition in which a hole develops through (*perforate*) an organ (*viscus*).

periodontal disease: disease of the area around (*peri*) the teeth (*dontal*).

portal hypertension: condition of high (*hyper*) blood pressure (*tension*) in the portal circulation of the liver.

proctitis: inflammation (*itis*) of the anus and/or rectum (*proct*).

prolapse of the rectum: weakened walls of the rectum fall (*lapse*) outward (*pro*) or downward.

pruritus ani: condition in which there is excessive itchiness (*pruritus*) around the anus (*ani*).

pyorrhea: flowing (*rrhea*) of pus (*pyo*) from infected gums.

rectocele: outpouching (*cele*) of the rectum (*recto*).

regurgitate: the rushing (*gurgi*) back (*re*) from the stomach of the food or drink recently swallowed.

retroperitoneal tumor: abnormal growth (*tumor*) in back of (*retro*) the peritoneum.

sialolithiasis: condition (*iasis*) in which there are stones (*lith*) in a salivary (*sial*) gland.

steatorrhea: flow (*rrhea*) of undigested fat (*steato*) through the digestive system.

stomatitis: inflammation (*itis*) of the mouth (*stomat*).

tenesmus: straining (*tenesmus*) or feeling the need to defecate without being able to do so.

volvulus: small (*ulus*) twisting or turning (*volv*) of the intestine that causes an obstruction.

vomit: to eject the contents of the stomach through the mouth. To throw up.

Diagnostic and Surgical Procedures

Analysis of selected terms related to diagnostic and surgical procedures done for diseases of the digestive system:

abdominal perineal resection: surgical procedure in which the anus, rectum, and sigmoid colon (which are organs in the perineal area) are cut out or resected, and the opening at the end of the descending colon is brought up to the abdominal wall where an opening, or colostomy, is created.

abdominocentesis: puncture (*centesis*) into the abdominal (*abdomino*) cavity to remove accumulated fluid.

analplasty: surgical repair (*plasty*) done in the anal (*anal*) region.

appendectomy: removal of (*ectomy*) the appendix (*append*).

balloon tamponade: procedure of inserting a long balloon into the esophagus to plug it (*tampon*). By inflating the balloon, direct pressure is exerted against the walls of the esophagus to control bleeding of the esophagus.

cholecystectomy: removal of (*ectomy*) the gallbladder [gall (*chole*), bladder (*cyst*)].

colectomy: removal of (*ectomy*) the colon. May be a hemicolectomy, which is the removal of one half (*hemi*) of the colon.

colostomy: procedure done in which an opening (*ostomy*) is made into the colon (*colo*) for the evacuation of bowel contents.

endoscopic papillotomy: procedure in which a viewing device (*scop*) is passed inside (*endo*) the body through the mouth, esophagus, stomach, and into the duodenum until it reaches the ampulla. At that point a wire that has been passed through the viewing device is passed into the ampulla (*papillo*) where a larger opening (*otomy*) of the ampulla is made to remove stones or allow for the drainage of bile.

esophagectomy: removal of (*ectomy*) the esophagus.

esophagoscopy: passing of a viewing instrument (*scopy*) for visualization of the esophagus.

exenteration: process of (*tion*) removing (*ex*) all of the intestines (*entera*).

exodontia: removal (*ex*) of teeth (*odontia*).

exploratory laparotomy: cutting into (*otomy*) the abdomen (*lapar*), usually for the purpose of exploring the abdominal cavity for disease.

extraction: act of pulling (*traction*) out (*ex*) teeth.

gastrectomy: removal of (*ectomy*) the stomach (*gastr*).

gastric lavage: procedure done to wash (*lavage*) the inside of the stomach (*gastric*).

gastroscopy: passing of a viewing instrument (*scopy*) for the purpose of visualizing the inside of the stomach (*gastro*).

gastrostomy: procedure done to make an opening (*ostomy*) into the stomach (*gastro*), usually for the purpose of inserting a tube for feeding.

gingivectomy: removal of (*ectomy*) the gums (*gingiv*).

glossectomy: removal of (*ectomy*) the tongue (*gloss*).

herniorrhaphy: repair of (*rraphy*) a hernia.

ileal conduit: procedure done in which a small segment of the ileum (*ileal*) is made into a tube (*conduit*) for the purpose of carrying urine to the outside. This procedure is done for disease of the urinary system.

ileostomy: procedure in which an opening (*ostomy*) is made into the ileum (*ile*) for the purpose of evacuation of digestive contents.

intestinal anastomosis: procedure done on the intestines in which two open ends (*stoma*) of different parts of the intestine are sewn together again (*ana*).

orthodontia: a branch of dentistry that is concerned with making teeth (*odont*) straight (*orth*).

pancreatectomy: removal of (*ectomy*) the pancreas (*pancreat*).

pancreaticojejunostomy: procedure done in which there is an opening (*ostomy*) made in the jejunum (*jejuno*) into which the pancreatic (*pancreatico*) duct is placed.

parotidectomy: removal of (*ectomy*) the parotid gland.

polypectomy: removal of (*ectomy*) polyps anywhere in the digestive tract.

proctoscopy: passing of a viewing device (*scopy*) into the anal and rectal region (*procto*).

sigmoidoscopy: passing of a viewing device (*scopy*) into the sigmoid (*sigmoido*) colon.

tracheostomy: formation of a somewhat permanent opening (*ostomy*) into the trachea (*trache*) at the throat.

tracheotomy: procedure done to cut into (*otomy*) the trachea (*trache*).

Drugs Used in Treatment

Analysis of selected terms related to drugs used in the treatment of diseases of the digestive system:

antacid: substance or medicine used against (*anti*) or to control the acid condition of the stomach.

antidiarrhetic: drug used against (*anti*) or to control diarrhea.

antiemetics: substances used against (*anti*) or to control vomiting (*emet*).

antiflatulents: drugs that work against (*anti*) the retention of air in the digestive system and allow for the release of air (*flatus*).

cathartic: substance used to cleanse the bowel, to induce bowel movement.

digestant: drug used to aid digestion.

emetic: substance used to induce or cause vomiting (*emet*).

laxative: substance used to loosen (*laxa*) the bowel to allow the contents of the bowel to be evacuated.

nutritional supplement: the taking in (*sup*) of a product meant to fill a person. These products pertain (*al*) to the nourishment (*nutrition*) of the person.

PRETEST/ POSTTEST FOR CHAPTER 14

1. The following terms are related to the digestive system as a whole. Briefly define each term.

   1. alimentary tract ______________________________
   2. bowel ______________________________
   3. celiac ______________________________
   4. digestion ______________________________
   5. entero ______________________________
   6. gastro ______________________________
   7. gastrointestinal system ______________________________

      ____

2. The following organs are part of the digestive system. Indicate their place in the sequence by numbering the organs from 1 to 14.

_____ oral cavity	_____ ileum
_____ stomach	_____ transverse colon
_____ rectum	_____ pharynx
_____ ascending colon	_____ cecum
_____ esophagus	_____ jejunum
_____ descending colon	_____ sigmoid colon
_____ anus	_____ duodenum

3. The following terms are related to the mouth. Match column A with column B.

Column A	Column B
1. _____ bucca	A. passage to the throat
2. _____ cheil	B. root word meaning tongue
3. _____ fauces	C. grapelike structure at the back of the mouth
4. _____ frenulum	D. inside of the cheek
5. _____ glossa; lingua	E. membrane holding the tongue in place
	F. roof of the mouth

Column A	Column B
6. _____ labia	G. opening into the mouth
7. _____ malar	H. the lips
8. _____ os, ora	I. root word meaning lip
9. _____ palate	J. cheek, including bones and flesh
10. _____ stoma	K. the mouth
11. _____ tonsil	L. oval mass of tissue on each side of the fauces
12. _____ uvula	

4. Complete the following statement:
The first set of teeth that develop is called baby teeth. They are also known as deciduous teeth because they ______________________________.

5. The following terms are related to the teeth. Match column A with column B.

Column A	Column B
1. _____ alveoli	A. root word meaning gum
2. _____ cementum	B. hard section of the tooth that forms major portion of the tooth
3. _____ crown	C. cavity in the root
4. _____ denti	D. bony sockets for the teeth
5. _____ dentin	E. hard, glossy covering
6. _____ enamel	F. narrow portion of the tooth
7. _____ gingiv	G. tissue holding the tooth firmly in place
8. _____ gum	H. central hollow cavity of the tooth
9. _____ neck	I. part of the tooth above the gum
10. _____ periodontal	J. portion of the tooth imbedded in the bony socket
11. _____ pulp cavity	K. firm, fleshy tissue covering the alveolar parts of the jaw
12. _____ root	L. root word meaning tooth
13. _____ root canal	M. fibrous connective tissues around the tooth

6. The following terms are related to the surfaces of a tooth. Match column A with column B.

Column A	Column B
1. _____ buccal surface	A. surface away from the midline of the jaw
2. _____ distal surface	B. surface that touches the tongue
	C. surface that touches the cheek

Column A	Column B
3. _____ labial surface	D. surface toward the midline of the jaw
4. _____ lingual surface	E. surface that touches the lips
5. _____ mesial surface	

7. The following terms are names of teeth. Match column A with column B.

Column A	Column B
1. _____ central incisor	A. wisdom tooth
2. _____ lateral incisor	B. tooth on the side of the first incisor
3. _____ canine	C. first tooth that grinds food
4. _____ first premolar	D. first tooth next to the midline
5. _____ second premolar	E. second bicuspid
6. _____ first molar	F. also known as the cuspid tooth
7. _____ second molar	G. first tooth in front of the molars
8. _____ third molar	H. second tooth that grinds food

8. The following terms are related to the salivary glands. Indicate the correct statement by circling the appropriate letter.

1. The root word meaning saliva is:
A. sail.
B. sial.

2. The names of the three pairs of salivary glands are:
A. parotid, submandibular, sublingual.
B. parotid, submaxillar, sublingual.
C. peripharyngeal, submandibular, sublingual.
D. parotid, submandibular, submaxillar.

9. The following terms are related to the pharynx. Fill in the blanks.

1. The adenoids are ____________________ masses of tissue in the nasopharynx.

2. The pharynx is a ____________________ that connects the oral and nasal cavities with the throat.

3. The term *nasopharynx* indicates the part of the pharynx that connects the ____________________ cavity with the esophagus and trachea.

4. The term *oropharynx* indicates the part of the pharynx that connects the ____________________ cavity with the esophagus and trachea.

5. The throat is a passageway for ____, ____________________ and ____________________.

10. Define the parts of the term *esophagus*:

eso ______________________

phagus ______________________

11. The following terms are related to the stomach. Match column A with column B.

Column A	Column B
1. _____ chyme	A. circular band and the entrance to the stomach
2. _____ pepsin	B. opening between the stomach and duodenum
3. _____ cardiac sphincter	C. liquid mass of food in the stomach
4. _____ fundus	D. the middle portion of the stomach
5. _____ body	E. entrance chamber to the duodenum
6. _____ rugae	F. upper portion toward the left
7. _____ antrum	G. circular band between the stomach and the duodenum
8. _____ pylorus	H. folds in the stomach that allow it to expand
9. _____ pyloric sphincter	I. digestive juice produced in the stomach

12. The following terms are related to the small intestine. Match column A with column B.

Column A	Column B
1. _____ duodenum	A. portion said to be empty after death
2. _____ ampulla (of Vater)	B. opening between the ileum and cecum
3. _____ jejunum	C. part that is said to be 12 finger-breadths long
4. _____ ileum	D. twisted portion
5. _____ ileocecal valve	E. opening into the duodenum from the common bile duct

13. The following terms are related to the large intestine. Match column A with column B.

Column A	Column B
1. _____ appendix	A. part of the colon shaped like the Greek letter sigma
2. _____ cecum	B. ringlike opening at the end of the alimentary tract
3. _____ colon	C. section of bowel that crosses over the abdomen
4. _____ ascending colon	D. root word meaning anus and rectum
5. _____ transverse colon	

Column A	Column B
6. ____ descending colon	E. term meaning large intestine
7. ____ sigmoid colon	F. section of bowel that moves downward
8. ____ rectum	G. part of the bowel that is straight
9. ____ anus	H. part of the colon with a blind pouch
10. ____ procto	I. organ hanging down from the cecum
	J. section of bowel that moves upward

14. There are three membranes in the abdominal cavity involved with holding the intestines in place. Write a brief definition of each term.

1. mesentery ____________________

____

2. omentum ____________________

____

3. peritoneum ____________________

____

15. The following terms are related to the activity of the digestive system. Select the best answer.

1. ________ is the release of air from the intestine.
   A. Peristalsis
   B. Flatus
   C. Both of the above
2. The act of eliminating waste from the body is called ________.
   A. defecation
   B. excretion
   C. both of the above
3. Absorption is the action by which the end products of digestion are
   A. taken into the lymphatic and blood systems.
   B. taken into the small intestine from the stomach.
4. The action in which the large intestine contracts to empty its contents is called ________.
   A. bowel movement
   B. defecation
   C. both of the above
5. The term for the waves of contractions along the walls of the digestive organs is ________.
   A. pericontractions
   B. peristalsis

16. Using the following terms, complete the statements:

mastication deglutition

1. The act of swallowing is called ____________________.
2. The act of chewing is called ____________________.

17. The following terms are related to the accessory organs, the liver, gallbladder, and pancreas. Match column A with column B.

Column A	Column B
1. _____ bile	A. produced by the liver
2. _____ chole	B. organ that appears to be all fleshy
3. _____ gall	C. root word meaning bile
4. _____ hepar	D. root word for liver
5. _____ cholecyst	E. another name for bile
6. _____ pancreas	F. gallbladder

18. The following terms are related to the accessory organ duct system. Match column A with column B.

Column A	Column B
1. _____ hepatic duct	A. opening into the duodenum from the duct system
2. _____ cystic duct	B. tube from the liver
3. _____ common bile	C. tube formed by the joining of the ducts from the liver and gallbladder
4. _____ pancreatic duct	D. tube from the pancreas
5. _____ hepatopancreatic ampulla	E. tube from the gallbladder

19. The following sets of terms are related to disease conditions of the digestive system, including terms related to signs and symptoms of disease. Match column A with column B. Be specific.

Set 1

Column A	Column B
1. _____ anorexia	A. inflammation of the gallbladder
2. _____ ascites	B. release of contents of the abdomen through a split in the abdominal wall
3. _____ appendicitis	C. difficulty in digestion; indigestion
4. _____ borborygmi	D. small tubular projections in the intestines
5. _____ caries	

Column A	Column B
6. ____ cholecystitis	E. loss of appetite
7. ____ choledocholithiasis	F. flow through of undigested food
8. ____ cholelithiasis	G. sore in the duodenum
9. ____ cirrhosis	H. inflammation of the appendix
10. ____ constipation	I. stones in the bile duct
11. ____ dehiscence	J. decay of teeth
12. ____ diarrhea	K. difficulty in the bowels
13. ____ diverticulosis	L. bowels packed with feces
14. ____ duodenal ulcer	M. difficulty in swallowing
15. ____ dysentery	N. bile stones
16. ____ dyspepsia	O. disease in which liver becomes dark yellow
17. ____ dysphagia	P. rumbling sounds made by movement of the intestines
	Q. accumulation of fluid in the stomach

Set 2

Column A	Column B
1. ____ emesis	A. vomiting blood
2. ____ eructation	B. protrusion of an organ out of its normal place
3. ____ evisceration	C. blockage in the intestinal tract
4. ____ gastritis	D. normal process of digestion not occurring
5. ____ hematemesis	E. burping or belching
6. ____ hemorrhoids	F. erosion of stomach or duodenum
7. ____ hepatitis	G. abdominal structures protruding out through an opening
8. ____ hernia	H. slipping of one section of intestine into another
9. ____ hyperacidity	I. vomiting
10. ____ indigestion	J. absence of peristalsis in the ileum
11. ____ intestinal obstruction	K. inflammation of the stomach
12. ____ intussusception	L. dilated veins near the anus
13. ____ jaundice	M. inflammation of the liver
14. ____ paralytic ileus	N. high amount of acid
15. ____ malocclusion	O. condition in which muscles of abdomen hang down
16. ____ pendulous abdomen	P. disease in which skin becomes yellow
17. ____ peptic ulcer	Q. teeth not coming together when the jaws are closed

Set 3

	Column A	Column B
1.	_____ perforated viscus	A. hole in an organ
2.	_____ periodontal disease	B. high blood pressure in the circulation to the liver
3.	_____ portal hypertension	C. flow of pus from the gums
4.	_____ proctitis	D. inflammation of the anus and rectum
5.	_____ prolapse of rectum	E. inflammation of the mouth
6.	_____ pruritus ani	F. to throw up
		G. itchiness around the anus
7.	_____ pyorrhea	H. disease around the teeth
8.	_____ rectocele	I. walls of rectum fallen downward
		J. rush back of food recently eaten
9.	_____ regurgitate	K. stones in a salivary gland
10.	_____ retroperitoneal tumor	L. straining to defecate
		M. flow of undigested fat
11.	_____ sialolithiasis	N. twisting of the intestines
12.	_____ steatorrhea	O. growth in back of peritoneum
		P. outpouching of the rectum
13.	_____ stomatitis	
14.	_____ tenesmus	
15.	_____ vomit	
16.	_____ volvulus	

20. The following sets of terms are related to diagnostic and surgical procedures done for diseases of the digestive system. Match column A with column B. Be specific.

Set 1

	Column A	Column B
1.	_____ abdominal perineal resection	A. formation of a somewhat permanent opening into the colon for evacuation of contents
2.	_____ abdominocentesis	B. removal of the appendix
3.	_____ analplasty	C. visualization of the esophagus
4.	_____ appendectomy	D. cutting out organs in perineal area
		E. removal of the esophagus
5.	_____ balloon tamponade	F. puncture of abdominal wall
6.	_____ cholecystectomy	G. removal of all of the intestines
		H. cutting into the abdomen to find disease
7.	_____ colectomy	I. removal of the gallbladder
8.	_____ colostomy	J. removal of the colon

Column A	Column B
9. ____ esophagectomy	K. repair of the anal region
10. ____ esophagoscopy	L. removal of teeth
11. ____ exenteration	M. insertion of balloon to plug the esophagus
12. ____ exodontia or extraction	
13. ____ exploratory laparotomy	

Set 2

Column A	Column B
1. ____ gastrectomy	A. removal of the gums
2. ____ gastric lavage	B. repair of a hernia
3. ____ gastroscopy	C. removal of the tongue
4. ____ gastrostomy	D. making a somewhat permanent opening into the stomach
5. ____ gingivectomy	E. washing of the inside of the stomach
6. ____ glossectomy	F. two ends of the intestinal tract are sewn together
7. ____ herniorrhaphy	G. visualizing the inside of the stomach
8. ____ ileal conduit	H. opening into the ileum
9. ____ ileostomy	I. using a segment of the small intestine to carry urine to the outside
10. ____ intestinal anastomosis	J. removal of the stomach

Set 3

Column A	Column B
1. ____ orthodontia	A. removal of a salivary gland
2. ____ pancreatectomy	B. visualization of the anal and rectal regions
3. ____ pancreaticojejunostomy	C. removal of a polyp
4. ____ endoscopic papillotomy	D. straightening of teeth
5. ____ parotidectomy	E. removal of the pancreas
6. ____ polypectomy	F. opening into the jejunum for the pancreatic duct
7. ____ proctoscopy	G. viewing device passed inside the body to enlarge the ampulla
8. ____ sigmoidoscopy	H. visualization of the sigmoid colon

21. The following terms are related to drugs used to treat diseases of the digestive system. Match column A with column B.

Column A

1. ____ antacid
2. ____ antidiarrhetic
3. ____ antiemetic
4. ____ antiflatulent
5. ____ cathartic
6. ____ digestant
7. ____ emetic
8. ____ laxative
9. ____ nutritional supplement

Column B

A. drug used to control vomiting
B. drug used to aid digestion
C. drug used to control acid condition
D. substance used to cleanse the bowel
E. substance used to loosen the bowel
F. drug used to control diarrhea
G. product used to aid nourishment
H. drug used to cause vomiting
I. drug that works against retention of air in the digestive system

PRETEST/ POSTTEST **ANSWERS** FOR CHAPTER **14**

1. **1.** the tract through which food passes
2. the intestines, the organs that look like little sausages
3. pertaining to contents of the belly
4. process by which food is changed so it can be absorbed
5. root word meaning intestine
6. root word meaning stomach
7. the system involving the stomach and intestines

2.

1	7
4	10
13	2
9	8
3	6
11	12
14	5

3. **1.** D **2.** I **3.** A **4.** E **5.** B **6.** H **7.** J **8.** G **9.** F **10.** K **11.** L **12.** C

4. normally fall out

5. **1.** D **2.** G **3.** I **4.** L **5.** B **6.** E **7.** A **8.** K **9.** F **10.** M **11.** H **12.** J **13.** C

6. **1.** C **2.** A **3.** E **4.** B **5.** D

7. **1.** D **2.** B **3.** F **4.** G **5.** E **6.** C **7.** H **8.** A

8. **1.** B **2.** A

9. **1.** glandlike
2. cavity or space
3. nasal
4. oral or mouth
5. food, drink, air

10. inner (eso), eating (phagus)

11. **1.** C **2.** I **3.** A **4.** F **5.** D **6.** H **7.** E **8.** B **9.** G

12. **1.** C **2.** E **3.** A **4.** D* **5.** B

13. **1.** I **2.** H **3.** E **4.** J **5.** C **6.** F **7.** A **8.** G **9.** B **10.** D

14. **1.** The mesentery is a membrane attached to the intestines (*entery*) that holds them in the middle (*meso*) of the abdominal cavity.
2. The omentum is a fold of peritoneum hanging like an apron from the stomach and adjacent organs.
3. The peritoneum is a membrane stretching around the abdominal contents.

15. **1.** B **2.** C **3.** A **4.** C **5.** B

16. **1.** deglutition
2. mastication

17. **1.** A **2.** C **3.** E **4.** D **5.** F **6.** B

18. **1.** B **2.** E **3.** C **4.** D **5.** A

19. **Set 1**
1. E **2.** Q **3.** H **4.** P **5.** J **6.** A **7.** I **8.** N **9.** O **10.** L **11.** B **12.** F **13.** D **14.** G **15.** K **16.** C **17.** M

Set 2
1. I **2.** E **3.** G **4.** K **5.** A **6.** L **7.** M **8.** B **9.** N **10.** D **11.** C **12.** H **13.** P **14.** J **15.** Q **16.** O **17.** F

---

* To avoid confusing the spelling of this ileum with the ilium of the hip bone, note that the letter *e* twists more than the little *i*. Therefore the *e* belongs to ileum which means "twisted."

Set 3

1. A	**4.** D	**7.** C	**9.** J	**11.** K	**13.** E	**15.** F
2. H	**5.** I	**8.** P	**10.** O	**12.** M	**14.** L	**16.** N
3. B	**6.** G					

20. **Set 1**

1. D	**3.** K	**5.** M	**7.** J	**9.** E	**11.** G	**13.** H
2. F	**4.** B	**6.** I	**8.** A	**10.** C	**12.** L	

Set 2

1. J	**3.** G	**5.** A	**7.** B	**8.** I	**9.** H	**10.** F
2. F	**4.** D	**6.** C				

Set 3

1. D	**3.** F	**4.** G	**5.** A	**6.** C	**7.** B	**8.** H
2. E						

21.

1. C	**3.** A	**5.** D	**6.** B	**7.** H	**8.** E	**9.** G
2. F	**4.** I					

15 THE URINARY SYSTEM

OBJECTIVES

At the end of this chapter you will be able to do the following:

1 List the organs in the urinary system.
2 Define terms related to the kidneys and the functioning unit of the kidney.
3 Define terms related to the formation of urine.
4 Define terms related to the ureter, bladder, and urethra.
5 Describe urination.
6 Analyze selected terms related to disease conditions of the urinary system.
7 Analyze selected terms related to diagnostic and surgical procedures done for diseases of the urinary system, including terms related to drugs.

THE URINARY SYSTEM

The organs in the urinary system are these (see Figure 15-1):

1 two kidneys
2 two ureters
3 one bladder
4 one urethra that extends down from the bladder

The chief function of the urinary system is the formation of urine. The kidney also produces substances that have an effect on other systems of the body; for example, the kidney releases renal erythropoietin that has an influence on the production of red blood cells.

The Kidneys

There are two kidneys in the body. They are bean-shaped organs lying against the muscles of the posterior abdominal wall just above the waistline.

Terms related to the anatomy of the kidney:

nephr: root word meaning "kidney."
pyelo: root word meaning "pelvis (*pyelo*) of the kidney."

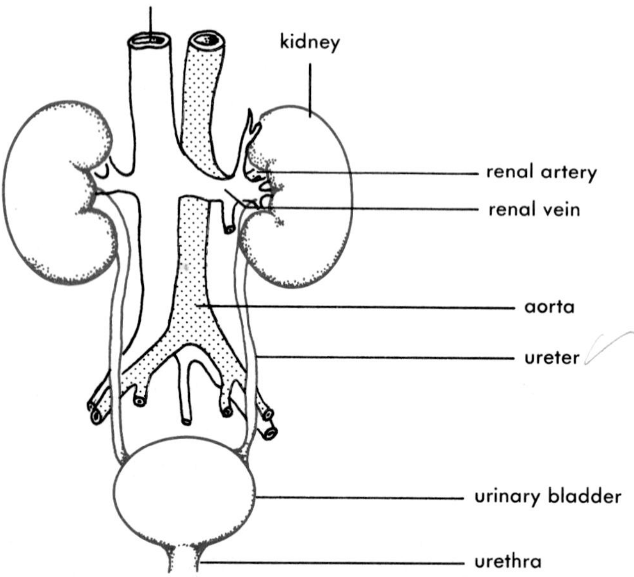

FIGURE 15-1
The urinary system.

renal: root word meaning pertaining to (*al*) the kidney (*ren*).
renal pelvis: basin (*pelvis*) or collection area within the kidney (*renal*).
ureter: tube that transports urine from the kidney to the bladder. The term derives from a word that means "to make water."
ureteropelvic junction: place (*junction*) where the ureter (*uretero*) leaves the renal pelvis (*pelvic*).

The functioning unit of the kidney is the *nephron.* Each nephron contains, among other things, a glomerulus and a collecting tubule that carries the urine to the kidney pelvis. There are about 1 million nephrons in each kidney.

Terms related to the nepron:

tubules: small (*ules*) tubes (*tub*) that are part of the nephron.
glomerulus: the collection of capillaries in the nephron that resembles a small (*ulus*) ball of yarn (*glomer*).
nephron: structural and functioning unit of the kidney (*nephr*).

Urine is formed in the kidney as it progresses through the nephron. The nephron of a healthy person has the ability to filter out and reabsorb the amount of water and other blood elements needed to meet the requirements of the body.

Terms related to urine formation in the kidneys:

clearance: term used to describe the efficiency with which the kidney excretes any substance.

glomerular filtration: process in which the glomerulus acts as a filter to begin the process of cleaning (*filtration*) the plasma.

tubular reabsorption and secretion: process in the system of tubules by which certain products are eliminated and certain products are reabsorbed. This is the area where concentration of particular elements occurs.

ur-: combining form meaning "urine."

The Ureters

A ureter is attached to each kidney at the base of the renal pelvis. The renal pelvis and ureter relationship may be compared to a funnel lying on its side. The pelvis is the basin-shaped part and the ureter is the narrowing tubelike structure draining the urine. The base of this long tube is attached to the urinary bladder where urine is stored.

The Bladder

The urinary bladder is a baglike organ whose main function is to store urine. Urine is being formed continuously. As it is being produced, it is transported to the bladder where it is stored. When a sufficient quantity is collected, the bladder is stretched, and a person gets the urge to empty the bladder. The bladder may be considered an organ of convenience because without it we would be constantly dripping urine.

Another important function of the bladder is to protect the kidney from outside bacteria. If the kidney, which is a very delicate organ, opened directly to the outside, as does the digestive system, it would become invaded and infected very easily.

Urinary bladder activity is controlled by the parasympathetic nervous system. The center of this activity is in the spinal cord.

Terms related to the urinary bladder:

bladder: sac or organ that is the receptacle for a fluid, in this case urine.

cysto: root word meaning "bladder."

trigone: triangular (*trigone*) internal surface of the posterior wall of the bladder. The three corners of the trigone are marked by the openings of the two ureters and the urethra.

ureteric orifice: small opening or mouth (*orifice*) of the ureter as it enters the bladder from the kidney. There are two of these openings.

urethral orifice: small opening or mouth (*orifice*) of the urethra as it leaves the bladder.

vesical: pertaining (*al*) to the bladder (*vesic*).

The Urethra

The urethra is the tube that carries urine to the outside of the body.

In the female the urethra only carries urine from the bladder to outside the body. The urethra is very short in the female, and lies anterior to the vaginal opening.

The urethra in the male has two separate functions. It conveys urine to outside the body, and also, at a different time, serves as a passageway for semen.

Because of the dual role of the urethra in the male and the embryology of the urinary and genital systems in both sexes, the urinary system is sometimes (particularly for the male) studied with the reproductive system under the heading of the genitourinary or urogenital system (see Chapter 17).

Terms related to the urethra:

genitourinary: system involving the reproductive (*genito*) and urinary (*urinary*) organs. Sometimes called the *urogenital system.*
urethra: tube from the bladder to outside the body that allows for the passage of urine, derived from a word meaning "to make water."
urethral meatus: opening (*meatus*) of the urethra to outside of the body.

Urination

The action of the urinary bladder is both voluntary and involuntary and is called *urination.*

As urine fills it, the bladder becomes stretched. When the pressure in the bladder rises, a person has the desire to urinate voluntarily. If the pressure continues to rise, urination then becomes involuntary. During urination urine flows into the urethra where it is channeled to the outside.

Terms related to urination:

diuresis: condition (*sis*) in which there is an increased amount of urine (*diure*) passed.
urinate: to pass urine from the urinary bladder to the outside.
micturate: to make water (*mict*), as in urination.
void: to empty (*void*) the bladder.

DISEASE CONDITIONS OF THE URINARY SYSTEM

Analysis of selected terms related to disease conditions of the urinary system including terms relating to signs and symptoms:

anuria: absence (*an*) of urine (*uria*).
cystitis: inflammation (*itis*) of the urinary bladder (*cyst*).
enuresis: A person involuntarily (*en,* variation of *in*) passes urine (*uresis*).
ESRD: end stage renal disease.
glomerulonephritis: inflammation (*itis*) of the glomeruli (*glomerulo*) of the kidneys (*nephr*).
glycosuria: condition in which there is sugar (*glycos*) in the urine (*uria*).
hematuria: condition in which there is blood (*hemat*) in the urine (*uria*).
hydroureter: overdistention of the ureter (*ureter*) from the backup of the water (*hydro*) of urine.
incontinent: pertaining to the condition in which there is a lack of (*in*) ability to contain (*continent*) or hold urine.
kidney agenesis: absence (*a*) of one kidney at birth (*genesis*).

nephrolithiasis: presence of stones (*lithiasis*) in the kidney (*nephro*). The stones are also called *renal calculi.*

nephroptosis: condition in which the kidney (*nephr*) has dropped (*ptosis*) from its normal place. Also called a "floating kidney."

neurogenic bladder: condition in which there is decreased functioning of the bladder caused by (*genic*) an injury to the nerves (*neuro*) to the bladder muscle.

nocturia: frequent urination (*uria*) during the night (*noct*).

nocturnal enuresis: involuntary urination that occurs at night. Also known as *bed-wetting*.

oliguria: scant or small amounts (*olig*) of urine (*uria*) are produced.

pyelonephritis: inflammation (*itis*) of the kidney (*nephr*) pelvis (*pyelo*).

polydipsia: condition of excessive thirst that usually accompanies polyuria.

polyuria: urinating (*uria*) many times (*poly*). Also known as frequency of urination.

renal calculi: kidney (*renal*) stones (*calculi*); also called *nephrolithiasis.*

renal failure or shutdown: kidney (*renal*) stops filtering or forming urine.

tubular necrosis: cellular death (*necrosis*) of the tubules of the kidney.

uremia: waste products normally found in urine (*ur*) are not filtered through the kidney, and thus remain in the blood (*emia*).

ureteral colic: severe pain (*colic*) from a stone or blood clot in the ureter.

ureteritis: inflammation (*itis*) of the ureter.

vesical fistulas: abnormal openings (*fistula*) between the bladder (*vesical*) and other nearby organs.

Diagnostic and Surgical Procedures and Drugs for Treatment

Analysis of selected terms related to diagnostic and surgical procedures done for diseases of the urinary system and terms related to drugs used:

cystectomy: removal (*ectomy*) of the bladder.

cystometry: the measurement (*etry*) of the efficiency and capacity of the urinary bladder (*cysto*).

cystoscopy: passing of a viewing scope (*scopy*) device into the bladder (*cyst*) for visualization of the inside of the bladder.

diuretic: drug used to cause an increased flow of urine (*diuresis*).

hemodialysis: procedure in which blood (*hemo*) from an individual is shunted through a special device in which waste products are separated out (*dialysis*) and taken out. The cleaned blood continues through the device and is sent back into the individual.

peritoneal dialysis: method of separating out (*dialysis*) waste products by special procedures utilizing the peritoneal cavity and membrane. Example: continuous ambulatory peritoneal dialysis (CAPD). There is a continuous flow of solution into and out of the peritoneal cavity. The person is not confined in bed (ambulatory) during this type of dialysis.

intravenous pyelogram (IVP): x-ray of the kidney pelvis (*pyelo*) following injection into a vein (*intravenous*) of a radiopaque substance.

kidney transplant: act of taking a kidney from a donor and surgically implanting it

Lithotripsis

in a recipient. A donor is one who (*or*) gives (*don*) a kidney. The recipient is one who receives the kidney. This is also called a *renal transplant (see Glossary of Terms Related to Transplantation).*

nephrectomy: removal (*ectomy*) of a kidney (*nephr*).

nephrolithotomy: cutting into (*otomy*) the kidney (*nephro*) for the removal of stones (*lith*).

nephropexy: surgical fixation (*pexy*) of a floating kidney (*nephro*).

nephrotoxic: a substance that potentially may cause damage (*toxic*) to the kidney (*nephro*); particularly used with regard to drugs.

ureterocystostomy: procedure done to make a new opening (*ostomy*) into the bladder (*cyst*) to which the ureter (*uretero*) is attached. This procedure is done when there is disease in the bladder near the natural openings near the ureters.

urinary diversion: surgical procedure done to divert the flow of urine away from the bladder. Example: ileal conduit (see Chapter 14).

PRETEST/ POSTTEST FOR CHAPTER 15

1. List the organs in the urinary system.

1. ____________________
2. ____________________
3. ____________________
4. ____________________

2. The following terms are related to the anatomy of the kidney. Match column A with column B.

Column A	Column B
1. _____ nephr	A. root word meaning kidney
2. _____ pyelo	B. collection area within the kidney
3. _____ renal	C. pertaining to the kidney
4. _____ renal pelvis	D. place where ureter joins the kidney
5. _____ ureter	E. root word meaning pelvis of the kidney
6. _____ ureteropelvic junction	F. small tubes that are part of the nephron
	G. functioning unit of the kidney
	H. ball of capillaries in the nephron
	I. tube that transports urine from the kidney to the bladder

Column A	Column B
7. ____ tubules	
8. ____ glomerulus	
9. ____ nephron	

3. The following terms are related to the process of urine formation. Select the correct statement.
   1. The term *clearance* refers to:
      A. the urine leaving the kidney by way of the ureter.
      B. the efficiency with which the kidney excretes any substance.
      C. both of the above.
   2. Glomerular filtration is:
      A. the process in which the glomerulus acts as a filtering device for plasma.
      B. the process by which urine is formed.
      C. both of the above.
   3. Tubular reabsorption and secretion constitute:
      A. the process by which some products are eliminated and other products reabsorbed.
      B. the process by which products are concentrated.
      C. both of the above.
   4. The combining form meaning urine is:
      A. urea-.
      B. ur-.
      C. both of the above.

4. The following terms are related to the ureter, bladder, and urethra. Match column A with column B. Be specific.

Column A	Column B
1. ____ ureter	A. root word meaning bladder
2. ____ bladder	B. opening of the tube from the kidney into the bladder
3. ____ cysto	C. another name for bladder
4. ____ trigone	D. opening to outside of the body
5. ____ ureteric orifice	E. tube to the bladder from the kidney
6. ____ urethral orifice	F. the reproductive and urinary organs
7. ____ vesical	G. opening of the tube from the bladder to the outside
8. ____ genitourinary	H. triangular internal surface of the back wall of the bladder
9. ____ urethra	I. receptacle for urine
10. ____ urethral meatus	J. tube leaving the bladder

5. The following terms are related to urination. Select the best answer.

1. The act of emptying the bladder is called ________________.
A. voiding
B. urinating
C. both of the above

2. The terms ________________ mean the same thing.
A. urinate and micturate
B. urinate and diuresis
C. micturate and diuresis
D. all of the above

3. A condition in which there is an increase in the amount of urine passed is called ________________.
A. diuresis
B. micturition
C. both of the above

6. The following sets of terms are related to disease conditions of the urinary system. Match column A with column B. Be specific.

Set 1

Column A	Column B
1. ____ anuria	A. sugar in the urine
2. ____ cystitis	B. inflammation of the bladder
3. ____ dysuria	C. decreased function of bladder because of nerve injury
4. ____ enuresis	D. absence of urine
5. ____ glomerulonephritis	E. overdistention of the ureter from the backup of urine
6. ____ glycosuria	F. difficulty in urination
7. ____ hematuria	G. involuntary urination
8. ____ hydroureter	H. lack of ability to hold urine
9. ____ incontinency	I. blood in the urine
10. ____ kidney agenesis	J. kidney stones
11. ____ nephrolithiasis	K. dropped kidney
12. ____ nephroptosis	L. absence of one kidney at birth
13. ____ neurogenic bladder	M. inflammation of the glomeruli

Set 2

Column A	Column B
1. _____ nocturia	A. kidney shutdown
2. _____ nocturnal enuresis	B. cellular death of the kidney tubules
3. _____ oliguria	C. frequent urination at night
4. _____ pyelonephritis	D. kidney stones
5. _____ polyuria	E. abnormal openings between the bladder and other nearby organs
6. _____ polydipsia	F. commonly called bed-wetting
7. _____ renal calculi	G. waste products remaining in the blood
8. _____ renal failure	H. inflammation of the kidney pelvis
9. _____ tubular necrosis	I. inflammation of the ureter
10. _____ uremia	J. scant or small amounts of urine
11. _____ ureteral colic	K. excessive thirst
12. _____ ureteritis	L. frequent urination
13. _____ vesical fistulas	M. severe pain from a blood clot or stone in the ureter

7. The following terms are related to the diagnosis and treatment of diseases of the urinary system, including terms related to drugs. Match column A with column B.

Column A	Column B
1. _____ cystectomy	A. viewing inside the bladder
2. _____ cystometry	B. separating waste products by use of the peritoneal membrane
3. _____ cystoscopy	C. putting a donor's kidney into a recipient
4. _____ diuretic	D. measurement of the capacity of the bladder
5. _____ hemodialysis	E. x-ray of the kidney pelvis
6. _____ peritoneal dialysis	F. surgical fixation of a dropped kidney
7. _____ intravenous pyelogram	G. removal of the bladder
8. _____ kidney transplant	H. cutting into a kidney to remove a stone
9. _____ nephrectomy	I. drug that causes an increased flow of urine
10. _____ nephrolithotomy	J. making a new opening in the bladder to attach the ureters
11. _____ nephropexy	K. drug that damages the kidneys
12. _____ nephrotoxic	L. removal of a kidney
13. _____ ureterocystostomy	

Column A	Column B
14. _____ urinary diversion	M. separating waste products directly from the blood
	N. diverting flow of urine away from the bladder

PRETEST/ POSTTEST **ANSWERS** FOR CHAPTER **15**

1. **1.** two kidneys
2. two ureters
3. one bladder
4. one urethra

2. **1.** A **2.** E **3.** C **4.** B **5.** I **6.** D **7.** F **8.** H **9.** G

3. **1.** B **2.** C **3.** C **4.** B

4. **1.** E **2.** I **3.** A **4.** H **5.** B **6.** G **7.** C **8.** F **9.** J **10.** D

5. **1.** C **2.** A **3.** A

6. **Set 1**
1. D **2.** B **3.** F **4.** G **5.** M **6.** A **7.** I **8.** E **9.** H **10.** L **11.** J **12.** K **13.** C

Set 2
1. C **2.** F **3.** J **4.** H **5.** L **6.** K **7.** D **8.** A **9.** B **10.** G **11.** M **12.** I **13.** E

7. **1.** G **2.** D **3.** A **4.** I **5.** M **6.** B **7.** E **8.** C **9.** L **10.** H **11.** F **12.** K **13.** J **14.** N

16 THE ENDOCRINE SYSTEM

OBJECTIVES

At the end of this chapter you will be able to do the following:

1. Describe an endocrine gland.
2. List the general functions of the endocrine system.
3. Define terms related to the endocrine system.
4. Name, describe the location, list, and define the hormones of each of the following structures that produce hormones:

    hypothalamus
    hypophysis or pituitary gland
    pineal gland
    thyroid gland
    parathyroid gland
    thymus gland
    pancreatic islets
    adrenal or suprarenal glands
    gonads: ovaries and testes
    placenta

5. Analyze terms related to disease conditions of the endocrine system, including terms related to signs and symptoms of disease.
6. Analyze terms related to the treatment of endocrine diseases including diagnostic, surgical, and drug-related terms.

THE ENDOCRINE SYSTEM

The endocrine system is made up of glands that produce hormones that are secreted directly into the bloodstream. This means that the blood vessels that enter the glands to supply them with blood also pick up the hormones produced in that gland.

The endocrine glands secrete their hormones into the bloodstream within the glands, as opposed to the exocrine glands, which excrete their products into ducts that lead to a specific area (for example, salivary glands excrete their hormones into ducts that lead to the mouth). Because of this difference, the endocrine glands are sometimes referred to as "ductless glands."

The functions of the endocrine system generally are these:

- to regulate or stimulate other body functions
- to maintain the body in a balanced state known as *homeostasis*

Each gland has specific functions that will be discussed separately.

The mechanism of action of hormones in the body is not totally understood. There are many ways in which hormones exert their effects. A hormone from one gland may act upon specific other glands, which are called *target organs,* or on cells located throughout the body.

Terms related to the endocrine system:

endocrine: type of gland that separates (*crine*), or produces, hormones that are secreted into the blood vessels within (*endo*) the gland.

exocrine: type of gland that separates (*crine*), or produces, a chemical substance that it secretes into a tube that carries the substance out (*ex*) of the gland to another location where it has a specific function.

gland: a true gland is an organ that produces a substance to be secreted. Some organs are called glands because they are similar in appearance, though not in function.

homeostasis: condition of the body in which a stable (*homeo*) balance (*stasis*) of all internal activities is maintained.

hormone: chemical substance produced by endocrine glands that stimulates cells in a specific way or sets a body function in motion.

regulate: to control or adjust body functions and responses.

stimulate: to excite or cause a part to function, as a goad (*stimul*) causes cattle to move.

The endocrine system is a very complex system and is not easily understood. For the purpose of study of terms related to the endocrine glands, this chapter will be divided into separate sections for each of the glands.

The following information will be briefly covered for each structure or gland that produces a hormone:

- the name
- the location
- the hormones and the definition of each hormone

Hypothalamus

The hypothalamus is the structure located under (*hypo*) the thalamus in the brain that has an endocrine function. Among other hypothalamic functions, it manufactures two hormones that are stored in the posterior pituitary gland. It also produces releasing and inhibitory factors that control the secretion of the anterior pituitary gland.

The releasing and inhibitory hormones and factors of the hypothalamus are the following:

- thyrotropin-releasing hormone (TRH)
- corticotropin-releasing factor (CRF)

gonadotropin-releasing hormone (GnRH)
growth hormone-releasing factor (GHRF)
growth-hormone release-inhibiting hormone (GHRIH)
prolactin-releasing factor (PRF)
prolactin-inhibitory factor (PIF)
melanocyte-stimulating hormone-releasing factor (MRF)
melanocyte-stimulating hormone-inhibitory factor (MIF)

The names of the two posterior pituitary hormones manufactured in the hypothalamus are covered in the section on the pituitary gland.

Terms related to the endocrine function of the hypothalamus:

inhibitory factor or hormone: substance (*factor*) that has the function of (*ory*) preventing (*inhibit*) the release of a specific hormone. Example: prolactin-inhibitory factor (PIF) prevents the release of the hormone prolactin.

releasing factor or hormone: substance (*factor*) that has the function of allowing hormones to be released into the bloodstream. Example: growth hormone-releasing factor (GHRF) allows growth hormone to get into the bloodstream.

Hypophysis or Pituitary Gland

The pituitary gland, or hypophysis, is a gland under the cerebrum in the skull. It lies in a bony place called the *sella turcica.* It is divided into anterior and posterior sections or lobes.

Terms related to the pituitary gland and its parts:

pituitary gland: name derived from an ancient belief that this gland produces spittle. The sound made when a person spits is somewhat like "ptu."

hypophysis: another name for the pituitary gland denoting the fact that it grows (*physis*) under (*hypo*) the cerebrum.

adenohypophysis: anterior lobe of the pituitary (*hypophysis*) that is a glandlike (*adeno*) structure.

neurohypophysis: posterior lobe of the pituitary (*hypophysis*) gland that is a neural (*neuro*) extension of the brain.

sella turcica: bony structure holding the hypophysis that resembles a Turkish (*turcica*) saddle (*sella*).

The following hormones are produced in the adenohypophysis (anterior lobe):

somatotropic hormone (*STH*) *or growth hormone* (*GH*): hormone that stimulates (*tropic*) the body (*somato*) to grow.

thyroid-stimulating hormone (*TSH*) *or thyrotropin:* hormone that stimulates (*tropin*) the thyroid (*thyro*) to produce thyroid hormones.

adrenocorticotropic hormone (*ACTH*) *or corticotropin:* hormone that stimulates (*tropic*) the adrenal (*adreno*) cortex (*cortico*).

gonadotropic hormones: the hormones that stimulate (*tropic*) the release of sex-related (*gonado*) hormones.

follicle-stimulating hormone (*FSH*): hormone that stimulates the small, baglike (*follicle*) structures that produce the egg in the female ovary and sperm in the male testes.

luteinizing hormone (LH): hormone that affects the yellow (*lute*) areas in the ovary of the female.

interstitial cell-stimulating hormone (*ICSH*): male hormone that corresponds to LH in the female and which controls the production of testosterone by the interstitial cells in the testes.

lactogenic hormone: hormone that stimulates the production (*genic*) of milk (*lacto*). Also called *prolactin,* or the hormone that favors (*pro*) the production of milk (*lact*).

melanocyte-stimulating hormone (*MSH*): hormone that stimulates the cells (*cyte*) that contain the dark (*melano*) pigment of the skin.

The release of many of these hormones is under control of the releasing and inhibitory factors of the hypothalamus.

The following hormones are produced in the hypothalamus but are stored in the neurohypophysis. They are usually considered as hormones of the neurohypophysis:

vasopressin: hormone (*in*) that helps maintain the pressure (*press*) in the blood vessels (*vaso*). This hormone works against (*anti*) the excessive flow of urine (*diuretic*) and helps maintain the volume of fluid in the bloodstream.

oxytocin: hormone (*in*) that causes a hastening (*oxy*) of the birth (*tocin*) of a child.

Pineal Gland

The name *pineal* comes from the pine-cone (*pineal*) shape of this gland. It is located at about the middle of the brain. It is also called the *epiphysis cerebri.*

Thyroid Gland

The thyroid gland is a gland that is so named because it is shaped like a shield. It is composed of two lobes, one on each side of the trachea in the neck.

The thyroid gland produces the following hormones:

thyroxine: hormone (*in*) of the thyroid (*thyrox*) gland.

triiodothyronine: hormone (*in*) of the thyroid (*thyron*) that has three (*tri*) iodine (*iodo*) atoms in its chemical structure.

thyrocalcitonin: hormone (*in*) of the thyroid (*thyro*) gland that helps to control (*ton*) the level of calcium (*calci*) in the blood.

The release of the first two hormones from the thyroid gland depends on the effect of the thyroid-stimulating hormone (TSH) from the adenohypophysis.

These thyroid hormones in general promote growth and have an effect on the rate of metabolism.

Parathyroid Glands

The parathyroid glands are four tiny glands situated around (*para*) the posterior surface of the thyroid gland (*thyroid*).

The parathyroid glands produce parathormone. This hormone is also called parathyroid hormone.

The main function of these glands is the regulation of the amount of calcium in the blood.

Thymus Gland

Only the name and located

The thymus gland is a gland that resembles a cluster of thyme, the garden herb.

The thymus gland has two lobes and is located near the trachea in the thoracic cavity. Its function as an endocrine gland is not totally understood. The gland originates before birth, reaches its greatest size at puberty, and then begins to atrophy or shrink. It does not disappear completely but remains evident throughout life. The hormones thymosin and thymin are secreted by the thymus gland.

thymosin: the hormone that appears to play an important part in the immune system (see Chapter 12).
thymin: a hormonelike substance that affects neuromuscular function.

Pancreatic Islets

The pancreatic islets are islandlike organs in the pancreas. The islets are also known as the *islands of Langerhans*. They contain the cells that produce two hormones, insulin and glucagon.

The pancreas is also an accessory organ to the digestive system (see Chapter 14).

The action of insulin produced in the pancreas, among other things, is to increase the use of glucose and aid in the storage of nutrients. It plays a vital role in carbohydrate metabolism.

The function of glucagon is opposite to that of insulin. It causes the release of nutrients stored in the liver and in fatty tissue.

The regulation of the production of insulin is dependent in part on the levels of glucose in the blood. After a person eats, insulin is secreted into the blood. This occurs as a result, in part, of the increased levels of glucose in the blood.

The regulation of glucagon is dependent on the level of glucose in the blood. When the blood sugar drops, either in response to insulin or because of the lack of food intake, glucagon is produced.

The hormones of the pancreatic islets:

insulin: one of the hormones (*in*) from the islets (*insul*) of the pancreas.
glucagon: hormone that produces (*gon,* variation of *gen*) the release of glucose (*gluca*) into the bloodstream.

Adrenal Glands

The adrenal glands are located in a position near or toward (*ad*) the kidneys (*renal*). They are sometimes referred to as *suprarenal glands* because of their location above (*supra*) the kidneys (*renal*).

There are two distinct parts to each adrenal gland. Each gland is made of an adrenal cortex and an adrenal medulla. The adrenal cortex is the outermost (*cortex*) part, and the adrenal medulla is the small (*ulla*) portion, more or less in the middle (*med*) of the gland.

The adrenal cortex produces three major groups of hormones called *steroids*.

The hormones of the adrenal cortex:

mineralocorticoids: steroid (*oid*) hormones of the adrenal cortex (*cortic*) that help regulate the mineral content of the blood. Aldosterone is the principal mineralocorticoid.

glucocorticoids: steroid hormones of the adrenal cortex (*cortic*) that have an effect on sugar (*gluco*) levels in the blood, among other things. Cortisol is the principal glucocorticoid.

The adrenal cortex also produces small amounts of the sex hormones. This is the third major group of steroid hormones.

Adrenal cortex activity is controlled by the adrenocorticotropic (ACTH) hormones of the adenohypophysis.

The adrenal medulla produces hormones referred to as *catecholamines*.

The hormones of the adrenal medulla:

adrenalin: hormone (*in*) from the adrenal (*adrenal*) gland. *Epinephrine* is another name for adrenalin. Epinephrine refers to the hormone (*ine*) produced in the gland over (*epi*) the kidney (*nephr*).

noradrenalin: hormone (*in*) that is similar to but has a different chemical (*nor*) form than adrenalin. It may also be referred to as *norepinephrine*.

These hormones function in conjunction with the sympathetic nervous system in certain types of stress situations. They are involved in the fight-or-flight response. These hormones increase the energy level during emergencies and allow a person extra energy to fight or extra energy to take flight or run away.

Gonads

The gonads are the sex-related [sex (*gon*), related (*ad*)] glands. In the female the sex-related endocrine glands are the *ovaries*. The ovaries are located in the pelvic cavity. The function of the hormones from the ovary pertains to (*aries*) the formation of the egg, or ovum (*ov*), and maintenance of the female reproductive cycle.

The hormones produced by the ovaries:

estrogen: hormone that produces (*gen*) the female characteristics and the female menstrual cycle (*estrus*). The term estrus means "gadfly," which comes from the ancient belief that during the menstrual cycle the female had characteristics of a pesty gadfly.

progesterone: hormone that favors (*pro*) pregnancy (*gest*) by preparing the uterus for implantation and maintenance of the fertilized ovum.

In the male, the sex-related endocrine glands are the *testes.* The testes are located in the scrotum. The function of the hormones from the testes involves the production of sperm and the development of secondary male sexual characteristics.

The hormone produced in the testes:

testosterone: the steroid (*sterone*) hormone produced in the interstitial cells of the testes (*testo*) that functions in the development and maintenance of the male sexual characteristics.

Terms related to testosterone:

androgenics: class of hormones that function in developing (*genic*) the male (*andro*) sexual characteristics.

interstitial cells: specialized cells within the testes that function to produce testosterone. The name for these cells is the *interstitial cells of Leydig.*

The production of the gonadal hormones depends on the influence of the gonadotropic hormones from the adenohypophysis (see also Chapters 17 and 18).

Placenta

The placenta, which is the structure that provides nourishment for a developing fetus, is considered an endocrine gland because its outermost layer produces hormones. This layer is called the *chorion*.

The hormones produced by the chorion act to help maintain the flow of other hormones necessary for a developing fetus.

The hormones of the chorion layers of the placenta are the following:

chorionic gonadotropin: hormone of the outermost layer (*chorionic*) of the placenta, which stimulates (*tropin*) the production of some of the sex-related (*gonado*) hormones needed during pregnancy.

estrogen and progesterone: varying amounts of estrogens and progesterone are also produced in the placenta. See also the section on the gonads in this chapter.

DISEASES OF THE ENDOCRINE GLANDS

Diseases of the endocrine glands are often interrelated. For example, a condition of the pituitary gland may also affect the thyroid gland, adrenal gland, and gonads. A symptom of a thyroid disease may in fact be a symptom of pituitary disease because of the close relationship of these two glands.

Since the amounts of hormones in the body are so delicately balanced, an undersecretion or oversecretion of any of the hormones causes an abnormal or disease condition.

Disease Conditions Including Signs and Symptoms

Analysis of selected terms related to disease conditions of the endocrine system including terms related to signs and symptoms of endocrine disease:

acromegaly: description of (*ly*) a condition in which the tips (*acro*) of the extremities become enlarged (*mega*).

adrenocortical insufficiency: condition related to the adrenal (*adreno*) cortex (*cortical*) in which insufficient amounts of the hormones are produced. Also known as *hypoadrenocorticism.*

adrenogenital syndrome: condition in which there are a group of symptoms (*syndrome*) that are caused by the overproduction of hormones of the adrenal (*adreno*) gland. Many of these symptoms are related to the premature development of the reproductive organs (*genital*).

cretinism: condition (*ism*) caused by an undersecretion of the thyroid gland and that is characterized, among other things, by physical deformity and mental retardation.

diabetes insipidus: disease in which large amounts of clear, almost colorless urine, which is urine without distinctive qualities (*insipid*), is passed (*betes*) through (*dia*), or excreted.

diabetes mellitus: disease in which one of the findings is sugar (*mellitus*) passing (*betes*) through (*dia*) in the urine. This finding is known as *glycosuria.*

dwarfism: condition in which a person does not grow normally and develops into a small, but well-proportioned human being. This person usually is not mentally retarded.

exophthalmic goiter: type of goiter disease that is characterized by the protrusion of the eyes (*ophthalmic*) out (*ex*) of their sockets.

giantism: condition (*ism*) caused by overproduction of the growth hormone in children. The child grows and becomes very large (*giant*).

goiter: term denoting an enlargement of the throat (*goiter*) caused by the enlargement of the thyroid gland.

hyperadrenocorticism: condition (*ism*) in which there is oversecretion [over (*hyper*)] of the hormones from the adrenal (*adreno*) cortex (*cortic*).

hyperaldosteronism: condition (*ism*) in which there is an increase (*hyper*) in the secretion of the mineralocorticoid hormone (*aldosteron*) from the adrenal cortex.

hyperthyroidism: condition (*ism*) in which there is oversecretion [over (*hyper*)] of the thyroid (*thyroid*) hormones.

hypothyroidism: condition (*ism*) in which there is undersecretion [under (*hypo*)] secretion of the thyroid (*thyroid*) hormones.

myxedema: condition resulting from hypothyroidism in which one of the signs is that the body is somewhat swollen (*edema*) by mucus (*myx*) deposits in the skin.

panhypopituitarism: condition (*ism*) in which all (*pan*) or most of the hormones of the pituitary (*pituitar*) gland are undersecreted [under (*hypo*)].

parathyroid tetany: state of intermittent severe muscle contractions (*tetany*) because of an undersecretion of the parathyroid hormone.

pheochromocytoma: tumor, usually of the adrenal medulla, in which the cells (*cyt*) become dusky (*pheo*) in color (*chroma*).

prognathism: condition (*ism*) in which the jaw (*gnath*) protrudes forward (*pro*).
thymoma: tumor (*oma*) of the thymus (*thym*) gland.
thyroiditis: inflammation of the thyroid gland.
thyrotoxicosis: condition (*osis*) in which the thyroid (*thyro*) gland oversecretes its hormones at such a rate as to act like a poison (*toxi*).

For terms related to diseases of the reproductive glands, see Chapters 17 and 18.

Treatment of Endocrine Diseases

Analysis of terms related to the treatment of endocrine diseases including diagnostic, surgical, and drug-related terms.

adrenalectomy: removal of (*ectomy*) the adrenal gland. A bilateral adrenalectomy is the removal of the adrenal glands on both (*bi*) sides (*lateral*) of the body.
antithyroid drugs: various types of drugs used to work against (*anti*) or to control the oversecretion or overproduction of the hormones from the thyroid gland.
hypoglycemic agents: drugs used in the treatment of diabetes mellitus. These drugs (*agents*) cause a lowering (*hypo*) of the sugar (*glyc*) content of blood (*emic*).
parathyroidectomy: removal of (*ectomy*) one or all four of the parathyroid glands.
replacement therapy: method of treatment (*therapy*) of endocrine diseases in which undersecretion of particular glands is treated by replacing the hormone with a natural or synthetic preparation of the hormone.
steroid therapy: treatment (*therapy*) of various diseases with hormones that are produced from the adrenal cortex (*steroids*).
thymectomy: removal of (*ectomy*) the thymus (*thym*) gland.
thyroidectomy: removal of (*ectomy*) the thyroid gland.
transsphenoidal hypophysectomy: removal of (*ectomy*) the pituitary (*hypophys*) gland by an incision across (*trans*) the sphenoid sinus (*sphenoid*).

PRETEST/ POSTTEST FOR CHAPTER 16

1. The following terms are related to the endocrine system. Complete the statements below by using terms from the following list.

endocrine	hormone
exocrine	regulate
gland	stimulate
homeostasis	

If you choose to make the test more difficult, cover the list of words.

1. A gland that secretes chemical substances into a tube that carries it out of the gland is called an ________ gland.
2. A ________ is an organ that produces hormones.
3. To excite or cause a part to function is to ________ the part.
4. The condition in which a stable balance of all internal activities is maintained is known as ________.
5. A gland that secretes hormones into the blood vessels within the gland is called an ________ gland.
6. To control or adjust body functions and responses is to ________ the part.
7. A substance that stimulates cells in a specific way or sets a body function in motion is called a ________.

2. The following statements are related to the hypothalamus. Select the word that best completes the following sentences.

1. The hypothalamus is located _____ the thalamus.
   A. under
   B. over
2. It produces factors that prevent the release of specific hormones. These factors are called _____ factors.
   A. inhibitory
   B. releasing
3. It also produces factors that permit the release of specific hormones. These factors are called _____ factors.
   A. inhibitory
   B. releasing
4. The hypothalamus produces two hormones that are stored in the _____.
   A. adenohypophysis
   B. neurohypophysis

3. The following terms are related to the pituitary gland. Select the terms that complete the following statements:

hypophysis adenohypophysis neurohypophysis

1. The anterior lobe of the pituitary gland is called the ________________.
2. ________________ means "growing under."
3. The posterior lobe of the pituitary gland is called the ________________.

4. The following terms are related to the pineal, thyroid, parathyroid, and thymus glands. Choose the correct completion of each statement.

1. The thyroid gland is located
  A. near the trachea in the neck.
  B. near the trachea in the thorax.

2. The name thyroid comes from the fact that the gland resembles
  A. a cluster of thyme.
  B. a shield.

3. The parathyroid glands are four tiny glands situated
  A. around the pineal gland.
  B. around the thyroid gland.

4. The thymus gland is located
  A. near the trachea in the neck.
  B. near the trachea in the thorax.

5. The pineal gland is located
  A. at the back of the brain.
  B. in the middle of the brain.

5. The following terms are related to the pancreatic islets. Mark the statements true, *T,* or false, *F.*

1. _____ The pancreas produces insulin and glucagon.

2. _____ Insulin is involved in the metabolism of glucose.

3. _____ Glucagon releases the hormones from the adrenal cortex.

6. The following terms are related to the adrenal glands. Select the terms that best complete the following statements.

adrenal cortex   adrenal medulla   suprarenal

1. The term meaning "above the kidney" is ____________________.

2. The outside portion of the adrenal gland is the ____________________.

3. The inside portion of the adrenal gland is the ____________________.

7. The following terms are related to the gonads and placenta. Mark the statements true, *T,* or false, *F.*

1. _____ The term *gonad* means "related to sex."

2. _____ Testosterone and progesterone are the same hormone.

3. _____ Chorionic gonadotropin is produced in the interstitial cells.

4. _____ The pituitary hormones that stimulate the sex glands are called gonadotropins.

8. The following list of terms is related to some hormones and factors of the endocrine system. Interpret the meaning of the name of the hormone or factor.

1. Somatotropic hormone: ____________________
2. Adrenalin: ____________________
3. Prolactin inhibitory factor: ____________________
4. Thyroxine: ____________________
5. Mineralocorticoid: ____________________
6. Oxytocin: ____________________
7. Testosterone: ____________________
8. Progesterone: ____________________
9. Adrenocorticotropic hormone: ____________________
10. Chorionic gonadotropin: ____________________
11. Insulin: ____________________
12. Parathormone: ____________________
13. Lactogenic hormone: ____________________
14. Thymin: ____________________

9. The following sets of terms are related to disease conditions of the endocrine system. Match column A with column B.

Set 1

Column A

1. _____ acromegaly
2. _____ adrenocortical insufficiency
3. _____ adrenogenital syndrome
4. _____ cretinism
5. _____ diabetes insipidus
6. _____ diabetes mellitus
7. _____ dwarf
8. _____ exophthalmic goiter
9. _____ giantism
10. _____ goiter
11. _____ hyperadreno-corticism

Column B

A. condition in which a person is physically deformed and mentally retarded
B. involves passing large amounts of clear urine
C. condition producing small, normally intelligent person
D. enlargement of the throat
E. tips of extremities become enlarged
F. also known as hypoadrenocorticism
G. includes symptoms of early development of the reproductive organs
H. sugar passed in the urine
I. caused by overproduction of the growth hormone
J. condition characterized by eyes protruding from their sockets
K. oversecretion of the hormones from the adrenal cortex

Set 2

	Column A	Column B
1.	____ hyperaldosteronism	A. severe muscle contractions because of hormone deficiency
2.	____ hyperthyroidism	B. undersecretion of thyroid hormones
3.	____ hypothyroidism	C. tumor of the thymus gland
4.	____ myxedema	D. inflammation of the thyroid gland
5.	____ panhypopituitarism	E. protruding jaw
6.	____ parathyroid tetany	F. increase in the production of the mineralocorticoid hormone
7.	____ pheochromocytoma	G. mucus deposits under the skin
8.	____ prognathism	H. oversecretion of thyroid hormones
9.	____ thymoma	I. decrease in all hormones of the hypophysis
10.	____ thyroiditis	J. toxicity caused by oversecretion of the thyroid gland
11.	____ thyrotoxicosis	K. tumor in which the involved cells become dusky in color

10. The following statements are related to the treatment of endocrine disorders. Mark the statement true, *T*, or false, *F*.

1. ____ The removal of the adrenal gland is called a corticectomy.
2. ____ Antithyroid drugs are used in the treatment of hypothyroidism.
3. ____ The basal metabolic rate is the rate at which the body uses energy.
4. ____ Hypoglycemic agents cause lowering of the blood sugar.
5. ____ Parathyroidectomy is a surgical procedure to remove a part of the thyroid gland.
6. ____ Replacement therapy uses natural or synthetic hormones to treat oversecretion by some glands.
7. ____ Steroid therapy involves the use of the hormones of the adrenal cortex.
8. ____ A thyroidectomy is the removal of part of the parathyroid gland.
9. ____ A thymectomy is the removal of the thyroid gland.
10. ____ A transsphenoidal hypophysectomy is a method of removing the pituitary gland.

PRETEST/ POSTTEST **ANSWERS** FOR CHAPTER **16**

1. **1.** exocrine **5.** endocrine
2. gland **6.** regulate
3. stimulate **7.** hormone
4. homeostasis

2. **1.** A **2.** A **3.** B **4.** B

3. **1.** adenohypophysis*
2. hypophysis
3. neurohypophysis*

4. **1.** A **2.** B **3.** B **4.** B **5.** B

5. **1.** T **2.** T **3.** F

6. **1.** suprarenal
2. adrenal cortex
3. adrenal medulla

7. **1.** T **2.** F **3.** F **4.** T

8.
1. Somatotropic hormone is the hormone that stimulates the body to grow.
2. Adrenalin is the hormone from the adrenal gland.
3. Prolactin inhibitory factor is the substance that prevents the release of prolactin.
4. Thyroxine is a hormone from the thyroid gland.
5. Mineralocorticoid is a steroid hormone of the adrenal cortex that helps regulate the mineral content of the blood.
6. Oxytocin is the hormone that causes a hastening of the birth of a child.
7. Testosterone is the hormone produced in the testes.
8. Progesterone is the hormone that favors pregnancy.
9. Adrenocorticotropic hormone is the hormone that stimulates the adrenal cortex. Also known as ACTH.
10. Chorionic gonadotropin is the hormone of the outermost layer of the placenta.
11. Insulin is the hormone from the pancreatic islets or islands of Langerhans.
12. Parathormone is the hormone from the parathyroid glands.
13. Lactogenic hormone is the hormone that stimulates the production of milk.
14. Thymin is the hormone from the thymus gland.

9. **Set 1**
1. E **3.** G **5.** B **7.** C **9.** I **10.** D **11.** K
2. F **4.** A **6.** H **8.** J

---

* To avoid confusing adenohypophysis with neurohypophysis associate the *a* in *a*nterior with the *a* in *a*denohypophysis.

Set 2

1. F **2.** H **3.** B **4.** G **5.** I **6.** A **7.** K **8.** E **9.** C **10.** D **11.** J

10. **1.** F **2.** F **3.** T **4.** T **5.** F **6.** F **7.** T **8.** F **9.** F **10.** T

17 THE MALE REPRODUCTIVE SYSTEM

OBJECTIVES

At the end of this chapter you will be able to do the following:

1 List the functions of the male reproductive organs.
2 List the organs and structures in the male reproductive system, and define terms related to each of them.
3 Analyze selected terms related to conditions and diseases of the male reproductive system.
4 Analyze selected terms related to the diagnosis and treatment of conditions and diseases of the male reproductive system.

THE MALE REPRODUCTIVE SYSTEM

The male reproductive system consists of organs that produce and store sperm and a duct system that carries sperm. A section of the duct system also transports urine to the outside.

Because this system has two functions, it is sometimes referred to as the *urogenital system.* The urogenital system is the group of organs that function to convey urine (*uro*) and are also related (*al*) to the reproductive (*genit*) system. Also known as the *genitourinary system* (see Chapter 15).

The male organs involved in the reproductive function include the following:

scrotum: contains the testes, epididymis, and the beginning of the vas deferens.
internal organs: the vas deferens, the seminal vesicles, the ejaculatory duct, the prostate gland, and the bulbourethral glands.
penis: contains the urethra.

The tube involved in transporting urine is the *urethra,* which extends from the urinary bladder through the prostate gland and through the penis to the outside (see Chapter 15).

Scrotum

The scrotum is a pouch of skin that hangs behind the penis. It is divided into two sections, each containing and supporting one of the testes.

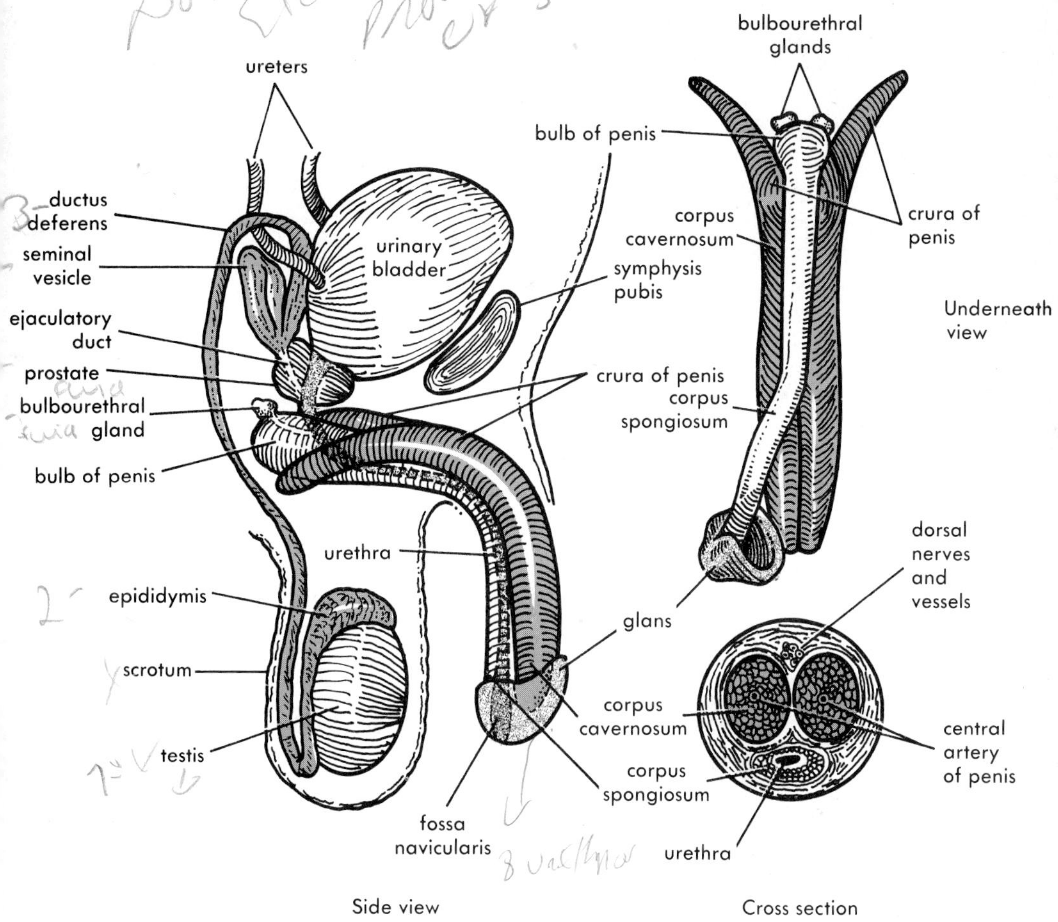

FIGURE 17-1
The male reproductive system.

The testes are the oval structures containing the reproductive cells that produce sperm. The interstitial cells of Leydig, which are responsible for the production of the male hormones, are also located in the testes (see Chapter 16).

Located on top and behind each testis is a structure called the *epididymis*. It is the first part of the system of tubes that carries sperm from the testes to the outside. The vas deferens leads off the epididymis and carries sperm to the seminal vesicle in the pelvic cavity.

Terms related to the scrotum, epididymis, and vas deferens:

scrotum: the bag (*scrotum*) covered with skin that hangs behind the penis.
testes: male sex glands named from the term *to testify*. The name is derived from an ancient practice of allowing persons to testify only if they were male.
orchido: root word meaning "testis," the organ that resembles the root of the orchid.

tunica albuginea: the white (*albuginea*) layer of tissue that makes up the outer layer (*tunica*) of the testis. Also known as the *tunica vaginalis* or the sheathlike [sheath (*vagina*)] covering (*tunica*). This structure is not labeled in Figure 17-1.

androgenic hormones: hormones involved in producing (*genic*) male characteristics (*andro*).

testosterone: hormone produced by the testes (*testo*).

epididymis: the pair (*didymis*) of tubelike structures located over (*epi*) the testes.

vas deferens: vessel (*vas*) that carries (*ferens*) sperm away (*de*) from the testis. Also known as the *ductus deferens* or the *seminal duct.*

spermatic cord: organ or structure that is made of the vas deferens, nerves, and lymphatic and blood vessels, whose main function is as a passageway for sperm en route to the seminal vesicle.

inguinal canal: space in the groin (*ingui*) where the spermatic cord enters the pelvic cavity.

Internal Organs

There are two seminal vesicles located in the pelvic cavity. These structures secrete seminal fluid, which is a thick, nutrient-containing fluid. The fluid nourishes the sperm to keep them alive until they reach the ovum in the female. The seminal vesicle ends in a straight and narrow tube that joins the vas deferens to form the ejaculatory duct.

During sexual arousal, seminal fluid is ejected into the urethra by the action of the ejaculatory duct.

The prostate gland surrounds the first part of the urethra, called the *prostatic urethra.* This gland functions to secrete a fluid that is part of semen.

The bulbourethral glands are located under the prostate on either side of the urethra. These glands produce a mucous secretion that lubricates the urethra before the ejaculatory duct expels the sperm and seminal fluids.

Semen is the thick, whitish fluid that is ejaculated during sexual arousal. It contains sperm from the testes, seminal fluid from the seminal vesicles, fluid from the prostate, and mucus from the bulbourethral glands.

Terms related to the internal male reproductive organs:

prostate gland: round, walnut-shaped gland of the male reproductive system. The name is derived from the ancient practice of males standing (*state*) up before (*pro*) a group to indicate their position as leaders.

prostatic urethra: section of the urethra that travels through the prostate (*prostatic*).

bulbourethral glands: two small, round (*bulbo*) glands on either side of the urethra. Also known as *Cowper's glands.*

seminal vesicle: elongated, saclike (*vesicle*) structure that produces seminal fluid.

ejaculatory duct: tube (*duct*) which functions to expel forcibly (*jacula*) semen from (*e,* variation of *ex*) the urethra.

semen: semiliquid fluid from the male reproductive organs that contains sperm or seeds (*semen*).

sperm: male seed that fertilizes the egg of the female.

Penis

The penis is the male organ of copulation. In its resting state it is said to be flaccid. It is composed of three columns of erectile tissue and covered with skin. During sexual arousal the columns of erectile tissue fill with blood, resulting in enlargement and hardening of the penis, known as erection. This change is necessary to allow the penis to penetrate the female vagina to deposit semen.

The penile urethra extends through the center of one of the columns of erectile tissue. This column enlarges at the end of the penis and forms the structure called the glans penis.

A fold of skin called the prepuce, or foreskin, covers the end of the penis.

The penis also functions in the process of urination. The urethra in the male extends from the urinary bladder to the glans penis at the end of the penis. During urination, urine passes from the bladder through the prostatic urethra, through the penile urethra to the outside.

Because of an intricate nervous control system, only urine or only semen can pass through the urethra at one time.

Terms related to the anatomy of the penis:

penis: male reproductive organ that hangs down (*pen,* variation of *pend*) from the pubic region; the organ of copulation.

phallo: root word meaning "penis."

shaft: long, slender part (*shaft*) of the penis; the body of the penis.

corpus cavernosum: the column of tissue along the body (*corpus*) of the penis that has many spaces (*cavern*) which fill with blood, resulting in erection. There is a corpus cavernosum situated on each side of the penis. The *crus* of the penis is the leglike (*crus*) part of each corpus cavernosum.

corpus spongiosum: the column of tissue situated between the corpora cavernosa (plural of corpus cavernosum) through which the penile urethra travels.

bulb region: the rounded (*bulb*) internal end of the corpus spongiosum column of the penis that is nearest the rectum.

corona: rounded ridge that is the proximal border of the glans penis.

glans penis: rounded mass (*glans*) of tissue at the end of the penis, sometimes referred to as the *head* of the penis.

balano: root word related to the glans penis.

penile urethra: section of the urethra that travels through the corpus spongiosum of the penis (*penile*) that transports semen or urine to the outside.

urethral meatus: opening (*meatus*) of the urethra (*urethral*) at the end of the penis. The *fossa navicularis* near this opening is so called because it is a cavity (*fossa*) in the urethra that resembles a boat (*navicularis*).

prepuce: fold of skin located in front of (*pre*) the end of the penis (*puce*). Commonly called the *foreskin,* or the skin at the front of (*fore*) the penis.

copulation: the act (*tion*) in which the male penis enters the female vagina and there is a sexual union (*copula*).

Terms related to the changes in the penis during erection:

erectile tissue: type of tissue that has spaces that, when filled with blood, make the tissue firm and straight (*erect*).

erection: condition of the penis after it has filled with blood and is firm and straight (*erect*).
flaccid: condition of the penis when it is soft and limp (*flaccid*).
tumescence: term related to the swelling of the penis.

DISEASES OF THE MALE REPRODUCTIVE SYSTEM

Analysis of selected terms related to conditions and diseases of the male reproductive system:

anorchism: condition (*ism*) in which the testes (*orch*) are absent (*an*).
balanitis: inflammation (*itis*) of the glans penis (*balan*).
benign prostatic hypertrophy: noncancerous (*benign*) condition characterized by the overgrowth [over (*hyper*), growth (*trophy*)] or enlargement of the prostate (*prostatic*) gland.
chancre: ulceration or sore on the genitals, often the first sign of the venereal disease syphilis.
cryptorchism: condition (*ism*) in which the testes (*orchid*) remain in the pelvic cavity and thus are hidden (*crypt*). Also known as *undescended testicles.* Also spelled cryptorchidism.
epididymitis: inflammation (*itis*) of the epididymis.
epididymoorchitis: inflammation (*itis*) of the epididymis and testes (*orch*).
epispadias: a condition in which the opening (*spadias*) of the urethra is on the top (*epi*) of the penis.
eunuchoidism: condition (*ism*) in which the male develops characteristics like (*oid*) those of a eunuch. A eunuch is a castrated male, or a male whose testes have been removed by a knife (*castr*).
hydrocele: an outpouching (*cele*) of the testis caused by an accumulation of fluid in the tunica albuginea.
hypogonadism: condition (*ism*) in which there is undersecretion [under (*hypo*)] of the sex-related (*gonad*) hormones.
hypospadias: condition in which the opening (*spadias*) of the urethra is on the underside (*hypo*) of the penis.
impotence: condition characterized by a lack of (*im,* variation of *in*) sexual power (*potence*). Said of a male who is unable to achieve an erection.
infertility: lack of (*in*) ability to fertilize (*fertil*) an ovum. Inability to cause conception.
inguinal hernia: protrusion (*hernia*) of abdominal contents through the inguinal canal into the region of the scrotum.
mumps orchitis: inflammation (*itis*) of the testes (*orch*) caused by the mumps virus.
oligospermia: condition (*ia*) in which only a small amount (*oligo*) of sperm is produced.
orchitis: inflammation (*itis*) of the testes (*orch*).
paraphimosis: condition (*osis*) in which the foreskin is tightly constricted (*phim*) around (*para*) the penis behind the glans.
phallitis: inflammation (*itis*) of the penis (*phall*).
phimosis: condition (*osis*) in which the foreskin is tightly constricted (*phim*) and cannot be retracted or pulled back over the glans penis.

priapism: condition (*ism*) characterized by the continuous erection of the penis (*priap*).
prostatitis: inflammation (*itis*) of the prostate (*prostat*) gland.
spermatocele: condition characterized by the bulging out (*cele*) of the epididymis that contains sperm (*spermato*).
strangury: condition in which urine (*ury*) flows painfully, drop by drop (*strang*).
teratoma: tumor (*oma*) of the testis that is made of a number of different types of tissue. The term refers to a monsterlike (*terato*) condition and is so applied because the teratonia tissue cannot be identified.
testicular torsion: painful condition in which the testicle (*testicular*) becomes twisted (*torsion*) in the scrotum.
varicocele: bulging (*cele*) because of a swelling of the veins (*varico*) of the testes. Varicose veins of the scrotum.
venereal disease: see Chapter 18.

Diagnosis and Treatment

Analysis of selected terms related to the diagnosis and treatment of conditions or diseases of the male reproductive system:

circumcision: surgical procedure in which a cut (*cision*) is made around (*circum*) the skin of the penis to remove the prepuce or foreskin.
epididymectomy: removal of (*ectomy*) an epididymis.
hydrocelectomy: removal of (*ectomy*) the membrane and fluid (*hydro*) causing a swelling (*cel*) around the testis.
meatotomy: procedure done to cut a larger opening (*otomy*) in the urethral meatus (*meat*).
orchiectomy: removal of (*ectomy*) one or both of the testes (*orchi*). Also spelled orchectomy, or orchidectomy.
orchiopexy: surgical procedure done to fasten (*pexy*) an undescended testicle (*orchio*) in the scrotum. Also spelled orchidopexy.
prostatectomy: removal (*ectomy*) of part or all of the prostate gland.
- *suprapubic prostatectomy:* removal (*ectomy*) of the prostate gland through an incision over (*supra*) the pubic bone (*pubic*).
- *transurethral prostatectomy:* prostatectomy done by passing a cutting catheter through (*trans*) the urethra (*urethral*).

spermatocelectomy: removal of (*ectomy*) a spermatocele.
transillumination: examination done in which a light (*illumination*) is directed across (*trans*) or through (*trans*) the scrotum to determine the presence of blood or fluid, a tumor, or a hernia. A hydrocele contains clear fluid, and therefore light (*lumin*) can pass through (*trans*) it.
varicocelectomy: removal of (*ectomy*) a varicocele (*varicocel*).
vasectomy: removal of (*ectomy*) a segment of the vas deferens (*vas*) to interrupt the flow of sperm. The semen of the male who has had a vasectomy does not contain sperm.

PRETEST/ POSTTEST FOR CHAPTER 17

1. The following terms are related to the scrotum, epididymis, and vas deferens. Using the list of terms, complete the statements which follow.

scrotum	epididymis
testis	vas deferens
orchido	spermatic cord
tunica albuginea	inguinal canal

1. The term meaning testes is ________________.
2. The sheath of tissue covering the testes is the ________________.
3. The ________________ is the tubelike structure located over the testes.
4. The space where the spermatic cord enters the pelvic cavity is called the ________________.
5. The ________________ is made up of the vas deferens, nerves, and lymphatic and blood vessels.
6. The ________________ is the vessel that carries sperm away from the testes.
7. The male sex gland is the ________________.
8. The sac of skin holding the testes is called the ________________.

2. The following terms are related to the internal male reproductive organs. Using the list of terms, complete the statements that follow.

prostate	seminal vesicle
prostatic urethra	semen
bulbourethral	sperm

1. A section of the tube carrying urine or semen is called the ________________.
2. Structure that produces seminal fluid is the ________________.
3. The two small glands on either side of the urethra are the ________________ glands.
4. The walnut-shaped gland in the pelvic cavity is the ________________ gland.
5. The semiliquid fluid from the male reproductive system is called ________________.

6. The male seed involved in fertilization is called ________________.

3. The following sets of terms are related to the penis. Match column A with column B. Choose the one best answer.

Set 1

Column A	Column B
1. ____ penis	A. rounded internal end of the corpus spongiosum
2. ____ shaft	B. column of tissue through which the urethra travels
3. ____ corpus cavernosum	C. head of the penis
4. ____ corpus spongiosum	D. long slender part of the penis; the body of the penis
5. ____ bulb region	E. opening at the end of the penis
6. ____ corona	F. long column on each side of the penis
7. ____ glans penis	G. the foreskin
8. ____ penile urethra	H. rounded ridge that is the proximal border of the glans
9. ____ urethral meatus	I. tube carrying urine or semen to the outside
10. ____ prepuce	J. organ of copulation

Set 2

In this set of terms related to the penis, use the following list to complete the statements:

phallo	erection
balano	flaccid
copulation	tumescence
erectile	

1. The type of tissue that has spaces that fill with blood is called ____________ tissue.
2. The act in which there is sexual union is known as ____________.
3. The root word for penis is ________________.
4. The condition of the penis when it is firm and hard is called ____________.
5. The penis is said to be ________________ when it is soft and limp.
6. The root word for the glans penis is ________________.
7. The term referring to the swelling of the penis is ________________.

4. The following sets of terms are related to diseases of the male reproductive system. Match column A with column B.

Set 1

Column A

1. ______ anorchism
2. ______ balanitis
3. ______ chancre
4. ______ cryptorchism
5. ______ epispadias
6. ______ epididymitis
7. ______ epididymoorchitis
8. ______ hydrocele
9. ______ hypogonadism
10. ______ hypospadias
11. ______ impotence
12. ______ infertility

Column B

A. opening of the urethra on the top surface of the penis
B. absent testes
C. inflammation of the epididymis and testes
D. collection of fluid around the testes
E. inflammation of the head of the penis
F. opening of the urethra on the underside of the penis
G. inability to cause conception
H. undersecretion of the sex-related hormones
I. inability to achieve erection
J. undescended testicles
K. sore on the genitals
L. inflammation of the epididymis

Set 2

Column A

1. ______ oligospermia
2. ______ orchitis
3. ______ paraphimosis
4. ______ phallitis
5. ______ phimosis
6. ______ priapism
7. ______ prostatitis
8. ______ spermatocele
9. ______ strangury
10. ______ teratoma
11. ______ varicocele

Column B

A. foreskin tightly constricted and cannot be pulled back over the head of the penis
B. varicose veins of the testes
C. inflammation of the testes
D. inflammation of the penis
E. slow and painful flow of urine
F. continuous erection of the penis
G. small amount of sperm produced
H. foreskin tightly constricted around the penis
I. tumor of the testis consisting of unidentifiable tissue
J. bulging out of the epididymis
K. inflammation of the prostate gland

Set 3

In this set, use the following list of terms to complete the statements:

benign prostatic hypertrophy
eunuchoidism
inguinal hernia
mumps orchitis
testicular torsion

1. A condition like that of a castrated male is called ________________.
2. A condition of the testes caused by a virus is called ________________.
3. The noncancerous enlargement of the prostate gland is called ________________ ________________.
4. The painful twisting of the testes in the scrotum is called ________________ ________________.
5. The protrusion of abdominal contents through the normal opening for the spermatic cord is called ________________.

5. The following terms are related to the diagnosis and treatment of diseases of the male reproductive system. Match column A with column B. Choose the one best answer.

Column A	Column B
1. _____ circumcision	A. procedure to fasten an undescended testicle in the scrotum
2. _____ epididymectomy	B. to cut around the skin of the penis to remove the foreskin
3. _____ hydrocelectomy	C. examination of the scrotum by the use of light
4. _____ meatotomy	D. procedure done to make a larger opening in the meatus
5. _____ orchiopexy	E. removal of all or part of the prostate gland
6. _____ orchiectomy	F. removal of an epididymis
7. _____ prostatectomy	G. removal of bulging veins
8. _____ spermatocelectomy	H. removal of one or both testes
9. _____ transillumination	I. removal of a section of the vas deferens
10. _____ varicocelectomy	J. removal of a protruding area containing sperm
11. _____ vasectomy	K. removal of the fluid and membrane around the testes

PRETEST/ POSTTEST **ANSWERS** FOR CHAPTER **17**

1.
1. orchido
2. tunica albuginea
3. epididymis
4. inguinal canal
5. spermatic cord
6. vas deferens
7. testis
8. scrotum

2.
1. prostatic urethra
2. seminal vesicle
3. bulbourethral
4. prostate
5. semen
6. sperm

3. **Set 1**

1. J **2.** D **3.** F **4.** B **5.** A **6.** H **7.** C **8.** I **9.** E **10.** G

Set 2
1. erectile
2. copulation
3. phallo
4. erection
5. flaccid
6. balano
7. tumescence

4. **Set 1**

1. B **2.** E **3.** K **4.** J **5.** A **6.** L **7.** C **8.** D **9.** H **10.** F **11.** I **12.** G

Set 2

1. G **2.** C **3.** H **4.** D **5.** A **6.** F **7.** K **8.** J **9.** E **10.** I **11.** B

Set 3
1. eunuchoidism
2. mumps orchitis
3. benign prostatic hypertrophy
4. testicular torsion
5. inguinal hernia

5. **1.** B **2.** F **3.** K **4.** D **5.** A **6.** H **7.** E **8.** J **9.** C **10.** G **11.** I

18 THE FEMALE REPRODUCTIVE SYSTEM

OBJECTIVES

At the end of this chapter you will be able to do the following:

1. List the external and internal organs in the female reproductive system, and define terms related to each organ.
2. Define the menstrual cycle.
3. Define ovulation.
4. Describe fertilization and implantation.
5. Define terms related to pregnancy.
6. Describe the stages of labor, and define terms related to labor and delivery.
7. Analyze selected terms related to gynecological conditions.
8. Analyze selected terms related to the diagnosis and treatment of gynecological conditions.
9. Analyze selected terms related to obstetrical conditions.
10. Analyze selected terms related to the treatment of obstetrical patients.

THE FEMALE REPRODUCTIVE SYSTEM

The female reproductive system is designed for the ultimate purpose of childbearing. The root word for female is *gyne* or *gyneco.*

The structures of the female reproductive system may be divided into the external and internal reproductive organs (see Table 18-1).

The mammary glands, or female breasts, are considered accessory reproductive organs because of their function in providing milk for newborn babies (see Chapter 19).

The external organs of the reproductive system are located in the part of the body called the *perineum.* The perineum is the inferior outlet of the pelvis, which includes the area from the symphysis pubis backward to the tip of the coccyx, or tailbone.

The openings in the female perineum include the urethra, the anus, and the opening of the vagina.

The term *perineum* means "the area around (*per,* variation of *peri*) the external openings in the floor of the pelvis where body contents are evacuated (*ineum*)."

TABLE 18-1
Female Reproductive Organs

External (vulva)	Internal
mons pubis	vagina
labia majora	uterus
labia minora	uterine tubes
clitoris	ovaries
vestibule	
various glands	
hymen	

The External Female Reproductive Organs

The *vulva,* or external female reproductive organs, includes the organs that cover or fold over the opening to the vagina.

The mons pubis is a cushionlike mass of adipose tissue that lies over the symphysis pubis and is covered by pubic hair.

The labia majora are the two larger folds of adipose tissue covered by skin and pubic hair that extend from the mons pubis back to encircle the entire vestibule.

The labia minora are the two smaller folds of skin lying inside the labia majora and also enclosing the vestibule. The labia minora join in front of the clitoris where they form the prepuce over the clitoris.

The clitoris is a pea-shaped structure that contains nerves and blood vessels in erectile tissue. The clitoris is a very sensitive structure and is important in the sexual excitation of the female.

The vestibule refers to the space at the opening of the vagina between the folds of the labia minora. Located in the vestibule are the urethral orifice, the paraurethral glands, the vaginal orifice, the greater vestibular glands, and the hymen.

Terms related to the structures of the vulva:

clitoris: a pea-shaped structure within the vulva. The term means "doortender," implying the link between the clitoris and the entrance to the vagina.

episio: root word meaning "vulva."

erectile tissue: tissue that is capable of becoming filled with blood and by so doing assumes a more straight (*erect*) and firm structure.

genitalia: the external organs of reproduction (*genit*).

greater vestibular glands: the somewhat larger (*greater*) glands that open into the vestibule. Also known as *Bartholin's glands.*

hymen: fold of membrane (*hymen*) across the opening of the vagina.

labia majora: large (*majora*) liplike (*labia*) folds of skin of the vulva.

labia minora: smaller (*minora*) liplike (*labia*) folds of skin of the vulva.

mons pubis: mound (*mons*) of adipose or fatty tissue covered with hair over the pubic (*pubis*) bone.

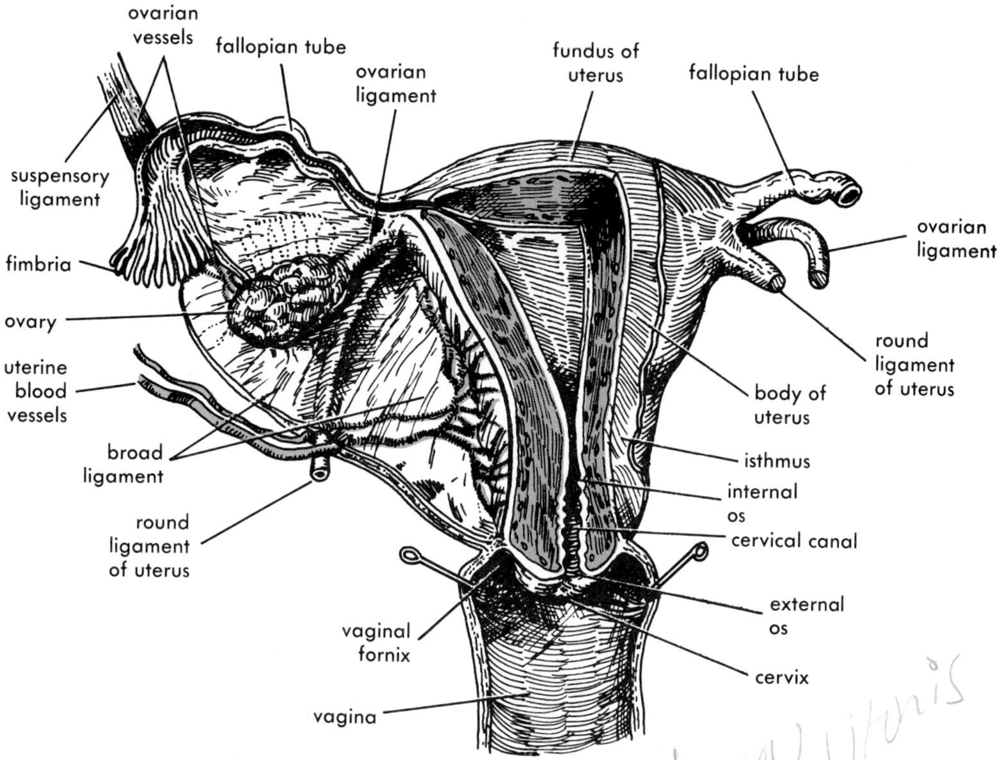

FIGURE 18-1
The internal female reproductive organs.

paraurethral glands: the glands near (*para*) the urethral opening. Also known as *Skene's glands.*
prepuce: fold of skin in front of the clitoris. The clitoris is the female counterpart to the male penis. The term prepuce means "the fold of skin in front of (*pre*) the small penis (*puce*) or the clitoris."
pudendal: pertaining to (*al*) the external genital organs. The term derives from a feeling of shame (*pudend*) resulting from exposure of the sex organs.
urethral orifice: opening (*orifice*) to the outside from the urethra, which is the tube that carries urine from the bladder.
vestibule: area in the perineum that is the entrance (*vestibule*) to the vagina or internal reproductive organs.
vulva: the external female reproductive organs.

The Internal Female Reproductive Organs

The internal reproductive organs of the female include the vagina, uterus, uterine tubes, and ovaries (Figure 18-1).

The vagina is the tube that leads to and from the uterus. This sheathlike organ is the structure in which the male penis deposits sperm during coitus. The sperm is able to enter the uterus by way of the vagina. The vagina also serves as the structure through which a child is born.

Terms related to the vagina:

birth canal: another name for the vagina, implying the fact that it is the tubular passageway (*canal*) through which a child is born (*birth*).
coitus: the act in which the male and female come together (*coitus*) or copulation.
colpo: root word meaning "vagina."
fornix: the area around the top of the vagina into which the cervix protrudes.
introitus: beginning (*introit*) or place at the entrance to the vagina.
virgin: person who has never engaged in sexual intercourse or coitus.

The uterus is an organ that resembles an inverted pear. It is located in the anterior part of the pelvic cavity between the urinary bladder and the rectum. The parts of the uterus, starting at the opening into the vagina, are the cervix, the isthmus, the body, and the fundus.

The uterus is covered by a layer of peritoneum and is attached to the pelvic cavity by several ligaments: the broad, round, cardinal, and uterosacral ligaments.

The walls of the uterus consist of three layers. The outside layer is peritoneal tissue. The middle layer, called the *myometrium,* is a thick muscular layer. The inside layer of mucous membrane is called the *endometrium.*

Changes occur in the lining of the uterus in a cycle of approximately every 28 days. This cycle is referred to as the *menstrual cycle.* This cycle is influenced by estrogens and progesterone. The cycle begins at puberty, the first cycle being referred to as the *menarche,* and continues until a stage in life called *menopause.*

The endometrium serves as a highly vascular place where a fertilized egg may implant and grow. If fertilization does not occur, the menstrual cycle continues; the endometrial lining is destroyed, and along with the blood from the increased vascular supply, flows out of the uterus through the vagina to the outside. This is referred to as the *menstrual flow.*

Terms related to the uterus:

hyster: root word meaning "uterus."
metro: root word meaning "uterus."
womb: common name for the uterus.
ligaments: structures tying (*ligament*) or holding the uterus in place.
cervix: the neck (*cervix*) of the uterus. The portion that opens into the vagina.
body: largest part of the uterus. The part of the body that is long and narrow is called the *isthmus* (long narrow channel).
fundus: the rounded part of the uterus that is opposite the opening (*fundus*). It is the uppermost part of the uterus.
external uterine orifice: the opening (*orifice*) from the uterus (*uterine*) to the outside (*external*) into the vagina. Also known as the *cervical os,* or the mouth (*os*) of the cervix (*cervical*).
myometrium: layer of muscle (*myo*) of the uterus (*metrium*).
endometrium: lining inside (*endo*) the uterus (*metrium*).

rectouterine pouch: space or pocket (*pouch*) between the anterior wall of the rectum (*recto*) and the posterior wall of the uterus (*uterine*). Also known as the *cul-de-sac.*

Terms related to menstruation:

menstrual cycle: regular occurrence (*cycle*) of menstruation (*menstrual*).
menstruation: act of (*ion*) vaginal bleeding on a monthly (*mens*) cycle.
menses: the monthly (*menses*) discharge of blood from the vagina. Commonly called "the period."
menarche: time in life when the monthly (*men*) cycles begin (*arche*).
menopause: stage in life when the monthly (*meno*) cycles stop (*pause*).

The uterine tubes are two flexible tubes extending from the uterus to the ovaries. They are held in place by a fold of the broad ligament.

The end of the tube near the ovaries has projections called fimbriae. These projections curve around the ovary but do not necessarily touch it. When an egg is released from the ovary, these fingerlike projections work to draw the egg into the uterine tube where it will travel toward the uterus.

Terms related to the uterine tube:

adnexa: a term meaning "attachments to a part." In relation to the female reproductive system the term means the uterine tubes and the ovaries collectively.
fimbriae: the fringed (*fimbriae*) border of the flared end of the uterine tube.
salpingo: root word for the uterine tube that means the "trumpetlike (*salping*) tube."
oviduct: another name for the uterine tube denoting its function to lead (*duct*) the egg (*ovi*) to the uterus. Also called the *fallopian tube.*

The ovaries are two oval-shaped structures located in the pelvic cavity on either side of the uterus. They are held in place by the suspensory ligament. They function to produce female hormones and to produce the ovum (*egg*) that is one of the essential elements in reproduction.

The endocrine function of the ovaries involves the production of estrogen and progesterone. Estrogen is the hormone that produces the female reproductive cycle called the *menses.* It is also responsible for the development of the secondary sex characteristics, or the sex-related features that are not directly involved in the reproductive process. The features are not of primary importance in reproduction; therefore they are secondary.

Progesterone is the female hormone that functions to prepare the uterus for implantation of the fertilized egg.

Ovulation

The production of an ovum by the ovary is referred to as *oogenesis.* The process of oogenesis occurs in a structure in the ovary called the ovarian follicle. This involves very complex interactions of the endocrine hormones.

Large amounts of follicle-stimulating hormone from the adenohypophysis at the onset of puberty initiate the process of oogenesis.

The production of an ovum by the ovary occurs in a cycle of approximately 28 days. This is referred to as the ovarian cycle.

Approximately in the middle of the 28-day cycle the ovum is released by the ovary in a process called *ovulation.* Once ovulation has occurred, the ovum is free to travel down the uterine tube into the uterus.

Terms related to the ovary and ovulation:

oophor: root word meaning "ovary" or "organ that is bearing (*phor*) ova (*oo*)."
ovary: organ which functions (*ary*) in the production of the egg (*ov*).
ovarian follicle: small (*cle*) saclike (*folli*) cavity in the ovary in which the ovum develops.
oo: root word meaning "egg" or "ovum."
oogenesis: action in the ovary in which an egg (*oo*) is produced (*genesis*).
ovum: the female reproduction cell, the egg (*ovum*).
ovulation: action (*ation*) that results in the release of an egg from the ovary.

Fertilization

Following ovulation the ovum begins to travel down the uterine tube toward the uterus. When the female has been impregnated with sperm, the sperm works its way up into the uterine tube where it meets the egg. If fertilization is to occur, one sperm enters the egg, and the fertilized ovum, called an *oosperm,* normally continues traveling down the uterine tube to the uterus. Here the fertilized ovum implants into the endometrium, and a pregnancy commences.

If a pregnancy occurs, the menstrual cycles are interrupted until the pregnancy is over. If a pregnancy does not occur, the cycles continue.

Terms related to fertilization:

fertilization: action resulting in the joining of the male and female reproductive elements.
implantation: event that occurs when the fertilized ovum buries (*implant*) itself into the highly vascularized endometrium.
oosperm: fertilized egg; an egg made from the union of an ovum (*oo*) and a sperm (*sperm*).
sperm: male reproductive cell. Also called the seed (see Chapter 17).

Pregnancy

If the ovum is fertilized and the oosperm is implanted into the endometrium, a woman is said to be pregnant or to have conceived a child. The fertilized ovum begins to grow and develops into an embryo. The embryo continues to grow, and at a certain stage, when the organs are recognizable, it is considered a fetus. The developing child is called a fetus until it is delivered.

Immediately following the implantation a structure called the placenta and fetal membranes begin to develop. The functions of the placenta include the nutrition and elimination of waste products of the fetus and protection for the fetus.

The placenta is a flat organ attached to the wall of the uterus. The side toward the fetus gives rise to the umbilical cord.

The fetal membrane, or amnionic sac, is made of two layers of tissue and is continuous with the placenta. The chorion is the layer on the outside, and the amnion is the layer on the inside closest to the fetus. This sac is filled with amnionic fluid that serves to cushion the developing fetus.

The period of time during which the development of a child is progressing is called the gestation period.

Terms related to pregnancy:

conceive: to become pregnant (*ceive*) with (*con*) a child.
conception: the act of (*tion*) taking in (*concept*), of becoming pregnant.
pregnancy: state of being pregnant. A time before (*pre*) a child is born (*gnan*).
antenatal: period of time before (*ante*) birth (*natal*).
gestation period: length of time (*period*) during which a child is carried (*gestation*) in the womb. The normal length of gestation is 280 days. The time may vary.
gravid: state of being pregnant or burdened (*gravid*) with a child.
embryo: a baby in its earliest stage of development at which time it appears to be a swelling (*bryo*) inside (*em*) the uterus.
fetus: term used to describe the unborn child (*fetus*) from about the time organs are distinguishable until it is born.
placenta: flat, cakelike (*placenta*) structure attached to the uterine wall through which the child is nourished.
umbilical cord: connection (*cord*) between the mother and child that is attached to the placenta at one end and the center (*umbilic*) of the abdomen of the fetus on the other end. The place of attachment of the cord to the abdomen of the fetus is also known as the *navel.*
fetal membranes: layers of tissue pertaining to (*al*) the fetus (*fet*).
  amnion: inside layer of fetal membranes, which is next to the fetus and is soft as a small (*ion*) lamb (*amn*).
  chorion: outside, skinlike (*chorion*) layer of the fetal membranes.
amnionic sac: fetal membranes. Commonly called "the bag of waters."
amnionic fluid: water (*fluid*) in the amnionic sac in which the fetus is cushioned.

Labor and Delivery

The process of giving birth is called labor and delivery, or parturition.

The reason for the onset of labor is poorly understood, but it is usually marked by the occurrence of uterine contractions. The hormone oxytocin has an influence on labor.

There are three stages of labor:

stage 1: the uterus is contracting regularly, the fetal membranes have ruptured, and the cervix of the uterus is dilated.

stage 2: the time from the complete dilation of the cervix until the actual delivery of the child.
stage 3: the time from the delivery of the neonate to the delivery of the placenta and fetal membranes or afterbirth.

Terms related to labor and delivery:

para: root word meaning "to bear" or "to give birth."
labor: term used to describe the hard, tiring work (*labor*) in the effort of giving birth to a child.
delivery: the birth process in which the child is set free (*deliver*) from its mother.
afterbirth: common name for the placenta and fetal membranes. It is so called because these organs are expelled after the birth of a baby.
contraction: action (*tion*) of the uterine muscles in which they pull (*tract*) the walls of the uterus together (*con*).
dilation of the cervix: process (*ation*) during which the neck of the uterus (*cervix*) is opening (*dilata*).
parturition: process (*ition*) of giving birth (*partur*).
postpartum: period of time shortly after (*post*) giving birth (*partum*).
neonate: newborn [new (*neo*) born (*nate*)] child.
lochia: pertaining to (*ia*) the flow of fluid from the uterus following childbirth (*loch*).
puerperal: pertaining to (*al*) the time of giving birth (*puerper*).

DISEASES OF THE FEMALE REPRODUCTIVE SYSTEM

Conditions or diseases of the female reproductive system may be divided into two separate categories that are gynecological and obstetrical.

Gynecological conditions are those conditions that are related to the female reproductive system. The term *gynecological* means "pertaining to (*al*) the study (*ologic*) of the female (*gynec*) reproductive system."

Obstetrical conditions are those conditions that are related to birth and pregnancy. The term *obstetric* means "a woman (*tric*) who stands (*ste*) before (*obs*) another woman who is giving birth." The term literally means midwife.

Obstetrics refers to the care of a pregnant female before, during, and after childbirth.

Gynecological Conditions

Analysis of selected terms related to gynecological conditions:

anovulation: condition in which ovulation does not (*an*) occur.
cervicitis: inflammation (*itis*) of the cervix (*cervic*).
cystocele: condition in which the wall of the urinary bladder (*cyst*) protrudes (*cele*) or bulges into the vagina.
dyspareunia: situation (*ia*) in which a woman experiences pain or difficulty (*dys*) during coitus with a partner (*pareun*).
endocervicitis: inflammation (*itis*) of the lining inside (*endo*) the cervix (*cervic*).

endometriosis: condition (*osis*) in which endometrial (*endometri*) tissue is found in the abdominal cavity.

fibromyoma: tumor (*oma*) composed of muscle (*myo*) of the uterus and fiber (*fibro*).

infertility: inability (*in*) of a woman to conceive (*fertil*) a child.

kraurosis of the vulva: condition (*osis*) in which the external reproductive organs (*vulva*) become dry (*kraur*).

leukoplakia of the vulva: condition in which white (*leuko*), thickened patches (*plakia*) develop on the vulva.

leukorrhea: condition in which there is a flow (*rrhea*) of white (*leuko*) mucus from the vagina.

menstrual disorder: condition in which the menstrual cycle is not (*dis*) what is considered normal (*order*).

- *amenorrhea:* lack of (*a*) the menstrual (*meno*) flow (*rrhea*).
- *dysmenorrhea:* difficult (*dys*) or painful menstrual flow (*menorrhea*).
- *hypomenorrhea:* menstrual flow (*menorrhea*) is decreased (*hypo*) from what is normal for that woman.
- *menorrhagia:* menstrual (*meno*) flow (*rrhagia*) is excessive.
- *metrorrhagia:* flow (*rrhagia*) of blood from the uterus (*metro*) occurs at irregular intervals.
- *oligomenorrhea:* condition in which the menstrual flow (*menorrhea*) decreases in frequency and the woman has fewer (*oligo*) menses.
- *postmenopausal bleeding:* recurrence of bleeding after (*post*) the menstrual cycles (*meno*) have ceased (*pausal*).

premenstrual tension: group of symptoms that occurs before (*pre*) the menses (*menstrual*) in which the woman may feel a degree of irritability and tension. Also known as premenstrual syndrome or PMS.

polycystic ovary: condition in which there are multiple (*poly*) little sacs of fluid (*cysts*) in the ovary.

prolapsed uterus: condition in which the uterus slips (*lapse*) outward (*pro*).

rectocele: condition in which the wall of the rectum (*recto*) protrudes (*cele*) or bulges into the vagina.

rectovaginal fistula: an abnormal, small (*ula*) passage (*fist*) between the rectum (*recto*) and the vagina (*vaginal*).

rigid hymen: condition in which the membrane (*hymen*) over the vagina is unyielding (*rigid*).

stenosis of the hymen: the normal opening in the membrane over the vagina (*hymen*) is narrowed (*stenosis*).

sterility: condition in which a man or woman is not capable of producing offspring.

Trichomonas vaginitis: inflammation (*itis*) of the vagina (*vagin*) caused by a parasite (*Trichomonas*).

uterine retroflexion: the uterus bends (*flexion*) backward (*retro*). Also known as a *retroverted uterus*.

vaginismus: condition (*ismus*) that is characterized by painful spasms of the walls of the vagina (*vagin*).

vaginitis: inflammation (*itis*) of the vagina.

venereal disease (*VD*): disease that is spread by the act of love (*vene,* variation of Venus) or by sexual contact.

gonorrhea: disease characterized by a flow (*rrhea*) of purulent discharge from the sexual (*gono*) organs.

syphilis: a venereal disease.

vesicovaginal fistula: an abnormal, small (*ula*) passage (*fist*) between the urinary bladder (*vesico*) and vagina (*vaginal*).

vulvitis: inflammation (*itis*) of the vulva (*vulv*).

vulvovaginitis: inflammation (*itis*) of the vulva (*vulvo*) and the vagina (*vagin*).

Treatment of Gynecological Conditions

Analysis of selected terms related to the treatment of gynecological conditions:

birth control: action taken to prevent (*control*) the birth of a child.

condom: sheath of material worn over the penis during sexual intercourse to prevent conception or transmission of venereal diseases. It is named after an 18th century physician who devised it.

intrauterine device (*IUD*): a product (*device*) that is placed inside (*intra*) the uterus (*uterine*) as a method of birth control.

oral contraceptive (*the Pill*): pill taken by mouth (*oral*) that acts against (*contra*) the conceiving (*ceptive*) of a child.

postcoital douche: directing of a flow of water (*douche*) into the vagina after (*post*) intercourse (*coital*).

spermicidal chemicals: preparations (*chemicals*) that are designed to kill (*cidal*) sperm (*spermi*).

sterilization: a procedure in which a person is rendered incapable of producing offspring.

tubal ligation: procedure done in which the uterine tubes (*tubal*) are tied (*ligation*) to block the passage of the egg toward the uterus.

vaginal diaphragm: mechanical device used to wall off (*diaphragm*) the opening of the cervix from the vagina (*vaginal*).

colpectomy: removal (*ectomy*) of the vagina (*colpo*).

colpocleisis: procedure done in which the vagina (*colpo*) is closed by sutures.

colporrhaphy: surgical repair (*rrhapy*) of the walls of the vagina (*colpo*). May be the anterior or posterior walls. Commonly referred to as an "A-P repair."

culdoscopy: passing of a viewing device (*scopy*) into the cul-de-sac (*culdo*) for the purpose of examination.

cytologic smear: test in which cells (*cyto*) from the cervix are studied (*logic*) by smearing them on a slide. Also known as a "Pap test," or Papanicolaou test.

dilatation and curettage (*D & C*): procedure done in which the opening of the cervix is widened (*dilatation*) and instruments are passed into the cervix to scrape (*curettage*) the lining of the uterus.

endometrial biopsy: microscopic examination (*biopsy*) of a section of the lining of the uterus (*endometri*).

hymenotomy: procedure done in which the hymen (*hymen*) is cut into (*otomy*).

hysterectomy: the removal (*ectomy*) of the uterus (*hyster*). A total *hysterectomy* usually implies the removal of all of the female reproductive organs except the vagina. Also called a *panhysterectomy*.
myomectomy: removal (*ectomy*) of a tumor (*om*) of the uterine muscle (*my*).
oophorectomy: removal of (*ectomy*) an ovary (*oophor*).
pelvic examination: procedure in which the internal female reproductive organs located in the pelvis are examined.
salpingectomy: the removal of a uterine tube (*salping*).
salpingo-oophorectomy: removal of (*ectomy*) an ovary (*oophor*) and a uterine tube (*salpingo*).
salpingorrhaphy: surgical repair (*rrhaphy*) of the uterine tube (*salpingo*).
vulvectomy: removal (*ectomy*) of the vulva.

OBSTETRICAL CONDITIONS

Analysis of selected terms related to obstetrical conditions:

abruptio placentae: situation in which the placenta breaks away (*abruptio*) prematurely from the uterus.
amnionitis: inflammation (*itis*) of the fetal membrane (*amnion*).
dystocia: situation in which there is an abnormal or difficult (*dys*) childbirth (*tocia*).
eclampsia: sudden development (*eclampsia*) in which a pregnant woman experiences convulsions and possibly coma.
ectopic pregnancy: pregnancy that is out (*ec*, variation of *ex*) of its normal place (*topic*). Most often refers to a pregnancy in one of the uterine tubes.
hydatidiform mole: abnormal pregnancy that results in the formation of a fleshy mass (*mole*) that looks like (*form*) a bunch of watery vesicles (*hydatid*) or grapes.
hyperemesis gravidarum: condition of pregnancy (*gravidarum*) in which the woman vomits (*emesis*) excessively (*hyper*).
intrauterine death: situation in which the fetus dies (*death*) while still inside (*intra*) the uterus.
placenta previa: situation in which the placenta is very close to the cervix, nearer the uterine outlet than the child (*previa*).
pregnancy history: the recording of the number of times a woman has been pregnant and the number of times she has given birth to a live child. Example: gravida 2, para 1 means a woman who has been pregnant twice and has given birth to one live child. This means that this woman has had one aborted (spontaneous or surgical) pregnancy.
- *multipara:* a woman who has given birth (*para*) more than once (*multi*).
- *nullipara:* a woman who has not (*nulli*) given birth (*para*).
- *primipara:* a woman giving birth (*para*) to her first (*primi*) child.

premature labor: labor starts before (*pre*) the child has been carried to full term (*mature*).
spontaneous abortion: loss of a fetus (*abort*) from natural, unplanned (*spontaneous*) causes. Commonly called a *miscarriage*.

TABLE 18-2
Other Types of Abortions

idiopathic: an abortion for which no cause can be found.

imminent: the expulsion of the fetus is about to occur.

incomplete: the contents of the uterus related to the pregancy are not completely expelled.

induced: an abortion that is intentionally started.

inevitable: an abortion that is in progress and will go to completion.

therapeutic: an abortion that is done to save the life or health of the pregnant woman.

threatened: an abortion that is in progress and may or may not go to completion.

tubal: an abortion in which the contents of the pregnancy extrude through the open end of the fallopian tube into the abdominal cavity.

stillborn: situation in which a child being delivered (*born*) has died before birth and thus does not move (*still*).

toxemia: condition in which substances capable of causing harm (*tox*) are in the blood (*emia*) of the mother.

Treatment of Obstetrical Conditions

Analysis of selected terms related to the treatment of obstetrical conditions:

abortion: removal of an embryo or fetus before it can live outside its mother.

amniocentesis: puncture (*centesis*) of the fetal membranes to withdraw amnionic (*amnio*) fluid, usually for study.

episiotomy: procedure done to cut into (*otomy*) the vulva (*episi*), specifically the perineum from the vagina backwards, to make the opening from the vagina larger to facilitate the birth of a baby.

evacuation of retained secundines (*ERS*): procedure done in which tissue remaining (*retained*) in the uterus from the afterbirth (*secundine*) is removed (*evacuated*).

hysterotomy: cutting into (*otomy*) the uterus (*hyster*) to remove a child. Commonly called a *cesarean section,* related to the fact that Julius Caesar was born by this method.

vaginal delivery: birth of a child (*delivery*) through the vagina. Commonly called a *normal delivery.*

PRETEST/ POSTTEST FOR CHAPTER 18

1. The following terms are related to the vulva. Use list of terms to fill in the blanks in the statements that follow.

clitoris	mons pubis
greater vestibular glands	paraurethral glands
hymen	prepuce
labia majora	urethral orifice
labia minora	vulva

1. The membrane across the opening of the vagina is called the ____________.
2. The small folds of skin in the vulva are ____________.
3. The opening through which urine passes is the ____________.
4. The ____________ is a term meaning external female reproductive organs.
5. The glands situated near the urethra are the ____________.
6. A pea-shaped structure within the vulva is the ____________.
7. The large folds of skin of the vulva are the ____________.
8. The ____________ is the fold of skin in front of the clitoris.
9. The mound of fatty tissue over the pubic bone is called the ____________.
10. The glands that open into the vestibule are the ____________.

2. Select the best answer.

1. Term(s) meaning the external reproductive organs is (are) _____.
   A. pudenda
   B. genitalia
   C. both of the above

2. Root word(s) meaning vulva is (are) _____.
   A. episio
   B. pudenda
   C. both of the above

3. Erectile tissue _____.
   A. becomes firm
   B. secretes a lubricant
   C. both of the above

4. The vestibule is ____.
   A. the entrance to the internal reproductive organs
   B. another name for the clitoris
   C. both of the above

3. The following terms are related to the vagina. Use the following terms to complete the statements below.

birth canal	colpo	introitus
coitus	fornix	virgin

1. Terms meaning vagina are ________ and ________.

2. Sexual intercourse is called ________.

3. The area around the top of the vagina is called the ________.

4. The area at the entrance to the vagina is called the ________.

5. A person who has never engaged in sexual intercourse is a ________.

4. The following statements are related to the uterus.

1. Root words meaning uterus are ____.
   A. hyster and metro
   B. womb and hyster
   C. all of the above

2. The structure(s) holding the uterus in place is called ____.
   A. ligaments
   B. myometrium
   C. both of the above

3. The neck of the uterus is the ____.
   A. cervix
   B. fundus
   C. both of the above

4. The external uterine orifice is ____.
   A. the opening into the vagina
   B. also called the cervical os
   C. both of the above

5. The muscle layer and inside layer of the uterus are the ____.
   A. fundus and endometrium
   B. myometrium and endometrium
   C. both of the above

6. The space between the rectum and vagina is called ____.
   A. the rectouterine pouch
   B. the cul-de-sac
   C. both of the above

5. Using the list of terms complete the statements.

menstrual cycle
menstruation
menses
menarche
menopause

1. The ________________ is the regular occurrence of menstruation.
2. ________________ is the time in life when the monthly cycle begins.
3. A term meaning monthly is ________________.
4. The occurrence of vaginal bleeding is called ________________.
5. ________________ is the time in life when the monthly cycle ends.

6. The following terms are related to the uterine tubes. Select the best answer.

1. Another term for the uterine tube is ____.
   A. oviduct
   B. salpingo
   C. both of the above
2. *Adnexa* refers to ____.
   A. the ovaries and tubes
   B. the uterine tubes
   C. all of the above
3. The ____ is (are) the fringed edge of the uterine tube.
   A. fimbriae
   B. oviduct
   C. both of the above

7. The following terms are related to the ovary. Using the list complete the following statements.

oophor
ovary
ovarian follicle
oo
oogenesis
ovum
ovulation

1. A term meaning bearing eggs is ________.
2. The organ which functions in the production of eggs is the ________.
3. Root words for egg are ________ and ________.
4. The small saclike cavity in the ovary is the ________.
5. The process by which an egg is formed is called ________.
6. The action in which an egg is released is called ________.

8. The following statements are related to fertilization. Mark the statements true, *T*, or false, *F*.

1. _____ Fertilization is the process resulting in the joining of the male and female reproductive elements.
2. _____ Implantation is the action of the sperm joining the egg.
3. _____ An oosperm is a fertilized egg.

9. The following statements are related to pregnancy. Select the best answer.

1. A term referring to becoming pregnant is _____.
   A. to conceive
   B. conception
   C. both of the above

2. The fetal membranes are _____.
   A. also called the amnionic sac.
   B. also called the embryo.
   C. both of the above.

3. The term fetus means _____.
   A. the child early in its development.
   B. the developing child later in the pregnancy.
   C. both of the above.

4. The placenta is the _____.
   A. structure containing amnionic fluid.
   B. structure through which a fetus is nourished.
   C. both of the above.

5. The umbilical cord connects _____.
   A. the abdomen of the baby and the placenta.
   B. the abdomen of the baby and the navel.
   C. both of the above.

6. The period of time before giving birth is called _____.
   A. the antenatal period.
   B. the gestation period.
   C. both of the above.

7. *Gravid* means _____.
   A. heavy with child.
   B. pregnant.
   C. both of the above.

10. The following terms are related to labor and delivery. Select the best answer.

1. A term meaning to give birth is _____.
   A. para.
   B. parturition.
   C. both of the above.

2. Labor and delivery involves the ____.
   A. birth of a child.
   B. expulsion of the afterbirth.
   C. both of the above.

3. Postpartum refers to the ____.
   A. time shortly after giving birth.
   B. time shortly before giving birth.
   C. both of the above.

4. A newborn child is referred to as ____.
   A. fetus.
   B. neonate.
   C. both of the above.

5. Lochia is the ____.
   A. flow of fluid after a child is born.
   B. afterbirth.
   C. both of the above.

11. The following terms are related to conditions or diseases of the female reproductive tract. Select the best answer.

1. Gynecological conditions are those conditions related to ____.
   A. the nonpregnant female.
   B. the pregnant female.
   C. both of the above.

2. Obstetrical conditions are those conditions that are related to ____.
   A. the nonpregnant female.
   B. the pregnant female.
   C. both of the above.

3. Obstetrical conditions include ____.
   A. labor and delivery.
   B. pregnancy.
   C. both of the above.

12. The following sets of terms are related to gynecological disorders. In each set match column A with column B. Be specific.

Set 1

Column A	Column B
1. ____ anovulation	A. pain during coitus
2. ____ cervicitis	B. white patches on the external reproductive organs
3. ____ cystocele	C. inflammation of the cervix
4. ____ dyspareunia	D. endometrial tissue found in the abdominal cavity

Column A	Column B
5. ____ endocervicitis	E. failure of ovulation to occur
6. ____ endometriosis	F. tumor of the uterine muscle and fiber
7. ____ fibromyoma	G. wall of the bladder protruding into the vagina
8. ____ infertility	H. flow of white mucus from the vagina
9. ____ kraurosis of the vulva	I. inability to conceive
10. ____ leukoplakia of the vulva	J. inflammation of the lining of the cervix
11. ____ leukorrhea	K. dryness of external reproductive organs

Set 2

Column A	Column B
1. ____ amenorrhea	A. bleeding after the menses have ceased
2. ____ dysmenorrhea	B. difficulty in menstruation
3. ____ hypomenorrhea	C. decrease in the frequency of menses
4. ____ menorrhagia	D. lack of menstrual flow
5. ____ metrorrhagia	E. excessive menstrual flow
6. ____ oligomenorrhea	F. flow of blood from the uterus at irregular intervals
7. ____ postmenopausal bleeding	G. irritability before the menses begin
8. ____ premenstrual tension	H. decreased menstrual flow

Set 3

Column A	Column B
1. ____ polycystic ovary	A. uterus has slipped out
2. ____ prolapsed uterus	B. inflammation of the vagina caused by a parasite
3. ____ rectocele	C. unyielding membrane over the vagina
4. ____ rectovaginal fistula	D. multiple little sacs of fluid in a structure
5. ____ rigid hymen	E. incapable of producing offspring
6. ____ stenosis of the hymen	F. an abnormal passage between the rectum and vagina
	G. narrowed normal opening in the membrane over the vagina
	H. the wall of the rectum protruding into the vagina

Column A	Column B
7. ____ sterility	
8. ____ *Trichomonas vaginalis*	

Set 4

Column A	Column B
1. ____ uterine retroflexion	A. painful spasms of the walls of the vagina
2. ____ vaginismus	B. inflammation of the vulva and vagina
3. ____ vaginitis	C. the uterus bent backward
4. ____ venereal disease	D. inflammation of the external female organs
5. ____ vesicovaginal fistula	E. disease spread by sexual contact
6. ____ vulvitis	F. abnormal passage between the bladder and vagina
7. ____ vulvovaginitis	G. inflammation of the vagina

13. Using the following list of terms related to diagnosis and treatment of gynecological conditions, complete the statements which follow.

birth control	cytologic smear
colpectomy	dilatation and curettage
colpocleisis	endometrial biopsy
colporrhaphy	pelvic examination
culdoscopy	

1. The action taken to prevent the birth of a child is called ____________.
2. The test in which cells from the cervix are studied is called ____________.
3. ____________ is a procedure to widen the opening of the cervix and scrape the lining of the uterus.
4. ____________ is the repair of the walls of the vagina.
5. ____________ is an examination of tissue from the lining of the uterus.
6. The removal of the vagina is called ____________.
7. Passing a viewing instrument into the cul-de-sac is called ____________.
8. The procedure to close the vagina by sutures is called ____________.
9. The procedure in which the internal female reproductive organs are examined is called a ____________.

14. The following terms are related to gynecological conditions. Match column A with column B. Choose the best answer.

Column A	Column B
1. ____ hymenotomy	A. removal of a tumor of the uterine muscle
2. ____ hysterectomy	B. removal of the vulva
3. ____ myomectomy	C. removal of the uterus
4. ____ oophorectomy	D. removal of the uterine tubes
5. ____ salpingectomy	E. surgical cutting into the membrane over the vagina
6. ____ salpingo-oophorectomy	F. repair of the uterine tubes
7. ____ salpingorrhaphy	G. removal of the uterine tubes and the ovaries
8. ____ vulvectomy	H. removal of the ovaries

15. The following two sets of terms are related to obstetrical conditions. Using the lists of terms complete the statements.

Set 1

abruptio placentae	intrauterine death
ectopic	placenta previa
hydatidiform mole	premature
hyperemesis gravidarum	spontaneous abortion

1. A pregnancy which develops out of its normal place is called (a) an ____________ pregnancy.
2. Labor that starts before the full term of pregnancy is complete is ____________ labor.
3. The formation of a fleshy mass from an abnormal pregnancy is called a (an) ____________.
4. ____________ means excessive vomiting during pregnancy.
5. ____________ is a situation in which the placenta breaks away prematurely from the uterus.
6. ____________ means the placenta is nearer to the uterine outlet than is the baby.
7. The loss of the fetus from natural, unplanned causes is called a ____________.
8. When a child dies before it is born, an ____________ has occurred.

Set 2

amnionitis	stillborn
dystocia	toxemia
eclampsia	

1. A difficult labor is called ________________.
2. The condition in which harmful substances are in the blood of the mother is called ________________.
3. A sudden development of convulsions in pregnancy is called ____________.
4. Inflammation of the amnion is called ________________.
5. A child who is born dead is called ________________.

16. The pregnancy history of a woman is expressed in special terms. Match column A with column B.

Column A	Column B
1. _____ gravida 2, para 1	A. woman who has given birth more than once
2. _____ multipara	B. woman giving birth to her first child
3. _____ nullipara	C. woman who has never had children
4. _____ primipara	D. woman who has been pregnant twice and has one living child

17. The following terms are related to the treatment of obstetrical problems. Select the best answer.

1. An abortion is _____.
   A. the loss of an embryo.
   B. another name for miscarriage.
   C. both of the above.
2. In amniocentesis _____.
   A. the fetal membranes are punctured.
   B. the amniotic sac is removed.
   C. both of the above.
3. A hysterotomy is _____.
   A. another name for a cesarean section.
   B. a cutting into the uterus.
   C. both of the above.
4. An episiotomy is _____.
   A. a cutting into the vulva.
   B. a cutting into the uterine tube.
   C. both of the above.

5. The procedure to remove the remaining pieces of afterbirth is called ____.
   A. a hysterectomy.
   B. evacuation of retained secundines.
   C. both of the above.

6. A normal delivery is sometimes called ____.
   A. a hysterectomy.
   B. a vaginal delivery.
   C. both of the above.

PRETEST/ POSTTEST **ANSWERS** FOR CHAPTER **18**

1. **1.** hymen **6.** clitoris
2. labia minora **7.** labia majora
3. urethral orifice **8.** prepuce
4. vulva **9.** mons pubis
5. paraurethral glands **10.** greater vestibular glands

2. **1.** C **2.** C **3.** A **4.** A

3. **1.** birth canal, colpo **4.** introitus
2. coitus **5.** virgin
3. fornix

4. **1.** C **2.** A **3.** A **4.** C **5.** B **6.** C

5. **1.** menstrual cycle **4.** menstruation
2. menarche **5.** menopause
3. menses

6. **1.** C **2.** A **3.** A

7. **1.** oophor **4.** ovarian follicle
2. ovary **5.** oogenesis
3. oo, ovum **6.** ovulation

8. **1.** T **2.** F **3.** T

9. **1.** C **2.** A **3.** B **4.** B **5.** A **6.** C **7.** C

10. **1.** C **2.** C **3.** A **4.** B **5.** A

11. **1.** A **2.** B **3.** C

12. **Set 1**
1. E **3.** G **5.** J **7.** F **9.** K **10.** B **11.** H
2. C **4.** A **6.** D **8.** I

Set 2
1. D **2.** B **3.** H **4.** E **5.** F **6.** C **7.** A **8.** G

Set 3
1. D **2.** A **3.** H **4.** F **5.** C **6.** G **7.** E **8.** B

Set 4
1. C **2.** A **3.** G **4.** E **5.** F **6.** D **7.** B

13.
1. birth control
2. cytologic smear
3. dilatation and curettage
4. colporrhaphy
5. endometrial biopsy
6. colpectomy
7. culdoscopy
8. culpocleisis
9. pelvic examination

14. **1.** E **2.** C **3.** A **4.** H **5.** D **6.** G **7.** F **8.** B

15. Set 1
1. ectopic
2. premature
3. hydatidiform mole
4. hyperemesis gravidarum
5. abruptio placentae
6. placenta previa
7. spontaneous abortion
8. intrauterine death

Set 2
1. dystocia
2. toxemia
3. eclampsia
4. amnionitis
5. stillborn

16. **1.** D **2.** A **3.** C **4.** B

17. **1.** C **2.** A **3.** C **4.** A **5.** B **6.** B

19 THE INTEGUMENTARY SYSTEM

OBJECTIVES

At the end of this chapter you will be able to do the following:

1 List the structures in the integumentary system.
2 Define terms related to skin, hair, sebaceous glands, nails, and breasts.
3 Analyze selected terms related to disease conditions of structures of the integumentary system.
4 Analyze selected terms related to the treatment of diseases of the integumentary system, including diagnostic, surgical, and drug-related terms.

THE INTEGUMENTARY SYSTEM

The integumentary system is composed of skin and various appendages. It is the natural covering of the body (Figure 19-1).

The appendages of the integumentary system include hair, sebaceous glands, sweat glands, nails, and breasts.

The Skin

The skin is the largest organ in the body. The functions of skin are as follows:

1 protection: it protects underlying tissues by preventing excessive loss of fluids, it shields the body from radiation from the sun, and it protects parts of the body from trauma.
2 sensation: the skin picks up sensations of pain, touch, pressure, and temperature.
3 regulation of heat.
4 secretion: sebum and sweat are secreted by the skin.
5 metabolism: skin plays a role in vitamin D metabolism.

Skin is composed of layers of tissue. Those layers are the epidermis, dermis, and subcutaneous tissue.

The epidermis is the outer layer of skin, and it contains many layers of tissue and the cells that give skin color, melanocytes.

The dermis, or dermal layer, lies directly under the epidermis and is often called

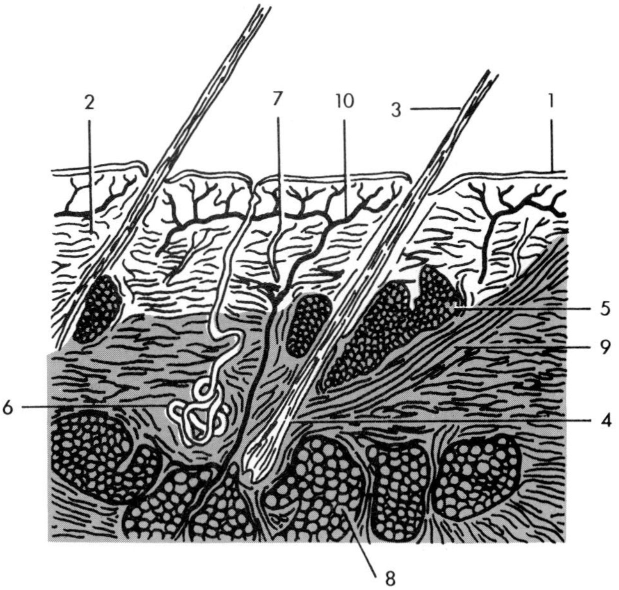

FIGURE 19-1
The skin in cross section: (1) epidermis, (2) dermis, (3) hair shaft, (4) hair follicle, (5) sebaceous gland and duct, (6) sweat gland and duct, (7) nerve ending, (8) fat, (9) arrector pili muscle, (10) blood vessel.

the *true skin*. It is made of connective tissue. Embedded in the dermis are the blood vessels, lymphatic vessels, hair follicles, and sweat glands.

Subcutaneous tissue attaches the dermis to the underlying structure. This tissue contains varying amounts of adipose tissue. This fatty tissue acts as insulation for the body.

Terms related to the skin:

adipose tissue: section of subcutaneous tissue that contains fat (*adipose*).
cutis: root word meaning "skin."
dermis: true skin (*derm*).
epidermis: layer of tissue that lies over (*epi*) the true skin (*derm*).
melanocyte: cell (*cyte*) producing melanin, which gives the skin its relatively dark (*melano*) color.
subcutaneous tissue: layer of tissue under (*sub*) the skin (*cutan*).

The Hair

Hair covers the entire body except for the palms of the hand, the soles of the feet, and parts of the external reproductive organs. Its main function is protection of delicate structures.

The development of body hair is linked to the development of sexual maturity.

Terms related to the anatomy of hair and the distribution of hair on the body:

arrector pili muscle: muscle that is attached to the hair follicle and causes the hair (*pili*) to stand straight (*rector*).
axillary hair: hair in the armpit (*axilla*).
cilia: hair on the edges of the eyelid. Eyelashes.
eyebrow: hair on the ridge (*brow*) over the eye.
hair follicle: small (*cle*) cavity (*folli*) in which the hair grows.
hair shaft: long polelike (*shaft*) portion of hair.
lanugo: fine hair on the body of a newborn baby.
pilus: root word meaning "hair."
pubic hair: hair over the pubic area.
tricho: root word meaning "hair."

Sebaceous Glands

Sebaceous glands are located in the skin and secrete an oily substance that gives skin and hair its glossy appearance. The oily substance secreted is called *sebum.*

Most of these glands open into the walls of hair follicles. There are also sebaceous glands at the corners of the mouth and around the external sex organs that open directly upon the surface of the skin.

Sweat Glands

Sweat glands are found in most areas of the body.

The most abundant type of sweat gland is called an eccrine sweat gland. These glands function to cool the body. The palms of the hands and soles of the feet contain large numbers of these glands. Sweat from these glands is odorless.

Another type of sweat gland is called an apocrine sweat gland. This type of gland is connected to hair follicles in the armpits and the pubic area and is also found at the navel and nipples. The secretion from these sweat glands increases in response to sexual stimulation. They function in lubricating the genital area and play a part in sexual arousal because of the mild odor.

Terms related to sweat glands:

apocrine sweat glands: glands that separate (*crine*) or produce a fluid that contains substances that have been separated (*apo*) from the hair follicle. This substance gives the somewhat viscid fluid from these glands a mild odor.
eccrine sweat gland: ordinary sweat gland that separates (*crine*) or produces sweat from (*ec,* variation of *ex*) most of the surface of the skin.
hidr: root word meaning "sweat."
perspiration: another name for sweating. The name comes from the fact that when the skin is wet, you can feel air blowing (*spir*) through (*per*) or past the skin.

Nails

The nail is a thin, hard, protective plate consisting of epidermal tissue. The nails are located on the upper surface of the ends of the fingers, thumbs, and toes.

Terms related to the nails:

cuticle: small (*cle*) area of dead skin (*cuti*) around the edge of the nail.
lunula: small (*ula*), white, moon-shaped [moon (*lun*)] area at the base of the nail.
onych: root word meaning "nail."
onyx: root word meaning "nail."
paronychial: pertaining to (*al*) the area around (*par*) the nail (*onych*).
subungual: pertaining to (*al*) the area under (*sub*) the nail (*ungual*).
ungual: root word meaning "nail."

The Breasts

The breasts are appendages of the integumentary system and are also accessory reproductive organs.

There are two breasts situated on the anterior wall of the thorax. The female breasts develop at the time of puberty and become active lactating glands after childbirth. The male breasts are flat, nonfunctioning organs.

Terms related to the breasts:

areola: small (*ola*) area (*are*) of color around the nipple.
galact, lacto: root words meaning "milk."
lactation: process of producing milk (*lacta*).
mammary gland: pertaining to (*ary*) the breast of the female (*mamma*), which is capable of secreting (*gland*) milk.
mast: root word meaning "breast."
nipple: tip or point (*nip*) of the breast.

DISEASES OF THE INTEGUMENTARY SYSTEM

Diseases or disorders of the integumentary system and the description of the signs and symptoms of diseases are numerous.

The skin is easily examined, and thus even subtle changes can be described. Many conditions of the integumentary system, especially the skin, are sometimes signs of diseases of other systems of the body.

Disease Conditions of the Integumentary System, Including Signs and Symptoms

Analysis of selected terms related to diseases of the integumentary system, including signs and symptoms:

abrasion: scraped (*rasion*) away (*ab*) portion of skin.
acne: disease condition of the skin in which there are pointed (*acne,* variation of *acme*), often pus-filled, eruptions on the skin.
  acne rosacea: form of acne in which the nose, forehead, and cheeks appear rose colored (*rosacea*).

acne vulgaris: common (*vulgar*) form of acne.
alopecia: condition (*ia*) in which there is loss of hair, similar to the loss of hair experienced by balding foxes (*alopec*). Commonly known as *baldness.*
amastia: congenital absence (*a*) of a breast (*mastia*).
angioma: tumor (*oma*) consisting mainly of blood vessels (*angi*) that appear on the skin. Also called *hemangioma.*
blackhead: discolored (*black*) plug at the opening (*head*) of a sebaceous gland.
boil: a bump (*boil*) on the skin resulting from an acute infection of the subcutaneous layers of the skin, gland, or hair follicle.
bulla: a large vesicle.
burn: skin trauma resulting from exposure to harmful substances such as chemicals, heat, sun, or wind.
callus: condition in which an area of the skin has become hardened (*callus*).
carbuncle: small (*cle*), painful inflammation of the skin, usually containing pus, which is reddened in a way similar to burning coal (*carbun,* variation of *carbon*).
cellulitis: inflammation (*itis*) of cellular (*cellul*) tissue.
cheilitis: inflammation (*itis*) of the lips (*cheil*).
clammy skin: situation in which the surface of the skin feels cold and damp, similar to the way cold mud (*clam*) might feel.
contusion: condition in which tissue beneath the skin is injured but the skin is not broken.
cutis anserina: condition of the skin (*cutis*) in which bumps appear and a texture like that of a plucked goose (*anserina*) develops. Also known as *gooseflesh* or *goosebumps.*
decubitus ulcer: sore (*ulcer*) on the skin of a person who has been lying down (*decub*); a bed sore.
dermatitis: inflammation (*itis*) of the skin (*derma*).
diaphoresis: condition (*sis*) in which there is an excessive amount of sweat carried (*phore*) through (*dia*) the skin.
ecthyma: skin condition in which fluid rushes (*thyma*) out (*ec,* variation of *ex*) of sores in the skin. Also called *ulcerative impetigo.*
eczema: condition in which there is a flowing out (*ecze*) of fluid from (*ec,* variation of *ex*) the affected skin.
epithelioma: tumor (*oma*) of epithelial (*epitheli*) tissue.
erysipelas: disease in which there is a spread of a deep red (*erysi,* variation of *erythro*) color to the skin (*pelas*).
erythema: abnormal redness of the skin.
erythema nodosum: condition in which reddened (*eryth*) lumps (*nodosum*) appear on the skin.
erythromelalgia: condition in which the skin of the extremities (*mel*) becomes red (*erythro*) and painful (*algia*).
eschar: a hard crust or scab (*eschar*) that forms after a traumatic injury.
excoriation: process (*tion*) in which there is removal of (*ex*) or loss of skin (*coria*) by trauma, burns, or other causes.
furuncle: another name for a boil. Associate the term *fur* with *furnace,* which is a place where water boils.

gangrene: condition in which soft tissue, including skin, is necrotic.
gynecomastia: condition (*ia*) in which the male breast (*mast*) enlarges to resemble the breast of a female (*gyneco*).
hidradenitis: inflammation (*itis*) of a sweat (*hidr*) gland (*aden*).
hirsute: condition in which there is excessive hairiness. The body is covered with shaggy (*hirsute*) hair.
hives: condition of the skin characterized by the appearance of very itchy, raised (*hives*) areas.
hyperhidrosis: condition (*osis*) in which there is excessive (*hyper*) sweating (*hidr*).
hypermastia: condition in which the female breast is abnormally large. Only one breast may be involved.
hypertrichosis: condition (*osis*) in which there is an excessive (*hyper*) amount of hair (*trich*).
hypomastia: condition in which there is an abnormally underdeveloped [under (*hypo*)] breast. May be on one or both sides.
ichthyosis: condition (*osis*) in which skin is dry and scaly like the skin of a fish (*ichthy*).
icterus: condition in which the skin becomes yellow (*icterus*). Another name for *jaundice.*
impetigo: condition in which the skin is invaded (*impetigo*) by bacteria, and superficial eruptions result.
intertrigo: superficial dermatitis between (*inter*) the folds of the skin usually caused by rubbing (*trigo*). Also known as *chafing.*
keloid: scar formation that is elevated and looks like (*oid*) a tumor (*kel*).
laceration: process (*tion*) in which a wound or irregular tear (*lacera*) of the skin or flesh occurs.
lichen: term describing a papular skin eruption. *Lichen planus* is a term describing flat (*planus*) papules (*lichen*).
lupus vulgaris: tuberculosis of the skin so named because it eats away the skin in wolflike (*lupus*) manner. It has a tendency to be chronic (*vulgaris*).
macula: a spot (*macula*) or blotch.
mastitis: inflammation (*itis*) of the breast (*mast*).
melanoma: tumor (*oma*) involving the melanocyte (*melan*) cells in the skin.
miliaria: rash with eruptions the size of very small millet seeds (*mili*). Also known as "heat rash" or "prickly heat."
mole: small spot (*mole*) on the skin, usually of dark color, slightly elevated, and often hairy.
mottled skin: condition in which the color of the skin created by underlying blood vessels is varied (*mottled*).
nevus: mark on the skin, including various types of birthmarks (*nevus*) and all types of moles.
nummular dermatitis: inflammation (*itis*) of the skin (*derma*) characterized by the formation of coin-shaped (*nummular*) lesions.
onychomycosis: disease (*osis*) of the nails (*onych*) because of fungus (*myc*).
peau d'orange: the appearance of the skin of the breast in which it resembles an orange peel (*peau d'orange*).

pediculosis: condition (*osis*) in which there is an infestation of lice (*pedicul*).
pediculosis pubis: a condition in which there are lice in the pubic (*pubis*) hair.
pediculosis capitis: condition known as "head (*capitis*) lice."
pediculosis corporis: condition known as "body (*corporis*) lice."
pemphigus: disease that is characterized by the appearance of vesicles and bullae that resemble bubbles (*pemphi*) under the skin.
petechia: small hemorrhage under the skin that appears as a small spot (*petechia*).
pilonidal cyst: a cyst filled with hair (*pilo*) that grows in a place (*nid,* a variation of nidus) where germs can grow easily. The place is usually at the base of the spine.
pimple: small, circumscribed swelling or elevation of the skin.
pityriasis rosea: skin disease (*iasis*) marked by shedding of reddish (*rosea*) branlike (*pityr*) scales of epidermis.
plantar keratosis: condition (*osis*) in which there is hardening (*kerat*) of the skin of the sole (*plantar*) of the foot.
pruritus: root word meaning "itchiness."
psoriasis: a chronic skin disease (*iasis*) characterized by scaly, itchy (*psor*) patches.
purpura: condition in which there are purple (*purpura*) spots under the skin or mucous membrane.
pustule: small (*ule*), circumscribed elevation of the skin containing pus (*pust*).
rhinophyma: condition in which the nose (*rhino*) grows (*phyma*) in size because of an increase in the thickness of the skin.
scab: crustation that forms over a sore or wound during healing.
scabies: skin disease caused by parasitic mites that burrow under the skin and cause a severe itchiness (*scabies*).
scar: the mark left by a healed wound.
scleroderma: condition that is characterized by the hardening (*sclera*) of the skin (*derma*).
sebaceous cyst: condition in which the sebaceous gland is closed and becomes a saclike (*cyst*) structure filled with sebum.
seborrheic dermatitis: inflammation (*itis*) of the skin (*derma*) in which there is an excessive flow (*orrh*) of sebum (*seb*).
superfluous hair: condition in which there is an overabundant (*superfluous*) amount of hair, especially on parts of the body that are not usually covered by hair.
supernumerary breasts: condition in which the individual has a greater (*super*) number (*numerary*) of breasts than is normal.
suppuration: process (*tion*) in which pus is produced (*suppur*).
telangiectasis: condition (*sis*) in which the ends (*tel*) of blood vessels (*angi*) are dilated (*ectasis*), especially the capillaries under the skin of the nose and face.
tinea: skin disease caused by fungus, also known as *ringworm (tinea)*.
tinea barbae: ringworm (*tinea*) of the face, particularly the area where the beard (*barbae*) grows.
tinea capitis: ringworm (*tinea*) of the head (*capitis*).
tinea corporis: ringworm (*tinea*) on the body (*corporis*) or trunk.
tinea pedis: ringworm (*tinea*) of the foot, also known as "athlete's foot."
tinea unguium: fungus infection (*tinea*) of the nails (*unguium*).

ulcer: open sore on the surface of the skin.
urticaria: skin reaction in which there is intense itchiness near pale, irregular raised patches of skin. Also known as "nettle (*urticar*) rash."
verruca: small, flat growths known commonly as warts (*verruca*).
vesicle: rounded area of the skin that is raised and contains fluid. Also known as a "blister."
vitiligo: smooth, white patch of skin (*vitiligo*) caused by loss of pigmentation.
wen: another name for a sebaceous cyst.

Treatment of Diseases of the Integumentary System

Terms related to the treatment of diseases of the integumentary system:

antipruritic drugs: medicines used against (*anti*) or to control itchiness (*pruritic*).
debridement: action which results in the removal of dead tissue which restrains (*bride*) the healing of a lesion. This can be done by surgical means or by the use of drugs.
depilatory: agent for the removal (*de*) of hair (*pila*).
dermabrasion: scraping (*abrasion*) of the skin (*derma*) usually to remove acne scars.
electrolysis: destruction (*lysis*) of hair follicles by means of an electrical (*electro*) current through a needle inserted into hair follicles.
emollient: medicinal preparation (*ent,* variation of *ment*) used to soften (*emolli*) the skin.
epilating wax: use of hot wax to pull out (*e,* variation of *ex*) hair (*pila*).
incision and drainage: procedure involving the cutting into (*incision*) of an inflamed area to remove (*drain*) pus.
keratolytic lotion: liquid preparation used to break down (*lytic*) a layer of hard skin (*kerato*).
lumpectomy: surgical removal (*ectomy*) of an isolated tumor (*lump*).
mammography: taking x-ray (*graphy*) pictures of the breast (*mammo*).
mammoplasty: plastic surgery (*plasty*) of the breast (*mammo*). Augmentation mammoplasty is the procedure done to increase (*augment*) the size of the breasts. Reduction mammoplasty is the procedure done to reduce (*reduct*) the size of the breasts.
mastectomy: removal (*ectomy*) of a breast (*mast*).
scabicide: preparation used to kill (*cide*) the organism that causes scabies (*scabi*).
skin graft: procedure done in which a living portion of skin from one part of the body is transplanted (*graft*) to another part of the body to replace lost skin (see Glossary of Terms Related to Transplantation).

PRETEST/ POSTTEST FOR CHAPTER 19

1. The following sentences are related to skin. Select the terms that best complete the statements.

   1. The term meaning tissue containing fat is ____.
      A. adipose tissue
      B. subcutaneous tissue

   2. The root word for skin is ____.
      A. pilus
      B. cutis

   3. The layer of tissue on the surface of the body is called ____.
      A. the epidermis
      B. the dermis

   4. The cells responsible for the relatively dark color of skin are ____.
      A. melanocytes
      B. dermatocytes

   5. The layer that is called the true skin is the ____.
      A. dermis
      B. epidermis

   6. The layer of tissue connecting the skin with the underlying structures is called ____.
      A. integument
      B. subcutaneous

2. The following sentences are related to hair. Select the terms that best complete the statements.

   1. The name of the muscle that allows the hair to stand on end is the ____ muscle.
      A. arrector pili
      B. follicular pili

   2. The hair ____ is the cavity in which the hair grows.
      A. follicle
      B. shaft

   3. The hair ____ is the long, polelike portion of a hair.
      A. follicle
      B. shaft

4. A root word meaning hair is ____.
   A. cilia and hidr
   B. pilus and tricho

3. Using the following terms, fill in the blanks in the statements.

cilia	pubic hair
axillary	eyebrow
lanugo	

1. Hair in the armpit is called ________.
2. The hairs on the edge of the eyelids are called ________.
3. ________ is the fine hair on the body of a newborn baby.
4. The hair over the pubic area is called ________.
5. The hair on the ridge of the forehead is called the ________.

4. The following terms are related to sebaceous glands and sweat glands. Match column A with column B.

Column A	Column B
1. ____ sebaceous glands	A. another name for sweat
2. ____ sebum	B. glands found in armpits and pubic area
3. ____ apocrine glands	C. oily glandular secretion which gives hair and skin its glossy appearance
4. ____ eccrine glands	D. glands found over most of the body, especially the hands and feet
5. ____ hidr	E. glands that open into hair follicles or directly onto the surface of the skin
6. ____ perspiration	F. root word meaning sweat

5. The following terms are related to the nails. Use them to fill in the blanks.

cuticle	paronychial
lunula	subungual
onych	ungual
onyx	

1. The moon-shaped white area at the base on the nail is called the ________.
2. The small area of dead skin around the edge of the nail is called the ________.
3. The area under the nail is called ________.
4. The area around the nail is called ________.
5. The three root words meaning nail are ________, ________, and ________.

6. The following terms are related to the breast.

areola	mammary gland	nipple
galact or lacto	mast	lactation

1. The tip or point of the breast is called the ________.

2. The small area of color around the nipple is called the ________.

3. The breast of the female is sometimes called the ________.

4. The process of producing milk is called ________.

5. The root word for milk is ________.

6. The root word for breast is ________.

7. The following sets of terms are related to diseases of the integumentary system, including signs and symptoms of disease. Match column A with column B. Choose the one best answer.

Set 1

Column A	Column B
1. _____ abrasion	A. large vesicle
2. _____ acne	B. discolored plug in sebaceous gland
3. _____ alopecia	C. bed sore
4. _____ amastia	D. bump resulting from an infection
5. _____ angioma	E. loss of hair
6. _____ blackhead	F. excessive sweating
7. _____ boil	G. congenital absence of a breast
8. _____ bulla	H. inflammation of the skin
9. _____ burn	I. pointed, pus-filled eruptions
10. _____ decubitus ulcer	J. tumor consisting of blood vessels
11. _____ dermatitis	K. scraped away portion of skin
12. _____ diaphoresis	L. skin trauma resulting from exposure to harmful substance

Set 2

Column A	Column B
1. _____ callus	A. inflammation of the lips
2. _____ carbuncle	B. goose bumps
3. _____ cellulitis	C. cold and wet feeling to skin surface
	D. injury to tissue under skin without skin being broken

Column A

4. _____ cheilitis
5. _____ clammy skin
6. _____ contusion
7. _____ cutis anserina
8. _____ eczema
9. _____ ecthyma
10. _____ epithelioma
11. _____ erythema
12. _____ erythema nodosum
13. _____ erythromelalgia
14. _____ erysipelas
15. _____ eschar
16. _____ excoriation

Column B

E. disease characterized by the spread of deep red color over skin
F. fluid rushing out of sores in the skin
G. redness of skin
H. loss of skin by trauma
I. hardened area of skin
J. inflammation of cellular tissue
K. painful, red sore containing pus
L. hard scab
M. tumor of epithelial tissue
N. flowing of fluid from affected area
O. skin over the extremities reddened and painful
P. red lumps appearing on the skin

Set 3

Column A

1. _____ furuncle
2. _____ gangrene
3. _____ gynecomastia
4. _____ hives
5. _____ hypermastia
6. _____ ichthyosis
7. _____ icterus
8. _____ impetigo
9. _____ intertrigo
10. _____ keloid
11. _____ lichen
12. _____ lupus vulgaris
13. _____ mastitis
14. _____ hidradenitis
15. _____ hirsute

Column B

A. enlarged male breast
B. tuberculosis of the skin
C. dry and scaly skin
D. papular skin eruption
E. very itchy raised patches
F. inflammation of the breast
G. elevated scar
H. chafing between folds of skin
I. inflammation of a sweat gland
J. yellowed skin
K. excessive hairiness
L. abnormally large breasts in the female
M. necrotic skin and soft tissue
N. bacterial invasion causing skin eruptions
O. another name for a boil

8. In the following four sets of phrases use the lists of terms to fill in the blanks.

Set 1

hyperhidrosis	melanoma
hypertrichosis	miliaria
hypomastia	mottled skin
laceration	nevus
macula	

1. A birthmark is called a ________.
2. Another name for a spot or a blotch is ________.
3. A wound in which there is an irregular tear is called a ________.
4. An excessive amount of sweating is called ________.
5. A term meaning very small, underdeveloped breasts is ________.
6. Another name for heat rash is ________.
7. A condition in which there is an excessive amount of hair is called ________.
8. A condition in which there is variation in the color of skin produced by the underlying blood vessels is called ________.
9. A tumor of the melanocyte cells is called a ________.

Set 2

onychomycosis	petechiae
peau d'orange	pilonidal cyst
nummular	pimple
pediculosis	pityriasis rosea
pemphigus	plantar keratosis

1. A skin disease marked by shedding of reddish, branlike scales is called ________.
2. A small circumscribed swelling or elevation of the skin is commonly called a ________.
3. Small, spotlike hemorrhages under the skin are called ________.
4. ________ is a disease of the nails because of a fungus.
5. An infestation with lice is called ________.
6. When the skin over the breast resembles an orange peel, the term used to describe the skin is ________.
7. A ________ lesion is coin-shaped.
8. Vesicles and bullae that resemble bubbles under the skin are characteristic of a condition called ________.

9. A ________________ is filled with hair and develops in places where germs grow easily.

10. ________________ is a condition in which the skin on the sole of the foot becomes hardened.

Set 3

pruritus	scab
purpura	scabies
psoriasis	scar
pustule	scleroderma
rhinophyma	sebaceous cyst

1. A skin disease characterized by severe itchiness is called ________________.
2. A ________________ is a crust that forms over a sore or wound.
3. ________________ means hardening of the skin.
4. A root word meaning itchiness is ________________.
5. A thickening of the skin of the nose is called ________________.
6. A purple spot under the skin or mucous membrane is called a ________________.
7. A saclike structure filled with sebum is called a ________________.
8. A ________________ is a small circumscribed elevation of the skin that contains pus.
9. A chronic skin disease that is characterized by scaly, itchy patches is ________________.
10. The mark left by a healed wound is called a ________________.

Set 4

superfluous hair	ulcer
supernumerary breasts	urticaria
suppuration	verruca
telangiectasis	vesicle
tinea	vitiligo
seborrheic dermatitis	wen

1. Another name for a sebaceous cyst is ________________.
2. An open sore on the surface of the skin is called an ________________.
3. ________________ indicates an overabundance of hair.
4. ________________ indicates more than the normal number of breasts.
5. Another name for a fungus infection commonly called ringworm is ________________.

6. A ________________ is commonly called a wart.

7. An action in which pus is formed is called ________________.

8. ________________ is a condition in which the ends of blood vessels are dilated.

9. A patch of depigmented skin is called ________________.

10. A rounded area of skin that is raised and contains fluid is called a ________ ________.

11. In ________________ excessive amounts of sebum are produced.

12. ________________ is a skin reaction in which there is intense itching near pale, irregular, raised patches of skin.

9. The following terms are related to the treatment of diseases of the integumentary system. Match column A with column B. Be specific.

Column A	Column B
1. _____ antipruritic drug	A. scraping skin to remove acne scars
2. _____ debridement	B. preparation used to soften skin
3. _____ dermabrasion	C. preparation used to pull hair out
4. _____ depilatory	D. preparation that controls itchiness
5. _____ electrolysis	E. cutting into a part and removing pus
6. _____ emollient	F. chemical preparation for removal of hair
7. _____ epilating wax	G. removal of isolated tumor
8. _____ keratolytic lotion	H. liquid preparation used to break down a layer of hard skin
9. _____ incision and drainage	I. removal of hair with electric current
10. _____ lumpectomy	J. procedure to remove dead tissue
11. _____ mammography	K. portion of living skin transplanted to replace lost skin
12. _____ mammoplasty	L. x-ray examination of breasts
13. _____ mastectomy	M. preparation that kills scabies germs
14. _____ scabicide	N. plastic surgery done on breasts
15. _____ skin graft	O. removal of a breast

PRETEST/ POSTTEST **ANSWERS** FOR CHAPTER **19**

1. **1.** A **2.** B **3.** A **4.** A **5.** A **6.** B

2. **1.** A **2.** A **3.** B **4.** B

3. **1.** axillary **2.** cilia **3.** lanugo **4.** pubic hair **5.** eyebrow

4. **1.** E **2.** C **3.** B **4.** D **5.** F **6.** A

5. **1.** lunula **2.** cuticle **3.** subungual **4.** paronychial **5.** onych, onyx, ungual

6. **1.** nipple **2.** areola **3.** mammary gland **4.** lactation **5.** galact, lacto **6.** mast

7. **Set 1**
1. K **2.** I **3.** E **4.** G **5.** J **6.** B **7.** D **8.** A **9.** L **10.** C **11.** H **12.** F

Set 2
1. I **2.** K **3.** J **4.** A **5.** C **6.** D **7.** B **8.** N or F **9.** F or N **10.** M **11.** G **12.** P **13.** O **14.** E **15.** L **16.** H

Set 3
1. O **2.** M **3.** A **4.** E **5.** L **6.** C **7.** J **8.** N **9.** H **10.** G **11.** D **12.** B **13.** F **14.** I **15.** K

8. **Set 1**
1. nevus
2. macula
3. laceration
4. hyperhidrosis
5. hypomastia
6. miliaria
7. hypertrichosis
8. mottled
9. melanoma

Set 2
1. pityriasis rosea
2. pimple
3. petechiae
4. onychomycosis
5. pediculosis
6. peau d'orange
7. nummular
8. pemphigus
9. pilonidal cyst
10. plantar keratosis

Set 3

1. scabies
2. scab
3. scleroderma
4. pruritus
5. rhinophyma
6. purpura
7. sebaceous cyst
8. pustule
9. psoriasis
10. scar

Set 4

1. wen
2. ulcer
3. superfluous hair
4. supernumerary breasts
5. tinea
6. verruca
7. suppuration
8. telangiectasis
9. vitiligo
10. vesicle
11. seborrheic dermatitis
12. urticaria

9. **1.** D **2.** J **3.** A **4.** F **5.** I **6.** B **7.** C **8.** H **9.** E **10.** G **11.** L **12.** N **13.** O **14.** M **15.** K

20 THE EYE

OBJECTIVES

At the end of this chapter you will be able to do the following:

1 Define terms related to the eye.
2 Define terms related to the external structure of the eye, including the orbital cavity, the extrinsic muscles, the eyelids, the conjunctiva, and the lacrimal apparatus.
3 Describe terms related to the internal structure of the eye, including the wall of the eyeball, the inside of the eyeball, the eye fluids, and the lens.
4 List terms related to the sense of vision, including those related to focusing, field of vision, depth perception, and the nerve pathway to the brain.
5 Analyze selected terms related to signs and symptoms and disease conditions of the structure of the eye and abnormal conditions of vision.
6 Analyze selected terms related to the diagnosis and treatment of conditions of the eye.

THE EYES

The eyes are very delicate, globular organs. They are the visual sensory organs that distinguish the size, shape, placement, color, and distance of an object.

Terms related to the eye:

bulb: rounded, onionlike (*bulb*) shape of the eye.
fundus oculi: the body of the eye or the portion of the eye (*oculi*) opposite the entrance (*fundus*), or the pupil.
globe: rounded (*globe*) part of the eye. Another name for eyeball.
oculo: combining form meaning "eye."
ophthalmo-: combining form meaning "eye."
opia, ops: root words meaning a condition of sight.
optic: pertaining to the eye or sight.

EXTERNAL STRUCTURE OF THE EYE

The external structure of the eye comprises all of the structures involved in holding, protecting, and moving the eyeball.

The external structures of the eye include the following:

orbital cavity
extrinsic muscles
eyelids
conjunctiva
lacrimal apparatus

Orbital Cavity

The eye is situated in the orbital cavity, which is a bony, cone-shaped space in the front of the skull. It is lined with fatty tissue to cushion the eye.

The optic nerve and ophthalmic artery enter the cavity through the optic canal.

Terms related to the orbital cavity:

orbital cavity: round (*orbit*) bony socket (*cavity*) that contains and protects the eyeball.
retrobulbar fat: the thick, fatty (*fat*) cushion of tissue in back of (*retro*) the eyeball (*bulbar*).

Extrinsic Muscles

The extrinsic muscles are attached to each eye. These six muscles control the movement of the eye.

There are four straight (*rectus*) muscles and two oblique muscles.

superior rectus: attaches to the top (*superior*) surface of the eye.
inferior rectus: attaches to the bottom (*inferior*) surface of the eye.
lateral rectus: attaches to the lateral side of the eye.
medial rectus: attaches to the medial side of the eye.
superior oblique: attaches to the top (*superior*) surface of the eye.
inferior oblique: attaches to the bottom (*inferior*) surface of the eye.

The muscles of the eyes are coordinated in such a way that normally both eyes move together. For example, when looking to the left the lateral muscle of the left eye and the medial muscle of the right eye contract so that both eyes move at once. This is termed *conjugate eye movement.* The eyes move as if they were yoked (*jug*) together (*con*).

Eyelids

The eyelids are two movable folds of tissue located in front of the eye. The eyelids protect the eye from intense light, dust, and impact.

The eyelids meet at the canthus. The edges of the eyelids are lined with two or three rows of eyelashes that also protect the eye.

A plate of fibrous tissue, the tarsus, is located at the edges of the eyelid. This gives the delicate skin of the eyelid shape and firmness.

The tarsal plate contains tarsal or meibomian glands that are a form of sebaceous gland.

Terms related to the eyelid:

blepharo: root word meaning "eyelid."
canthus: the angle made by the eyelids that is located at the corner (*canthus*) of each eye.
inner canthus: corner of (*canthus*) the eye toward (*inner*) the midline.
outer canthus: the corner (*canthus*) of the eye away from (*outer*) the midline.
caruncle: small (*cle*) piece of flesh (*carun*) at the inner corner of the eyelids.
cilia: the eyelashes.
palpebra: term meaning "eyelid."
tarsus: flat (*tarsus*) cartilage of the eyelid.
tarsal glands: glands in the tarsal plate that secrete an oily substance that acts as a barrier to keep tears in the eyes. Also called *meibomian glands.*

Conjunctiva

The conjunctiva is a thin layer of mucous membrane that lines the inner surface of each eyelid and covers the exposed surface of each eyeball. The conjunctiva is a continuous membrane with opposed surfaces that slide past each other when the eyelids close and open. It is the membrane that serves to connect (*conjunct*) the globe of the eye to the eyelids.

Lacrimal Apparatus

The lacrimal apparatus functions to produce tears that lubricate and wash the eyes.

Tears are produced in the lacrimal gland, which is lateral and superior to the eyeball.

As the fluid drains from the lacrimal gland, it washes over the conjunctiva to the inner canthus. There it drains into two openings: the superior and inferior lacrimal puncta. These openings lead to the superior and inferior lacrimal canaliculi, to the lacrimal sac, into the nasolacrimal duct, and finally into the nose.

Terms related to the lacrimal apparatus listed in order from the lacrimal gland to the nose:

lacrimal gland: tissue mass (*gland*) that secretes tears (*lacrimal*).
lacrimal punctum: hole (*punctum*) at the inner angle of the eye through which tears drain.
lacrimal canaliculi: small (*uli*) canals that transport tears from the eye to the duct in the nose.
lacrimal sac: pouchlike (*sac*) area at the beginning of the nasolacrimal duct.
nasolacrimal duct: tube (*duct*) that transports tears (*lacrimal*) down the nose (*naso*).
dacryo-: combining form meaning "tears."
lacrimal fluid: fluid from the lacrimal glands; tears.
lacrimation: act of (*tion*) shedding tears (*lacrima*).

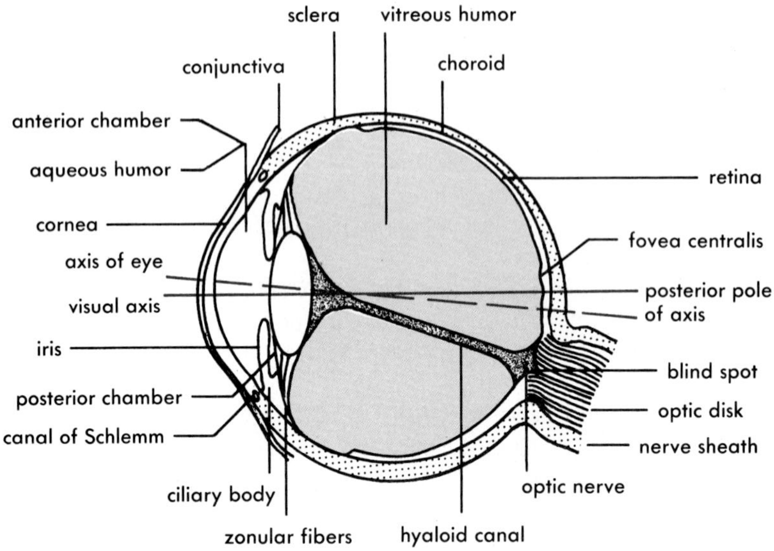

FIGURE 20-1
Horizontal section through the eye.

INTERNAL STRUCTURES OF THE EYE

The internal structures of the eye involve the globe of the eyeball. They are considered internal structures because they are all housed within the orbital cavity.

The internal structures include the following (Figure 20-1):

wall of the eyeball
inside of the eyeball
eye fluids (aqueous and vitreous humor)
lens

Wall of the Eyeball

The eyeball is covered by three separate layers (Table 20-1).

Outer layer

The sclera covers approximately three-quarters of the eyeball. It is the white, fibrous, and relatively tough layer of the eye. The optic nerve, central artery, and vein penetrate the sclera at the back of the eye.

The cornea is a transparent circular segment covering the iris and pupil. It has a slight outward curvature.

The sclera and cornea are joined at the sclerocorneal junction or limbus. Close to this juncture in the sclera is an opening called the venous sinus or canal of Schlemm. This sinus is the place where the excess eye fluids leave the eyeball and drain into the venous system.

TABLE 20-1
Layers of the Eye

Outer Layer	Middle Layer	Inner Layer
sclera	uvea or uveal tract, consisting of three sections from	vision receptor layer,
cornea	back to front: the choroid, the ciliary body, the iris	the retina

Terms related to the outer layer of the eye:

cornea: transparent circular structure covering the front of the eye. It covers the iris and pupil.
kerato: root word denoting relationship to the cornea.
limbus: circular edge (*limbus*) where the sclera joins the cornea.
sclera: white, dense, relatively hard (*scler*) covering of the eye. The white of the eye.
sclerocorneal junction: circular area where the sclera (*sclera*) joins (*junction*) the cornea (*corneal*). Same as limbus.
venous sinus: space (*sinus*) through the sclera where the inside fluids of the eye drain into the venous system. Excess aqueous humor is drained through this space. Also known as the canal of Schlemm.

Middle layer

The middle layer, also known as the uvea or uveal tract, consists of three segments: the choroid, the ciliary body, and the iris.

The choroid segment is a dark, thin membrane that contains the arteries and veins nourishing the eye. It surrounds the back three-quarters of the eye and is continuous with the ciliary body.

The ciliary body is a circular band of muscle and fiber. The muscle suspends and controls the shape and curvature of the lens. The ciliary body is attached to the lens.

The iris is a circular, pigmented, muscular diaphragm in the front of the eye. The diaphragm opening is called the pupil. The size of the opening varies according to the amount of light needed to focus. An open pupil is dilated, and a relatively closed pupil is constricted.

Terms related to the middle layer:

choroid: membrane (*chor*) layer of the eye that contains the blood vessels.
ciliary body: circular band of muscle and fiber that controls the shape and curvature of the lens.
irido-: combining form meaning "iris."
iris: circular, pigmented, muscular organ in the front of the eye. The term *iris* means "rainbow" and is used because the colors of the iris vary.
pupil: expanding or contracting opening in the center of the iris. The term means "little doll" and is used because of the small images reflected on the pupil.
uveal tract: middle layer of the eye. If the outer layer were peeled off, exposing the middle layer, the eye would resemble a grape (*uv*).

Inside layer

The retina is the inside layer of the eye. It is composed chiefly of nervous tissue and is the part of the eye that receives impulses or images of external objects.

The retina is continuous with the optic nerve at the back of the eye and continues around the eye to the front, where it attaches to the ciliary body.

The retina is a soft, semitransparent tissue with many layers of nerve cells. It contains layers of rods and cones, which are the nerve receptors for light.

The point at which the optic nerve enters the eyeball and becomes continuous with the retina is called the optic disk. This area does not contain rods or cones and is also called the "blind spot."

Close to the disk in the exact center of the back part of the retina is an oval area called the macula lutea (see Figure 20-1, referring to the line indicating the visual axis). In the center of the macula lutea is a depression called the fovea centralis. The fovea contains only cones. This is the area of keenest vision.

Terms related to the retina or inside layer:

fovea centralis: small pit (*fovea*) or depression in the center (*centralis*) of the macula in the back of the eye.
macula lutea: yellow (*lutea*) spot (*macula*) at the back of the eye.
optic disk: circular area (*disk*) at the back of the eye (*optic*) where the optic nerve and blood vessels enter the eye.
papilla-: combining form denoting the nipplelike (*papilla*) appearance at the optic disk.
retina: inside layer of the eye that receives images of external objects.
rods and cones: receptors of light in the retina.

Inside of the Eyeball

The inside of the eyeball is divided by the lens into two sections, the front section and the back section.

The front section contains the aqueous humor. It is divided into two chambers: The *anterior chamber* is the space between the iris and the cornea. The *posterior chamber* is between the iris and the lens.

The lens comes next, and then the back section of the eyeball, which contains the vitreous humor.

Fluids of the Eye

There are two fluids or humors of the eye: aqueous and vitreous.

Aqueous humor is the watery fluid in the front section of the eye.

Vitreous humor is the transparent gelatinous substance in the back section of the eye behind the lens. It is sometimes called the vitreous body because it is a physical mass. It gives the eyeball shape and helps hold the retina in place. The hyaloid canal is a tubelike space in the glasslike (*hyaloid*) vitreous humor. It functions in the development of the eye in the embryo.

Terms related to the fluids of the eye:

aqueous humor: watery (*aqueous*) circulating fluid (*humor*) in the front part of the eye.

vitreous humor: fluid (*humor*) in the back section of the eye that is as transparent as glass (*vitreous*).

VISION

The eye functions as the sensory organ of sight. Vision includes the following:

focusing
field of vision and depth perception
nerve pathway to the brain

Focusing

For a conscious awareness of the sense of vision the image of external objects must be focused, or formed on the retina.

Focus is the point at which rays of light meet. The focusing of rays of light by the lens that makes an image on the retina is called accommodation.

The rays of light that enter the eye are bent as they pass through the cornea, lens, and fluids of the eye. This bending of light rays is called refraction.

Terms related to focusing:

accommodation: action (*tion*) of adjusting (*accommoda*) the thickness of the lens to focus the image on the retina.

emmetropia: the measure (*metr*) of the distance from the lens to the focused image in the eye (*opia*) is correct for normal vision, because the image lies on (*em*) the retina.

refraction: act of (*action*) breaking (*fract*) up light rays as they enter the eye, and redirecting (*re*) the angle of the rays so that they focus on the retina.

Field of Vision

The measurement of how far the eye can see in all directions marks the field of vision. When the eye is in a fixed position, it is capable of viewing objects directly in front of it and in an area around that point. This is called peripheral vision.

The action of the muscles allows the eye to rotate and pick up images at different angles without the need to move the head.

Depth Perception

The eyes are so situated that the fields of vision of the two eyes overlap, with each eye receiving a slightly different view.

The design of having two slightly different views is called binocular vision. Because there are two different views transmitted to the brain, the brain is able to take the views and fuse them together to create perception of the third dimension.

Terms related to field of vision and depth perception:

binocular: involving both (*bin*) eyes (*ocular*).
orthoptic: condition in which there is normal position of the eyes, or vision in which the eyes (*optic*) are straight (*orth*) and not turned inward or outward.
peripheral vision: the area around (*peripheral*) the point directly in front that is visible without moving the eye.
scopic: root word pertaining to (*ic*) vision (*scop*).

Nerve Pathway to the Brain

When the image is focused on the retina, the rods and cones become stimulated. The light rays are converted to nerve impulses.

These impulses are picked up and sent to the optic nerve at the optic disk. Fibers of the optic nerve leave the eyes and extend to the optic chiasm. The optic chiasm is the area in the brain where there is a crossover of some of the optic nerve fibers from left to right. The crossover of the fibers results in a formation resembling the Greek letter *chi* (χ).

At the optic chiasm the nerves from each eye split into nerve tracts, and parts of each nerve continue to the visual center of the brain that is the occipital lobe of the cerebrum.

DISEASE CONDITIONS OF THE EYE

Analysis of selected terms related to disease or abnormal conditions of the eye:

amblyopia: term meaning dull (*ambly*) vision (*opia*). Also known as "lazy eye" because the dullness of vision results from not using (*lazy*) the eye.
ametropia: general term denoting a refractive disorder. The measure (*metr*) of the distance from the lens to the focused image does not (*a*) correspond to the distance to the retina, where the focused image should be.
anisometropia: condition in which the focusing ability of each eye is different. There is unequal (*aniso*) vision.
anopia: condition (*ia*) in which there is no (*an*) vision (*op*); usually in one eye.
aphakia: condition in which there is no (*a*) lens (*phakia*) either from birth or after surgery for removal of a cataract.
arcus senilis: appearance of a ring (*arcus*) of white cloud around the cornea in elderly persons.
astigmatism: condition (*ism*) in which light rays do not (*a*) converge to a point (*stigmat*). An image is not focused clearly on any spot.
blepharitis: inflammation (*itis*) of the eyelid (*blephar*).
blepharoptosis: drooping (*ptosis*) eyelids (*blepharo*).
cataract: lens becomes opaque as if flooded with a rush of water (*cataract*), and thus the amount of light that will pass through it is diminished.
chalazion: lump (*chalazion*) formed in the tarsal or meibomian glands of the eyelid.
color blindness: state of (*ness*) being unable to see (*blind*) or to distinguish some colors.

conjunctivitis: inflammation (*itis*) of the conjunctiva (*conjunctiv*).
corneal ulcers: sores (*ulcers*) on the cornea (*corneal*).
dacryoadenitis: inflammation (*itis*) of the tear (*dacryo*) gland (*aden*).
dacryocystitis: inflammation (*itis*) of the tear (*dacryo*) sac (*cyst*).
detached retina: condition in which the retina is pulled (*tach*) away (*de*) from the choroid and is floating in the vitreous humor.
diplopia: condition (*ia*) in which there is double (*dipl*) vision (*op*).
ectropion: condition in which the eyelid is turned (*tropion*) out (*ec*) and does not protect the eye.
enophthalmia: inward (*en*) or sunken-in condition (*ia*) of the eye (*ophthalm*).
entropion: condition in which the eyelid is turned (*tropion*) inward (*en*).
epicanthus: condition in which a vertical fold of skin covers over (*epi*) the inner angle (*canthus*) of the eye.
epiphora: condition in which there is excessive tearing. The tears are brought (*phor*) on (*epi*) the cheek.
episcleritis: inflammation (*itis*) of the tissue over (*epi*) the sclera (*scler*).
esotropia: "cross-eyed"; a turning (*tropia*) in (*eso*) of the eyes.
exophthalmia: an outward (*ex*) or protruding condition (*ia*) of the eye (*ophthalm*).
exotropia: "wall-eyed"; a turning (*tropia*) out (*exo*) of the eyes.
glaucoma: disease condition which is characterized by an increase in the pressure within the eye.
hemianopia: condition (*ia*) of loss (*an*) of vision (*op*) in one half (*hemi*) of the visual field.
hordeolum: eruption resembling a small (*olum*) barley seed (*horde*) on the edge of the eyelid. Also called a "stye."
hyperopia: the distance to the focused image from the lens is greater (*hyper*) than the length of the eye (*opia*). The image is focused in back of the retina. Also known as *hypermetropia* or *farsightedness.*
hypopyon: presence of pus (*pyo*) under (*hypo*) the cornea in the anterior chamber.
iridocyclitis: inflammation (*itis*) of the iris (*irido*) and the ciliary body (*cycl*).
iridodialysis: splitting (*lysis*) through (*dia*) of the iris (*irido*). The circular ring of the iris (*irido*) is broken or split (*lysis*) through (*dia*).
keratitis: inflammation (*itis*) of the cornea (*kerat*).
keratoconjunctivitis: inflammation (*itis*) of the cornea (*kerato*) and conjunctiva (*conjunctiv*).
keratoconus: conelike (*conus*) bulging of the cornea (*kerato*).
leukoma: dense, white (*leuk*) opacity of the cornea.
mydriasis: dilation of the pupil.
myopia: condition in which the object being viewed is focused in front of the retina. The term literally means a squinting (*my*) of the eye (*opia*). A myopic person squints the eye (*myopia*) in attempting to see a distant object. Also called *nearsightedness* because objects that are near are clearly seen.
myosis: condition characterized by a small (*myo*) or constricted pupil.
nebula: faint, cloudlike (*nebula*) opacity of the cornea.
nyctalopia: condition (*ia*) in which there is blindness or poor (*al*) vision (*op*) at night (*nyct*). Also called "night blindness."

nystagmus: an involuntary oscillation or swinging movement of the eyeball, usually from side to side, but sometimes up and down or around.
ophthalmoplegia: paralysis (*plegia*) of one or more of the muscles of the eye (*ophthalm*).
optic neuritis: inflammation (*itis*) of the optic nerve (*neur*).
papilledema: swelling (*edema*) around the papilla at the optic disk.
papillitis: inflammation (*itis*) of the papilla at the optic disk.
photophobia: an intolerance or dread (*phobia*) of light.
presbyopia: refractive disorder of the eye (*opia*) associated with older (*presby*) persons.
proptosis: a falling (*ptosis*) forward (*pro*) of the eyeball from its socket; a bulging of the eye.
pterygium: a small (*ium*), winglike (*pteryg*) fold of conjunctiva extending from the inner corner of the eye laterally over the eye.
refractive disorders: the parallel light rays entering the eye are bent (*fract*) at such an angle that the rays do not focus on the retina.
retinitis: inflammation (*itis*) of the retina.
retinopathy: general term for diseases (*pathy*) of the retina (*retino*).
scleritis: inflammation (*itis*) of the sclera (*scler*).
scotoma: loss of vision in part of the visual field; a blind spot or dark spot (*scotoma*) is seen.
squint: a partial closing of the eye in an attempt to focus.
strabismus: disorder of vision because of the turning of one or both eyes from their normal position so that both are not aimed in the same direction.
subconjunctival hemorrhage: bleeding (*hemorrhage*) under (*sub*) the conjunctiva.
sympathetic ophthalmia: condition (*ia*) in one eye (*ophthalm*) that occurs when the other eye has been injured. The noninjured eye suffers (*pathy*) with (*sym*) the injured eye.
trachoma: disease in which rough (*trach*) swellings (*oma*) appear on the surface of the eye.
trichiasis: condition (*iasis*) in which the hairs (*trich*) of the eyelid grow inward.
uveitis: inflammation (*itis*) of the uveal tract (*uv*), or middle layer of the eyeball.

Diagnosis and Treatment

Analysis of selected terms related to the diagnosis and treatment of conditions of the eye:

blepharoplasty: surgical procedure (*plasty*) done on the eyelid (*blepharo*).
corneal transplant: transplant of a cornea from one person to another.
cyclodialysis: surgical procedure in which a split (*lysis*) in the ciliary body (*cyclo*) is made around the iris to treat glaucoma.
dacryocystorhinostomy: surgical procedure in which an opening (*ostomy*) is made through the side of the nose (*rhin*) to drain the sac (*cysto*) that stores tears (*dacryo*).
enucleation: action (*ation*) that results in the removal of the eyeball. The eyeball is removed in total like a nut (*nucle*) from its shell.

gonioscope: device (*scope*) that measures the angle (*gonio*) between the corneoscleral junction and the iris.

intraocular surgery: any surgical procedure involving structures inside (*intra*) the eyeball (*ocular*).

iridectomy: the removal of (*ectomy*) part of the iris (*irid*).

keratoplasty: surgical procedure (*plasty*) performed on the cornea (*kerato*), including a corneal transplant.

keratoscope: device (*scope*) that measures the curves of the cornea (*kerato*).

laser photocoagulation: use of laser light (*photo*) rays to coagulate (*coagulate*) tissue to treat a detached retina.

miotic: a drug that causes the pupil to constrict or shut (*myo*). Also spelled *myotic.*

mydriatic: a drug that is used to dilate the pupil.

ophthalmoscope: instrument used to view (*oscope*) the inside of the eyeball (*ophthalm*).

orthoptic training: instructions in exercises aimed at straightening (*orth*) the direction of the eyes (*optic*).

phacoemulsification: surgical procedure in which the lens of the eye (*phaco*) is made (*fica*) somewhat liquid (*emulsi*) and thus can be easily removed through a needle.

refraction: changing of the direction (*refraction*) of light rays by means of an artificial lens to ensure the formation of the image on the retina.

- *concave lens:* lens that is curved inward, thus bending the light rays to a lesser degree, allowing the image to be focused at a longer distance. Used for the correction of myopia or nearsightedness.
- *convex lens:* lens that is rounded outward, thus bending the light rays to a greater degree and allowing the image to be focused at a shorter distance. Used in the correction of hyperopia or farsightedness.
- *contact lens:* refractive lens that comes in direct contact with the eyeball.
- *irregular lens:* refractive lens that is neither concave nor convex, but a combination (*irregular*) to accommodate the refractive condition of astigmatism.

repair of strabismus: surgical procedure for extrinsic ocular muscles that are not permitting both eyes to move in a conjugated manner.

scleral buckling operation: removal of a strip of sclera (*scleral*) near the site of a detached retina, followed by placement of a device and tightening around the device to buckle the sclera.

sclerotomy: cutting into (*otomy*) the sclera (*scler*).

scotometry: use of special charts to measure (*metry*) blind spots (*scoto*) in the field of vision.

surgical orbital decompression: surgical procedure done on the orbit of the eye (*orbital*) to reduce (*de*) the pressure (*compression*) on the eye and allow it to return to a normal place in the orbit.

tarsorrhaphy: procedure done to suture (*rrhaphy*) the eyelids (*tarso*) together.

tonometer: device used to measure (*meter*) the degree of tension (*tono*) or pressure in the eyeball.

vitrectomy: removal of (*ectomy*) some of the vitreous (*vitr*) humor.

PRETEST/ POSTTEST FOR CHAPTER 20

1. The following terms are related to the eye. Select the best answer.

   1. The terms meaning eye are ____.
      A. ocular, ophthalmo
      B. opia, optic
      C. all of the above

   2. The ____ is the rounded part of the eye.
      A. bulb
      B. globe
      C. both of the above

   3. The fundus oculi is ____.
      A. the body of the eye
      B. the portion of the eye opposite the pupil
      C. both of the above

   4. *Ops* is a root word meaning ____.
      A. a condition of sight
      B. eyeball
      C. both of the above

2. The following terms are related to the external structures of the eye. Select the best answer.

   1. The orbital cavity is the ____.
      A. bony socket that contains the eyeball
      B. space inside the eye
      C. both of the above

   2. The thick cushion of tissue in back of the eyeball is the ____.
      A. sclerocorneal junction
      B. retrobulbar fat
      C. both of the above

   3. The muscles of the eye move in such a way that they conjugate; in other words, they ____.
      A. both move together
      B. move as if they were yoked together
      C. both of the above

3. The following terms are related to the extrinsic muscles of the eye. Match column A with column B. Choose the one best answer.

Column A	Column B
1. ____ superior rectus	A. straight muscle that attaches to the bottom surface of the eye
2. ____ inferior rectus	B. oblique muscle that is attached to the bottom of the eye
3. ____ lateral rectus	C. straight muscle that attaches to the lateral side of the eye
4. ____ medial rectus	D. oblique muscle that is attached to the top of the eye
5. ____ superior oblique	E. straight muscle attached to the medial side of the eye
6. ____ inferior oblique	F. straight muscle that attaches to the top surface of the eye

4. The following terms are related to the eyelid. Match column A with column B.

Column A	Column B
1. ____ blepharo	A. root word meaning eyelid
2. ____ canthus	B. small piece of flesh in the inner corner of the eye
3. ____ caruncle	C. flat cartilage of the eyelid
4. ____ cilia	D. corner of the eyelid
5. ____ tarsus	E. eyelashes

5. The ________ is a term meaning eyelids.
   A. retrobulbar
   B. palpebrae
   C. both of the above
6. The conjunctiva is a thin membrane that:
   A. covers the exposed surface of the eyeball.
   B. lines the inner surface of eyelid.
   C. both of the above.
7. The following terms are related to the lacrimal apparatus. Match column A with column B. Choose the one best answer.

Column A	Column B
1. ____ lacrimal fluid	A. tissue that secretes tears
2. ____ lacrimal apparatus	B. small canals that transport tears from the eyes to the nose
3. ____ lacrimal gland	C. tube that carries tears down the nose

Column A	Column B
4. _____ lacrimal punctum	D. group of structures involved in lacrimation
5. _____ lacrimal canaliculus	E. pouchlike area at the beginning of the duct in the nose
6. _____ lacrimal sac	F. hole at the inner angle of the eye
7. _____ nasolacrimal duct	G. tears

8. The following terms are related to the outer layer of the eyeball.

1. The _____ is a transparent circular structure covering the front of the eye.
   A. sclera
   B. cornea
   C. both of the above

2. The _____ is the circular edge where the sclera joins the cornea.
   A. limbus
   B. sclerocorneal junction
   C. both of the above

3. The venous sinus is the space through the sclera where the aqueous humor _____.
   A. drains into the venous system
   B. drains into the nasal sinuses

4. The sclera is _____.
   A. the white of the eye
   B. the covering over the back of the eye
   C. both of the above

5. A root word denoting relationship to the cornea is _____.
   A. kerato
   B. sclerato
   C. both of the above

9. The following terms are related to the middle layer of the eye. Using them, complete the sentences.

choroid	irido
ciliary body	pupil
iris	uveal tract

1. The __________ is in the center of the iris.
2. A root word meaning iris is __________.
3. The circular band of pigmented tissue is the __________.
4. The membrane of the middle layer of the eye that covers the back three-quarters of the eye is called the __________.

5. Another name for the middle layer of the wall of the eye is the __________.

6. The circular band of tissue holding the lens is called the __________.

10. The following terms are related to the inside layer of the eye. Match column A with column B. Choose the one best answer.

Column A	Column B
1. ____ fovea centralis	A. yellow spot in the back of the eye
2. ____ macula lutea	B. receptors of light
3. ____ optic disk	C. term describing the nipplelike form at the back of the eye at the optic disk
4. ____ papilla	D. small pit in the center back of the eye
5. ____ retina	E. membrane lining the inside of the eye
6. ____ rods and cones	F. circular area where the optic nerve and blood vessels enter the eye

11. The following terms are related to the fluids of the eye and the lens. Mark the statements true, *T*, or false, *F*.

1. ____ The front section of the eye contains vitreous humor.
2. ____ The front section is divided into anterior and posterior chambers.
3. ____ Aqueous humor is the watery circulating fluid of the anterior chamber.
4. ____ The lens is held in place by the cornea.
5. ____ A zonule is a small band of tissue attached to the ciliary body.
6. ____ The term *biconvex* means caved in on both sides.
7. ____ The term *phaco* means the lens.

12. The following terms are related to vision. Select the best completions for the sentences.

1. Accommodation means the action of adjusting the:
   A. thickness of the lens.
   B. distance of the object.
   C. both of the above.
2. Emmetropia means:
   A. normal vision.
   B. blindness.
   C. neither of the above.
3. Refraction is the:
   A. reflection off the pupil.
   B. breaking and redirecting of light rays.
   C. both of the above.
4. Peripheral vision is:
   A. the view from one eye.
   B. the area visible without moving the eyes.
   C. both of the above.

5. Binocular:
   A. refers to both eyes.
   B. implies there is half vision in each eye.
   C. both of the above.
6. A term related to vision is:
   A. scopic.
   B. optic.
   C. both of the above.
7. The optic chiasm in the brain:
   A. is the place where the optic nerve fibers cross.
   B. is the place that resembles the letter *X*.
   C. both of the above.

13. The following five sets of terms are related to diseases or abnormal conditions of the eye. In each set match column A with column B. Choose the one best answer.

Set 1

Column A	Column B
1. ____ amblyopia	A. no vision, usually in one eye
2. ____ ametropia	B. image not focused clearly on any spot
3. ____ anisometropia	C. dull vision or "lazy eye"
4. ____ anopia	D. opaque lens
5. ____ aphakia	E. general term meaning a refractive disorder
6. ____ arcus senilis	F. drooping eyelid
7. ____ astigmatism	G. lump in the eyelid
8. ____ blepharitis	H. white, cloudlike ring around the cornea in elderly persons
9. ____ blepharoptosis	I. inability to distinguish some colors
10. ____ cataract	J. inflammation of the eyelid
11. ____ chalazion	K. different focusing ability in each eye
12. ____ color blindness	L. no lens

Set 2

Column A	Column B
1. ____ conjunctivitis	A. inflammation of tissue over the sclera
2. ____ corneal ulcers	B. inflammation of the tear gland
3. ____ dacryoadenitis	C. inside lining of the eye pulled away
4. ____ dacryocystitis	D. fold of skin over the corner of the eye
5. ____ detached retina	E. inflammation of the tear sac
	F. eye appearing to be sunken into the orbit

Column A	Column B
6. ____ diplopia	G. sores on the cornea
7. ____ ectropion	H. the eyelid turned outward
8. ____ enophthalmia	I. inflammation of the conjunctiva
9. ____ entropion	J. excessive tearing
10. ____ epicanthus	K. eyelid turned inward
11. ____ epiphora	L. double vision
12. ____ episcleritis	

Set 3

Column A	Column B
1. ____ esotropia	A. farsightedness
2. ____ exophthalmia	B. turning out of the eyes; wall-eyed
3. ____ exotropia	C. conelike bulging of the cornea
4. ____ glaucoma	D. protruding eyes
5. ____ hemianopia	E. pus under the cornea
6. ____ hordeolum	F. a stye
7. ____ hyperopia	G. inflammation of the iris and ciliary body
8. ____ hypopyon	H. turning in of the eyes; cross-eyed
9. ____ iridocyclitis	I. increased pressure in the eye
10. ____ iridodialysis	J. splitting of the iris
11. ____ keratitis	K. inflammation of the cornea and conjunctiva
12. ____ keratoconus	L. inflammation of the cornea
13. ____ keratoconjunctivitis	M. loss of vision in one half of the visual field

Set 4

Column A	Column B
1. ____ leukoma	A. nearsightedness
2. ____ mydriasis	B. involuntary movement of the eyeball
3. ____ myopia	C. inflammation around the optic disk
4. ____ myosis	D. dense, white opacity of the cornea
5. ____ nebula	E. paralysis of eye muscles
	F. constriction of the pupil
	G. inflammation of the optic nerve

Column A	Column B
6. ____ nyctalopia	H. swelling around the optic disk
7. ____ nystagmus	I. dilation of the pupil
8. ____ optic neuritis	J. night blindness
9. ____ ophthalmoplegia	K. faint, cloudlike opacity of the cornea
10. ____ papilledema	L. a bulging eye
11. ____ papillitis	M. refractive disorder associated with older persons
12. ____ presbyopia	
13. ____ proptosis	

Set 5

Column A	Column B
1. ____ pterygium	A. blind or dark spot in the field of vision
2. ____ refractive disorder	B. noninjured eye suffering with the injured eye
3. ____ retinitis	C. hairs of the eyelid growing inward
4. ____ retinopathy	D. vision not normal because light rays do not focus on the retina
5. ____ scleritis	E. looking with eyes partially closed
6. ____ scotoma	F. winglike fold of conjunctiva extending over the eye
7. ____ squinting	G. bleeding under the conjunctiva
8. ____ strabismus	H. inflammation of the retina
9. ____ subconjunctival hemorrhage	I. rough swelling on the eye
10. ____ sympathetic ophthalmia	J. inflammation of the sclera
11. ____ trachoma	K. both eyes not aimed in the same direction
12. ____ trichiasis	L. inflammation of the middle layer of the eyeball
13. ____ uveitis	M. general term meaning disease of the retina

14. The following four sets of statements are related to the diagnosis and treatment of conditions of the eye.
Using the list of words for each set, complete the statements.

Set 1

blepharoplasty	dacryocystorhinostomy
cyclodialysis	iridectomy

keratoplasty
phacoemulsification
tarsorrhaphy
vitrectomy

1. The surgical procedure in which the lens is more or less liquified is called ________________.
2. The removal of the iris is called ________________.
3. A procedure in which a slit is made around the iris is called ____________.
4. ________________ is a procedure done on the tear sac by going through the nose.
5. An example of ________________ is corneal transplant.
6. ________________ is plastic surgery performed on the eyelid.
7. The removal of some of the vitreous humor is called ________________.
8. The surgical procedure to suture the eyelids together is called ____________.

Set 2

enucleation
intraocular surgery
laser photocoagulation
orthoptic training
surgical orbital decompression
repair of strabismus
scleral buckling operation

1. The instruction in exercises done to straighten the eyes is called ____________.
2. The extrinsic muscles of the eye are operated on in a ________________.
3. The use of special light beams to correct a detached retina is called ________.
4. A procedure done inside the eyeball is called ________________.
5. ________________ is done to allow the eye to return to its normal place in the orbit.
6. The application of a device that is tightened around the sclera is called the ________________.
7. The removal of the eyeball itself is called ________________.

Set 3

gonioscope
keratoscope
ophthalmoscope
scotometry
tonometer

1. ________________ is done to measure blind spots.
2. The device used to measure the degree of pressure in the eyeball is called a ________________.
3. A ________________ measures the angle between the corneoscleral junction and the iris.

4. The instrument used to view the inside of the eye is called the ________ ________.

5. A device used to measure the curves on the cornea is called a ________.

Set 4

miotic	convex lens
mydriatic	contact lens
concave lens	irregular lens

1. A lens that comes in direct contact with the eyeball is called a ________.
2. A lens used to treat astigmatism is called an ________.
3. A lens that curves inward is called a ________.
4. A lens that is rounded outward is called a ________.
5. A drug that dilates the pupil is called a ________ drug.
6. A drug that constricts the pupil is called a ________ drug.

PRETEST/ POSTTEST **ANSWERS** FOR CHAPTER **20**

1.	**1.** A	**2.** C	**3.** C	**4.** A			
2.	**1.** A	**2.** B	**3.** C				
3.	**1.** F	**2.** A	**3.** C	**4.** E	**5.** D	**6.** B	
4.	**1.** A	**2.** D	**3.** B	**4.** E	**5.** C		
5.	B						
6.	C						
7.	**1.** G	**2.** D	**3.** A	**4.** F	**5.** B	**6.** E	**7.** C
8.	**1.** B	**2.** C	**3.** A	**4.** C	**5.** A		
9.	**1.** pupil **2.** irido **3.** iris	**4.** choroid **5.** uveal tract **6.** ciliary body					
10.	**1.** D	**2.** A	**3.** F	**4.** C	**5.** E	**6.** B	
11.	**1.** F	**2.** T	**3.** T	**4.** F	**5.** T	**6.** F	**7.** T
12.	**1.** A	**2.** A	**3.** B	**4.** B	**5.** A	**6.** C	**7.** C

13. Set 1

1. C	3. K	5. L	7. B	9. F	11. G	12. I
2. E	4. A	6. H	8. J	10. D		

Set 2

1. I	3. B	5. C	7. H	9. K	11. J	12. A
2. G	4. E	6. L	8. F	10. D		

Set 3

1. H	3. B	5. M	7. A	9. G	11. L	13. K
2. D	4. I	6. F	8. E	10. J	12. C	

Set 4

1. D	3. A	5. K	7. B	9. E	11. C	13. L
2. I*	4. F*	6. J	8. G	10. H	12. M	

Set 5

1. F	3. H	5. J	7. E	9. G	11. I	13. L
2. D	4. M	6. A	8. K	10. B	12. C	

14. Set 1

1. phacoemulsification
2. iridectomy
3. cyclodialysis
4. dacryocystorhinostomy
5. keratoplasty
6. blepharoplasty
7. vitrectomy
8. tarsorrhaphy

Set 2

1. orthoptic training
2. repair of strabismus
3. laser photocoagulation
4. intraocular surgery
5. surgical orbital decompression
6. scleral buckling operation
7. enucleation

Set 3

1. scotometry
2. tonometer
3. gonioscope
4. ophthalmoscope
5. keratoscope

Set 4

1. contact lens
2. irregular lens
3. concave lens**
4. convex lens**
5. mydriatic†
6. miotic†

---

* To avoid confusing mydriasis with myosis, remember the term that means *d*ilation has a *d* in it, my*d*riasis.

** To avoid confusing concave and convex, remember the concave lens is caved in.

† Refer to question 13-4.

21 THE EAR

OBJECTIVES

At the end of this chapter you will be able to do the following:

1 Define terms related to the external, middle, and inner ear.
2 Define terms related to hearing and equilibrium.
3 Analyze terms related to disease conditions of the ear and related structures.
4 Analyze terms related to the diagnosis and treatment of diseases of the ear.
5 Analyze terms associated with disorders of the sense of hearing.
6 Analyze terms related to the diagnosis of hearing loss.

THE EAR

The ear functions as the organ of the sense of hearing and the sense of balance, or equilibrium. The ears are located in the temporal bone near the mastoid process. The ear consists of three portions: external ear, middle ear, and inner ear (Figure 21-1).

The external ear consists of the auricle and the external auditory meatus. The middle ear consists of the tympanic membrane, the auditory ossicles, the round window, the oval window, the opening into the mastoid process, and the auditory tube. The inner ear consists of the vestibule, the cochlea, and the semicircular canals.

Terms related to the ear:

acoustic: pertaining to the sense of hearing or the organs of hearing.
auri: root word meaning "ear."
ot, oto: root words meaning "ear."

The External Ear

The external ear functions to collect sound waves and channel them into the external auditory meatus, which leads to the tympanic membrane. The auricle has ridges and hollow spaces so that it can direct sound waves into the meatus.

Terms related to the structure of the external ear:

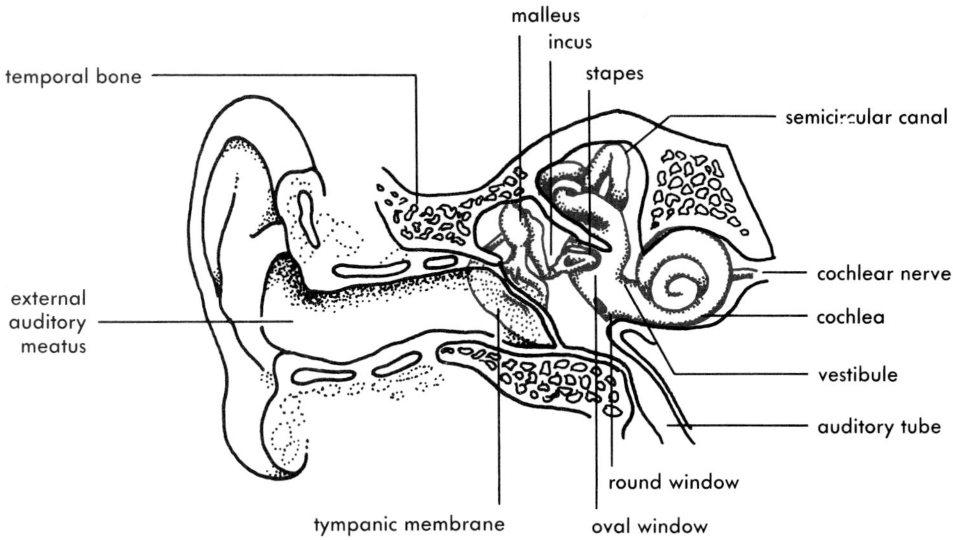

FIGURE 21-1
The ear.

auricle: small (*cle*)—in relation to the head—projecting, outer part of the ear (*auri*).
pinna: winglike [wing (*pinna*)] projection of the ear. Another name for auricle.
helix: curved, rolled (*helix*) fold of cartilage and skin forming the rim of the ear.
concha: shell-shaped [shell (*concha*)] depression at the opening of the ear.
tragus: fleshy prominence at the front of the opening into the ear. It sometimes has hairs on it; therefore it is called the hairy (*tragus*) part of the ear .
lobule: small (*ule*), rounded (*lob*) projection of tissue hanging down from the ear. Commonly known as the *earlobe.*
external auditory meatus: outside (*external*) opening and passage through which sound (*audit*) waves pass to the ear canal.
cerumen: wax (*ceru*) found in the external meatus of the ear.

The Middle Ear

The middle ear is a tiny cavity within the temporal bone. It contains the tympanic membrane and the three auditory ossicles; the malleus, the incus, and the stapes.

The auditory tube extends from the middle ear to the nasopharynx. The round window and oval window open into the inner ear.

The middle ear has three functions. It transmits sound waves from the external ear to the inner ear. It protects the inner ear from loud noises. It allows the pressure on both sides of the tympanic membrane to be equal.

Terms related to the middle ear:

tympanic membrane: tissue (*membrane*) between the external and middle ear that vibrates like a drum (*tympan*) in response to sound waves.

tympanic cavity: another name for the middle ear. It means the space (*cavity*) behind the tympanic membrane.
myringo: root word meaning "tympanic membrane."
eardrum: common name for the tympanic membrane.
auditory ossicles: small (*cle*) bones (*ossi*) that transmit sound waves for hearing (*auditory*).
malleus: first ossicle, which resembles a hammer (*malleus*).
incus: second ossicle, which looks like an anvil (*incus*).
stapes: third ossicle, which resembles a stirrup (*stapes*).
oval window: opening (*window*) into the inner ear to which the oval end of the stapes is connected.
round window: round opening (*window*) through which some sound waves travel into the inner ear.
auditory tube: tube that leads from the middle ear to the nasopharynx. It equalizes the pressure in the middle ear with the external pressure that is important in hearing (*auditory*). It is also called the *eustachian tube.*
salpingo: root word for a tube shaped like a trumpet (*salpingo*). The tube has a narrow end and an opposite end that flares. This term also refers to the tubes attached to the uterus (see Chapter 18).

The Inner Ear

The inner ear consists of the vestibule, the cochlea, and the semicircular canals. The inner ear is sometimes referred to as the *labyrinth* because of the combination of passages from which there is no exit.

The labyrinth consists of membranous tissue lying inside a bony labyrinth. The membranous labyrinth contains a fluid called endolymph.

The bony labyrinth consists of a series of canals hollowed out of the temporal bone.

The cochlea is the organ of hearing. The semicircular canals are the organs of equilibrium.

Terms related to the inner ear:

labyrinth: another name for the structures in the inner ear.
vestibule: chamber at the entrance (*vestibule*) to the inner ear.
cochlea: snail-shaped (*cochlea*) organ that is the organ of hearing.
semicircular canals: three half-circle [half (*semi*), circle (*circular*)] organs in the inner ear that are the organs of balance or equilibrium.
bony labyrinth: outside layer of tissue of the structures in the inner ear.
membranous labyrinth: membrane (*membranous*) layer of tissue inside the bony labyrinth.
endolymph: fluid (*lymph*) inside (*endo*) the labyrinth of the inner ear.

Hearing

The sense of hearing is one of the major senses of the body.

The sensation of sound is produced by vibrations from the outside striking the tympanic membrane. The vibrations, or sound waves, create vibrations of the tympanic membrane, which is attached to the malleus. The ossicles of the middle ear carry the sound waves to the oval window, where they are transmitted to the cochlear membrane. The sensation of sound waves is sent to the brain by way of the cochlear branch of the eighth cranial nerve, or auditory nerve, and the sound sensations are translated by the brain into the sense of hearing.

Terms related to the sense of sound:

audio: term related to the production and transmission of sound.
auditory: pertaining to hearing, to the sense of hearing, or to the organs of hearing.
auditory nerve: the nerve responsible for the sensation of hearing (*auditory*). It also functions in the sense of balance.

Balance

The sense of balance or equilibrium is controlled by nerves in the semicircular canals in the inner ear.

The lining of the canals contains hairs that respond to movement of the fluid inside the canals. The sensation of balance is sent to the brain by way of the vestibular branch of the auditory nerve.

DISEASES OF THE EAR

Diseases of the Ear, Including Signs and Symptoms

Analysis of selected terms related to diseases of the ear, including terms related to signs and symptoms of disease:

aural barotrauma: injury (*trauma*) to the ear (*aural*) resulting from a change in air pressure (*baro*), as in ascent or descent during air travel.
bilateral otitis media: inflammation (*itis*) of the middle (*media*) ear (*ot*). The condition exists on both (*bi*) sides (*lateral*), or in both ears.
endolymphatic hydrops: condition characterized by an abnormal accumulation of the fluid (*hydrops*) inside the membranous labyrinth (*endolymph*) in the inner ear. Commonly known as Ménière's disease.
eustachian salpingitis: inflammation (*itis*) of the tube (*salping*) from the middle ear to the nasopharynx (*eustachian*).
external otitis: inflammation (*itis*) of the external ear (*ot*).
furunculosis: condition (*osis*) of the external ear in which one or more furuncles (*furunculo*) are present.
impacted cerumen: condition in which wax (*cerumen*) is tightly packed (*impacted*) in the ear.
inspissated cerumen: wax (*cerumen*) in the ear becomes very thick (*inspissated*).
labyrinthitis: inflammation (*itis*) of the inner ear (*labyrinth*).
mastoiditis: inflammation (*itis*) of the mastoid process of the temporal bone.
meatal atresia: condition in which the normal opening into the ear (*meatal*) is closed (*atresia*).

myringitis: inflammation (*itis*) of the tympanic membrane.
otalgia: pain (*algia*) in the ear (*ot*).
otorrhagia: bursting (*rrhagia*) of blood vessels in the ear (*oto*). Bleeding from the ear.
otorrhea: discharge (*rhea*) of fluid from the ear (*oto*).
otosclerosis: condition (*osis*) in which hard (*scler*) new bone develops around the oval window.
perforated tympanic membrane: condition in which there is a hole (*fora*) through (*per*) the eardrum (*tympanic membrane*). Commonly called *ruptured eardrum.*
preauricular node: presence of a lump (*node*) in front of (*pre*) the ear (*auricular*).
tinnitus: sensation of noises in the ear, including hissing, ringing, buzzing, thumping, whistling, or roaring.
vertigo: sensation of turning (*vert*) while immobile. Also known as *dizziness.*

Diagnosis and Treatment

Analysis of terms related to the diagnosis and treatment of diseases of the ear:

ceruminolytic: substance used to dissolve (*lytic*) earwax (*cerumino*).
mastoidectomy: removal of (*ectomy*) parts of the mastoid process of the temporal bone.
myringoplasty: surgical (*plasty*) procedure done on the tympanic membrane (*myringo*).
myringotomy: cutting into (*otomy*) the tympanic membrane (*myring*).
otoplasty: surgical (*plasty*) procedure done on the external ear.
otoscope: instrument (*scope*) used to look into the ear (*oto*). This instrument is equipped with a speculum. A *speculum* is a cone-shaped attachment used to make it easier to see (*spec*) inside a part by widening its opening.
stapedectomy: removal of (*ectomy*) the third ossicle (*stape*) in the middle ear.

Disorders of the Sense of Hearing

Analysis of terms related to disorders of the sense of hearing:

anacusis: condition (*sis*) in which there is a complete loss (*an*) of hearing (*acu*).
deafness: condition in which a person is unable to hear.
- *total deafness:* person is unable to hear anything.
- *partial deafness:* person is able to hear some selected sounds.
- *progressive deafness:* amount of partial deafness is increasing and may be total eventually.
- *conductive deafness:* loss of hearing (*deafness*) caused by a problem in the transmission (*conduction*) of sound waves through the ear to the cochlea.
- *perceptive deafness:* loss of hearing (*deafness*) that results from a problem in the inner ear, or from nerves involved in the sensation (*percept*) of hearing. This type of deafness is also called *sensory-neural hearing loss.*

hyperacusia: condition (*sis*) in which there is an increase (*hyper*) in the sharpness of the sense of hearing (*acus*).

presbycusis: condition (*sis*) in which there is impaired hearing (*cu,* variation of *acu*) because of old age (*presby*).

Diagnosis of Hearing Loss

Analysis of selected terms related to the diagnosis of hearing loss:

audiometry: test done to measure (*metry*) the ability to hear sounds (*audio*).
- *pure tone audiometry:* type of test to evaluate hearing (*audiometry*) in which an electrical instrument is used to produce clear (*pure*) sounds (*tone*).
- *speech audiometry:* test of hearing done using the spoken word (*speech*).
- *testing of auditory acuity:* test of the sharpness (*acuity*) or the quality of hearing (*auditory*).

air conduction test: hearing test done by the transmission of sound waves through the air to the tympanic membrane and through the middle ear to the cochlea.

bone conduction test: hearing test in which sound waves are transmitted through the mastoid process (*bone*) or other skull bones to the cochlea.

electrocochleography: recording (*ography*) of electrical (*electro*) activity in the cochlea (*cochle*).

PRETEST/ POSTTEST FOR CHAPTER 21

1. The following terms are related to the ear.
   1. A term meaning ear is:
      A. auri.
      B. ot, oto.
      C. both of the above.
   2. The term *acoustic* means:
      A. pertaining to the sense of hearing.
      B. pertaining to the organs of hearing.
      C. both of the above.

2. The following terms are related to the external ear. Match column A with column B.

Column A	Column B
1. _____ helix	A. depression at the opening of the ear
2. _____ concha	B. fleshy prominence at the opening of the ear
	C. the ear lobe

Column A	Column B
3. ____ tragus	D. rim of the ear
4. ____ lobule	

3. Mark the following statements true, *T,* or false, *F:*
   1. ____ Auricle refers to the organ of hearing.
   2. ____ Pinna means the projecting part of the ear.
   3. ____ External auditory meatus is the passageway into the ear.
   4. ____ Cerumen is the organ sometimes covered by hairs.

4. The following terms are related to the middle ear. Match column A with column B. Choose the one best answer.

Column A	Column B
1. ____ tympanic membrane	A. bones of the middle ear
2. ____ myringo	B. also known as the eardrum
3. ____ auditory ossicles	C. root word meaning a trumpetlike tube
4. ____ auditory tube	D. extends from the middle ear to the pharynx
5. ____ salpingo	E. root word meaning tympanic membrane

5. Select the best answer to complete the following statements.
   1. The tympanic cavity is another name for:
      A. the external ear canal.
      B. the middle ear.
      C. the inner ear.
   2. The malleus is the ____ ossicle of the middle ear.
      A. first
      B. second
      C. third
   3. The incus is shaped like a:
      A. hammer.
      B. anvil.
      C. stirrup.
   4. The stapes is attached to the:
      A. inner ear.
      B. tympanic membrane.
      C. both of the above.
   5. A window that opens into the inner ear is:
      A. the oval window.

B. the round window.
C. both of the above.

6. The following terms are related to the inner ear. Use them to complete the statements.

labyrinth	bony labyrinth
vestibule	membranous labyrinth
cochlea	endolymph
semicircular canals	

1. The ________ is (are) the organ of balance or equilibrium.
2. Another name for the inner ear is ________.
3. The organ of hearing is the ________.
4. The ________ is the outside layer of tissue.
5. The ________ is the chamber at the entrance to the inner ear.
6. The ________ is the inside layer of tissue.
7. A name for the fluid in the inner ear is ________.

7. The following statements are related to the sense of sound and balance. Mark the statements true, *T,* or false, *F.*

1. ____ The term *audio* means hearing.
2. ____ Auditory refers to hearing.
3. ____ Equilibrium means a state of equal balance.
4. ____ The semicircular canals are shell-shaped tubes in the inner ear.

8. The following sets of terms are related to diseases of the ear. Match column A with column B. Choose the one best answer

Set 1

Column A	Column B
1. ____ aural barotrauma	A. thickened earwax
2. ____ bilateral otitis media	B. inflammation of the auditory tube
3. ____ endolymphatic hydrops	C. earwax tightly packed in the ear
4. ____ eustachian salpingitis	D. condition in which many furuncles are present
5. ____ external otitis	E. injury to the ear resulting from a change in air pressure
6. ____ furunculosis	F. inflammation of the inner ear
7. ____ impacted cerumen	G. abnormal accumulation of fluid in the labyrinth
	H. middle ear inflammation on both sides

Column A	Column B
8. _____ inspissated cerumen	I. inflammation of the bony process of the temporal bone
9. _____ labyrinthitis	J. inflammation of the external ear
10. _____ mastoiditis	

Set 2

Column A	Column B
1. _____ meatal atresia	A. ruptured eardrum
2. _____ myringitis	B. ringing in the ears
3. _____ otosclerosis	C. dizziness
4. _____ perforated tympanic membrane	D. bleeding from the ear
5. _____ preauricular node	E. presence of a lump in front of the ear
6. _____ tinnitus	F. closure of the normal opening into the ear
7. _____ otalgia	G. inflammation of the tympanic membrane
8. _____ otorrhagia	H. pain in the ear
9. _____ otorrhea	I. condition in which hard new bone develops around the oval window
10. _____ vertigo	J. flow of fluid from the ear

9. The following terms are related to the diagnosis and treatment of diseases of the ear. Match column A with column B. Be specific.

Column A	Column B
1. _____ ceruminolytic	A. removal of part of the bony process of the temporal bone
2. _____ mastoidectomy	B. cutting into the tympanic membrane
3. _____ myringoplasty	C. device used to look into the ear
4. _____ myringotomy	D. surgery on the external ear
5. _____ otoscope	E. substance used to dissolve earwax
6. _____ otoplasty	F. removal of the third ossicle of the middle ear
7. _____ stapedectomy	G. surgical repair of the tympanic membrane

10. The following terms are related to disorders of the sense of hearing. Select the best answer.

1. In _____ the person is unable to hear.
   A. anacusis
   B. total deafness
   C. both of the above

2. In _____ the loss of hearing is caused by a problem in the transmission of sound waves through the ear to the cochlea.
   A. conductive deafness
   B. sensory-neural deafness
   C. both of the above

3. In _____ the loss of hearing results from a problem in the inner ear or nerves involved in hearing.
   A. perceptive deafness
   B. sensory-neural deafness
   C. both of the above

4. An increase in the sharpness of hearing is called _____.
   A. hyperacusia
   B. bone conduction
   C. both of the above

5. Presbycusis is a condition in which there is _____.
   A. bone conduction before air conduction
   B. impaired hearing because of old age
   C. both of the above

11. The following terms are related to the diagnosis of hearing loss. Select the best answer.

1. An air conduction test is a test done by transmitting sound waves:
   A. through the tympanic membrane.
   B. through the middle ear.
   C. both of the above.
2. Electrocochleography is a test done to record the electrical activity:
   A. through the ossicles to the cochlea.
   B. from the cochlea.
   C. both of the above.
3. A bone conduction test is done by transmitting sound waves:
   A. through the bones in the skull.
   B. through the bones in the middle ear.
   C. both of the above.
4. Audiometry is a test that measures:
   A. the ability to hear sound.
   B. the sharpness of hearing.
   C. both of the above.

PRETEST/ POSTTEST **ANSWERS** FOR CHAPTER **21**

1. **1.** C **2.** C

2. **1.** D **2.** A **3.** B **4.** C

3. **1.** F **2.** T **3.** T **4.** F

4. **1.** B **2.** E **3.** A **4.** D **5.** C

5. **1.** B **2.** A **3.** B **4.** A **5.** C

6. **1.** semicircular canals
2. labyrinth
3. cochlea
4. bony labyrinth
5. vestibule
6. membranous labyrinth
7. endolymph

7. **1.** F **2.** T **3.** T **4.** F

8. **Set 1**
1. E **2.** H **3.** G **4.** B **5.** J **6.** D **7.** C **8.** A **9.** F **10.** I

Set 2
1. F **2.** G **3.** I **4.** A **5.** E **6.** B **7.** H **8.** D **9.** J **10.** C

9. **1.** E **2.** A **3.** G **4.** B **5.** C **6.** D **7.** F

10. **1.** C **2.** A **3.** C **4.** A **5.** B

11. **1.** C **2.** B **3.** A **4.** C

22 THINKING AND FEELING

OBJECTIVES

At the end of this chapter you will be able to do the following:

1 Describe factors involved in defining mental health.
2 Define terms related to the following types of mental disorders:
  mental retardation
  organic brain syndrome
  psychoses: the major mental illnesses
  psychoneuroses: the minor mental illnesses
  personality disorders
3 Analyze miscellaneous terms related to mental activity.
4 Analyze selected terms related to defense mechanisms.
5 Analyze selected terms related to the diagnosis and treatment of mental disorders.

MENTAL HEALTH

Each person who is conscious has some level of mental activity. There are degrees of mental health and mental illness. It is difficult, if not impossible, to classify terms descriptive of mental states in one category or another because there is lack of agreement concerning what constitutes mental health and mental illness.

Mental health is a positive condition in which a person's ongoing thinking, feeling, and actions are appropriate to his or her role in life and environment.

The following points may be considered in defining the state of mental health:

1 Attitudes toward self: people with self-esteem, self-respect, and a sense of personal worth have a healthy attitude toward themselves.
2 Self-actualization: the choice of what people plan to do with their abilities and what they (*self*) actually do (*actualization*) in relation to their ability is an important factor in mental health.
3 Integrative capacity: the ability (*capacity*) to tolerate anxiety and frustration and bring together (*integrative*) a balance of mental forces.
4 Autonomous behavior: the actions of people who make their decisions independent (*autonomous*) of outside influence. The ability to refuse to conform, even under social pressure, to an action (*behavior*) that is against personal values.

5 Perception of realities: the ability to have an accurate view (*percept*) of what is happening (*reality*) and to be able to react to what is seen without losing self-control.

6 Mastery of the environment: the ability to adapt, adjust, and behave, or be in control (*mastery*) of the surroundings (*environment*) so that satisfaction is achieved in love, work, play, and interpersonal reactions.

Mental illnesses, or mental disorders, are very complex conditions in which a person demonstrates behavior that is considered to be a deviation from the normal, or different from what is expected. The cause of many mental disorders is unknown.

Terms related to various categories of mental illness are covered in the following groups:

1 mental retardation
2 organic brain syndrome
3 psychoses: the major mental illnesses
4 psychoneuroses: the minor mental illnesses
5 personality disorders

Mental Retardation

Mental retardation involves a slowness or limitation in understanding, emotional development, and intelligence. In the United States, this term is preferred over mental deficiency. There are degrees of retardation. The following terms related to retardation are listed from the least to the most severe degree of retardation.

mild retardation: A mildly retarded person can usually master social and vocational skills and be self-supporting with some guidance.

moderate retardation: A moderately retarded person may be able to do semiskilled work under supervision.

severe retardation: A severely retarded person may be capable of partial self-care under supervision.

profound retardation: A profoundly retarded person may achieve some limited self-care but needs constant help.

Organic Brain Syndrome (OBS)

An organic brain syndrome is a group of signs and symptoms (*syndrome*) that can be related to a physical change in the organic structure of the brain. The physical change may be from chronic alcoholism, aging, intracranial infection, brain trauma, tumors, toxins, degenerative diseases, or conditions of other systems of the body that influence the brain.

Organic brain syndrome is sometimes accompanied by a psychosis. See "Psychoses" later in this chapter.

Selected terms related to organic brain syndrome:

alcoholic dementia: condition (*ia*) in which a person loses (*de*) mental (*ment*) capabilities because of a prolonged use of alcohol.

senile dementia: condition (*ia*) in which old persons (*senile*) lose (*de*) their mental (*ment*) capabilities.

Psychoses: The Major Mental Illnesses

A psychosis is a major or severe condition (*osis*) of the mind (*psycho*). A psychosis may involve loss of contact with reality, bizarre thinking and behavior, delusions, hallucinations, regression, or disorientation.

Selected terms related to psychoses:

involutional melancholia: psychotic state of depression in which the person's feelings turn (*volu*) inward (*in*). The term *melancholia* means dark (*melan*) bile (*cholia*), which in early times was thought to be the cause of the illness. Involution is the process of decline that normally occurs after middle life, and involutional melancholia is a severe depressive mental disorder occurring at this time in life.

manic-depressive illness: a condition characterized by mood swings from excitement (*manic*) to depression.

paranoia: psychotic condition (*ia*) in which the mind (*no,* variation of *nous*) is put aside (*para*). A characteristic of this psychosis is the projection of hostility. Paranoid people fear that others are out to get them.

psychotic depressive reaction: psychotic reaction involving severe depression and loss of contact with reality.

schizophrenia: psychotic condition (*ia*) in which it is said that the mind (*phren*) is split (*schizo*). There may be withdrawal from reality, misinterpretation of reality, and inappropriate actions and moods. Commonly known as "split personality."

Psychoneuroses: The Minor Mental Illnesses

A psychoneurosis is an impairment of personality in which excessive energy is directed to nonproductive activity. A psychoneurosis does not necessarily interfere with a person's contact with reality.

A psychoneurosis is a state of mind (*psycho*) that appears as a nervous (*neur*) condition (*osis*). These states of mind are sometimes referred to as *neuroses.*

Examples of types of psychoneuroses:

anxiety: uneasy feeling caused by the fear of danger or misfortune.

depersonalization: state in which the individual no longer (*de*) perceives the reality of self (*personal*) or surroundings.

depression: state of emotional withdrawal in which an individual feels sadness (*depress*) greater than what might be expected.

hypochondria: an expression of emotional disturbance through the imagining of ills. The term is related to the area under (*hypo*) the ribs (*chondr*) where persons with this neurosis often complain of discomfort. The term is used to describe the state of people who are overly concerned about their health, believing that they are gravely ill when no evidence of disease can be found.

hysteria: psychoneurotic disorder characterized by violent emotional outbreaks. The term is related to the term for uterus (*hyster*) because of an ancient belief that hysteria was observed only in women.

neurasthenia: general weakness (*asthenia*) as a result of nervous (*neur*) exhaustion. Commonly known as a "nervous breakdown."

obsessive-compulsive neurosis: anxiety characterized by a preoccupation (*obsessive*) with a persistent idea accompanied by (*com*) a strong impulse (*puls*) to perform a related act.

phobia: condition (*ia*) in which a fear (*phob*) that has no basis exists. For example, *claustrophobia* is the fear (*phobia*) of confined places (*claustro*), and *phobophobia* is the fear (*phobia*) of fear (*phobo*) itself.

Personality Disorders

Personality is the total of the physical, mental, emotional, and social characteristics of an individual. It is the quality of being a person. A personality disorder is a situation in which an aspect of personality is out of control and dominates the individual's behavior.

Examples of personality disorders:

antisocial behavior: behavior that is usually against (*anti*) or contrary to normal social (*social*) standards. This was formerly referred to as "sociopathic."

asthenic personality: a weak-willed [weak (*asthenic*)] person with low energy levels and difficulty in developing a sense of enjoyment.

cyclothymia: mild form of a manic-depressive state in which there is a cycle (*cyclo*) of feeling (*thym*), such as exhilaration alternating with depression.

explosive behavior: sudden outbursts (*explosive*) of rage with verbal or physical aggressiveness.

hysterical personality: pertaining to (*al*) hysteria (*hysteri*). A mild form of the same condition described in "Psychoneuroses." This personality trait is characterized by attention-seeking behavior, excitability, and emotional instability.

inadequacy: personality disorder in which responses to any form of stress are not (*in*) suitable (*adequate*) to the situation.

obsessive-compulsive personality: mild form of the same condition described in "Psychoneuroses." The personality trait is characterized by a concern for perfection and orderliness.

paranoid personality: condition resembling (*oid*) but not as severe as paranoia (*paran*).

passive-aggressive personality: disorder characterized by first inefficiency and sullenness, and later aggressive and undermining activity, once the person has decided to act.

schizoid personality: character exhibiting behavior that resembles (*oid*), but is not as severe as, schizophrenia (*schiz*).

Sexual deviation

There are certain personality traits that are associated with sexual behavior that may be considered a deviation from normal.

Examples of sexual deviation:

exhibitionism: practice (*ism*) of the showing (*exhibition*) of one's genitals to achieve sexual gratification.
fetishism: practice of (*ism*) using a favorite object (*fetish*) or a part of the body as a psychological stimulus to achieve sexual gratification.
homosexuality: situation in which an individual derives sexual pleasure from being with a person of the same (*homo*) sex. A heterosexual individual derives sexual pleasure from being with a person of the opposite (*hetero*) sex.
incest: sexual relations between closely related family members.
masochism: practice (*ism*) of achieving sexual pleasure by the infliction of suffering, pain, or humiliation. The pain may be imposed on oneself or be inflicted by others. Named for the novelist Sacher Masoch (*masoch*) whose work contained descriptions of the above behavior.
pedophilia: condition (*ia*) in which an adult has sexual desire (*philia*) for a child (*pedo*).
sadism: practice (*ism*) of deriving sexual pleasure from causing physical pain and humiliation. Named for the Marquis de Sade (*sad*) who was involved in this practice.
transsexualism: condition (*ism*) characterized by the desire to be of the opposite (*trans*) sex (*sexual*).
transvestism: practice of (*ism*) wearing the clothing (*vest*) of the opposite (*trans*) sex.
voyeurism: practice of gaining sexual gratification from secretly viewing (*voyeur*) sexual acts or objects.

Drug dependence and drug abuse

Drug dependence and drug abuse are considered personality disorders. A drug-dependent person is unable to face everyday existence without drugs. A drug abuser is a person who uses drugs for a purpose for which the drug was not intended. There are various classifications for addictive drugs.

Examples of types of preparations that may cause psychic (*mental*) and/or physical dependence:

antidepressants: a group of drugs that work against (*anti*) or control depression.
hallucinogens: group of drugs that produce (*gen*) the effect of inducing the experiencing of something that does not exist (*hallucin*).
hypnotics: preparations that have an effect of causing sleep (*hypno*).
psychostimulants: drugs that increase (*stimulant*) awareness of the activity of the mind (*psycho*).
psychotropic drugs: class of preparations that change (*tropic*) the psychological (*psycho*) or mental activity of the individual.

sedatives: preparations that have an ability to calm (*sedate*).
tranquilizers: preparations that produce a feeling of well-being (*tranquil*).

TERMS RELATED TO MENTAL ACTIVITY

Analysis of miscellaneous terms related to mental activity:

addiction: the state (*ion*) of being fixed (*dict*) to (*ad*) or dependent on a particular substance.
ambivalence: mental condition in which a person's feelings are strong (*valence*) in two (*ambi*) opposing directions. Good and bad feelings toward a person or object exist at the same time; for example, love and hate.
amnesia: condition (*ia*) in which there is a lack (*a*) or loss of memory (*mnes*).
anorexia nervosa: condition (*ia*) characterized by a loss (*an*) of the desire to eat (*orex*) caused by a nervous (*nervosa*) reaction.
apathy: lack of (*a*) feeling (*pathy*) or emotion; indifference.
autism: condition (*ism*) of being wholly self-centered (*aut*) in thought and behavior, shut off from other people and animate objects.
autosuggestion: the mental activity of making a suggestion to oneself (*auto*), either consciously or subconsciously, to effect a change in behavior.
consciousness: state of being aware of one's own existence, thoughts, or actions. The act of having, or being with (*con*), knowledge (*sci*) about oneself.
subconsciousness: the state in which activity is carried out below (*sub*) the level of awareness (*conscious*). Actions and mental processes are performed of which the individual is unaware.
unconsciousness: the state of being unaware (*un*) of one's own existence.
déjà vu: illusion of having previously experienced something that has never occurred before.
delirium tremens: state of violent excitement (*delirium*) accompanied by tremors (*tremens*).
delusion: mental condition in which a false, or not (*de*) true, idea is portrayed (*lus*) as true.
dependence: state of needing something for aid or support. The term means to hang (*pend*) from (*de*) something. In drug dependence a person needs a particular drug or combination of drugs to function.
physical drug dependence: in this condition a substance has been used repeatedly to the point where the user's body (*physical*) has become accustomed to its presence. Stopping the drug will cause a physical illness called *withdrawal syndrome.* A withdrawal syndrome is the group of symptoms (*syndrome*) that occurs when a drug is taken away (*withdraw*).
psychic drug dependence: in this condition a substance has been used repeatedly so that the dependent person considers the mental (*psychic*) state it induces as normal.
dipsomania: irresistible craving (*mania*) for an intoxicating drink to satisfy thirst (*dips*).

disorientation: situation in which a person does not (*dis*) realize time, place, or personal identity (*orientation*).
dyslexia: impairment or difficulty (*dys*) with reading words (*lexia*).
egocentric: self-centered [self (*ego*), centered (*centric*)].
empathy: ability to understand another person's feelings because you take the feeling (*pathy*) into (*em*) yourself.
extrovert: an outgoing person, one whose feelings are turned (*vert*) outward (*extro*).
fixation: condition (*ation*) in which an individual's mental development has stopped (*fix*) at an early point in life or at the point at which a severe traumatic event occurred.
hallucination: mental act (*ion*) that occurs while a person is awake, in which something that does not exist except in the wanderings of the mind (*hallucina*) is experienced. *Dreams* are the occurrences of mental images or thought during sleep.
hyperactivity: condition in which an individual has excessive (*hyper*) energy and moves around (*active*) to a great degree.
insomnia: condition (*ia*) in which there is an inability (*in*) to sleep (*somn*).
introvert: description of the mental activity in which feelings are turned (*vert*) inward (*intro*).
kleptomania: irresistible impulse (*mania*) to be a thief (*klepto*) and steal something for the sake of stealing.
malingering: situation in which a person pretends to have bad (*mal*) health and appears to be more or less haggard (*linger*) or worn out.
narcissism: practice (*ism*) in which an individual demonstrates self-love. This condition is named for a mythological character, Narcissus.
negativism: practice (*ism*) by individuals in which there is a tendency to resist command, or to do the opposite (*negative*) of what is requested, or to do nothing (*negative*).
nymphomania: abnormal and uncontrollable (*mania*) sexual desire in women (*nymph*).
perversion: condition in which an individual is said to turn (*vers*) away from (*per*) what is considered to be normal.
psychosomatic illness: an illness of the body (*soma*) that is influenced by the mind (*psycho*).
pyromania: irresistible urge (*mania*) to set things on fire (*pyro*).
somnambulism: practice of (*ism*) walking (*ambul*) during sleep (*somn*).

Defense Mechanisms

In an attempt to deal with anxiety or depression an individual may utilize mental activities called *defense mechanisms.*

A defense mechanism is an unconscious mental process used to seek relief from emotional conflict and anxiety. Following is an analysis of selected terms related to defense mechanisms:

compensation: effort to counterbalance (*compensate*) a deficiency or fault by stressing an attribute or quality.

conversion: the act of (*ion*) changing (*conver*) a mental problem into a physical illness.

denial: pertaining (*al*) to the mechanism of refusing to believe (*deni*) that something stressful exists.

displacement: mental activity of transferring an emotion from (*dis*) one object (*place*) to another.

fantasize: to engage in making up (*ize*) extravagant daydreams (*fantas*).

idealization: mechanism (*ation*) in which a person overestimates the qualities (*ideal*) of another individual.

identification: process (*ion*) by which a person identifies the qualities of another person as his or her own qualities.

introjection: the subconscious process (*tion*) of turning (*ject*) toward (*intro*) oneself the feelings one has for another person.

projection: mental activity of introducing (*jection*) one's own faults or qualities into (*pro*) one's understanding of another person.

rationalization: act of (*tion*) deciding that a behavior is acceptable (*rational*). An attempt to defend or justify unacceptable attitudes, feelings, or behaviors so that they appear rational.

regression: the act (*ion*) of going backward (*regress*) to an earlier level of development. Acting like a child.

repression: mental act of pushing (*press*) back (*re*) into the subconscious a painful idea or memory.

sublimation: the act (*ation*) of diverting energy from pursuit of an immediate goal to achievement of a higher (*sublim*) goal.

substitution: the act (*ation*) of making up for an area of deficiency by concentrating on another (*substitute*) goal that is more easily attainable so as to reduce frustration.

suppression: action (*ion*) of stopping (*suppress*) an impulse, feeling, or painful thought.

Diagnosis and Treatment of Mental Disorders

Analysis of selected terms related to the diagnosis and treatment of mental disorders:

conjoint therapy: treatment (*therapy*) aimed at both (*conjoint*) of two individuals involved in a problem.

crisis-intervention therapy: treatment (*therapy*) aimed at helping an individual to come through (*intervention*) a crisis successfully.

family therapy: form of treatment (*therapy*) involving the whole family.

group therapy: form of treatment (*therapy*) in which several persons (*group*) with problems are involved.

hypnosis: inducing of a sleeplike (*hypn*) condition (*osis*) during which an individual is highly susceptible to suggestions.

milieu therapy: form of treatment (*therapy*) in which an individual's environment (*milieu*) is controlled.

psychoanalysis: systematic review (*analysis*) of the thought (*psycho*) processes of an individual.

psychodrama: form of group therapy in which persons assume and act out (*drama*) roles of suggested characters to better understand their own mental (*psycho*) processes.

psychosurgery: the treatment of mental disorders by using surgical techniques. Example: frontal lobotomy, the cutting into (*otomy*) of the frontal lobe (*lob*) of the brain.

psychotherapy: general term meaning the treatment (*therapy*) of mental (*psycho*) disorders.

psychotropic drugs: preparations (*drugs*) used to change (*tropic*) the mental (*psycho*) reactions of an individual. See the discussion of drug dependence earlier in this chapter.

reality-oriented therapy: treatment (*therapy*) aimed at familiarizing (*orient*) a person with the real (*reality*) world.

shock therapy: form of treatment (*therapy*) in which the individual is shocked (*shock*) with or by chemicals or electrical current.

transactional analysis: method of treatment in which an attempt is made to understand (*analysis*) the interplay (*action*) between (*trans*) individuals.

PRETEST/ POSTTEST FOR CHAPTER 22

1. The following phrases are related to mental health. Match the phrase to the statement.

   A. attitude toward self
   B. self-actualization
   C. integrative capacity
   D. autonomous behavior
   E. perception of reality
   F. mastery of environment

   1. _____ The actions of people who make their own decisions.

   2. _____ Being in control of the surroundings so that satisfaction is achieved.

   3. _____ The ability to tolerate anxiety.

   4. _____ The ability to have an accurate view of what is happening.

   5. _____ Health constitutes self-esteem, self-respect, and a sense of personal worth.

6. _____ What people plan to do with their ability in relation to what they actually do.

2. The following sentences are related to categories of mental illnesses.
   1. In mental retardation there is a slowness in:
      A. understanding and intelligence.
      B. physical growth.
      C. both of the above.
   2. A moderately retarded person:
      A. may be capable of self-care under supervision.
      B. may be able to do semiskilled work under supervision.
      C. both of the above.
   3. Organic brain syndrome:
      A. is caused by physical changes in the brain.
      B. is another name for personality disorder.
      C. both of the above.
   4. Senile dementia:
      A. occurs in old age.
      B. results in loss of mental capabilities.
      C. both of the above.
   5. A psychosis is:
      A. a major mental illness.
      B. a minor mental illness.
      C. both of the above.
   6. A psychoneurosis is:
      A. also known as a neurosis.
      B. a minor mental illness.
      C. both of the above.
   7. A personality disorder is a:
      A. psychotic characteristic.
      B. condition in which one aspect of the personality is out of control.
      C. both of the above.

3. The following terms are related to psychoses. Match column A with column B.

Column A	Column B
1. _____ schizophrenia	A. feelings turned inward in depressed person
2. _____ involutional melancholia	B. split personality
3. _____ manic-depression	C. fear of others' intentions resulting in hostile behavior
4. _____ paranoia	D. severe depression in which the person loses touch with reality
5. _____ psychotic depressive reaction	E. severe mood swings

4. The following terms are related to psychoneuroses. Match column A with column B. Choose the one best answer.

Column A	Column B
1. ____ anxiety	A. emotional outbreak
2. ____ depersonalization	B. uneasy feeling of danger
3. ____ depression	C. illusion of having a serious illness
4. ____ hypochondria	D. fear with no basis for that fear
5. ____ hysteria	E. loss of perception of the reality of self
6. ____ neurasthenia	F. persistent idea with a strong desire to perform and act
7. ____ obsessive-compulsion	G. nervous breakdown
8. ____ phobia	H. emotional withdrawal and sadness

5. The following terms are related to personality disorders. Using the list of terms complete the following statements.

antisocial	inadequate
asthenic	obsessive-compulsive
cyclothymic	paranoid
explosive	passive-aggressive
hysterical	schizoid

1. A condition resembling paranoia is called ____________.
2. A personality trait characterized by attention-seeking behavior and excitability and emotional instability is called ____________.
3. Sudden outbursts of rage are characteristic of an ____________ personality.
4. Behavior that resembles schizophrenia is termed ____________.
5. A person who appears to agree to do a task, yet undermines the completion of the task, is said to have a ____________ personality.
6. A mild form of manic-depressive psychosis is called a ____________ personality disorder.
7. Behavior that is contrary to normal social standards is called ____________ behavior.
8. An ____________ personality does not respond suitably to situations.
9. ____________ personalities are characterized by a concern for perfection and orderliness.
10. A weak-willed person with low energy levels and difficulty developing a sense of enjoyment is said to be ____________.

6. The following terms are related to sexual behavior. Use them to complete the statements that follow.

exhibitionism	pedophilia
fetishism	sadism
homosexuality	transsexualism
incest	transvestism
masochism	voyeurism

1. The practice of achieving sexual pleasure by the infliction of pain or suffering on another person is called ________________.
2. Sexual relations between immediate family members is called ________.
3. ________________ is the practice of gaining sexual pleasure from secretly viewing sexual acts or objects.
4. The practice of wearing the clothing of the opposite sex is called ________.
5. Showing one's genitals to achieve sexual pleasure is called ____________.
6. Gaining sexual pleasure by inflicting pain or suffering on one's own self is called ________________.
7. In ________________ an individual has the desire to be of the opposite sex.
8. The practice of using a favorite object to achieve sexual gratification is termed ________________.
9. ________________ is a condition in which an adult has sexual desire for a child.
10. A condition in which a person derives pleasure from being with a person of the same sex is called ________________.

7. The following terms are related to drugs which may be abused. Match column A with column B. Be specific.

Column A	Column B
1. ____ antidepressant	A. drug that causes sleep
2. ____ hallucinogen	B. class of preparations that change mental activity
3. ____ hypnotic	C. drug that produces feeling of well-being
4. ____ psychostimulant	D. drug that causes the experience of something that does not exist
5. ____ psychotropic	E. preparation that has an ability to calm
6. ____ sedative	F. preparation that increases the activity of the mind
7. ____ tranquilizer	G. preparation used to control depression

8. The following three sets of terms are miscellaneous terms related to mental activity. In each set, match column A with column B. Be specific.

Set 1

Column A	Column B
1. _____ addiction	A. loss of the desire to eat
2. _____ ambivalence	B. self-centered obliviousness to other people or animate objects
3. _____ amnesia	C. state of being dependent on a substance
4. _____ anorexia nervosa	D. illusion of having previously experienced something that has not yet occurred
5. _____ apathy	E. loss of memory
6. _____ autism	F. awareness of one's own existence
7. _____ autosuggestion	G. indifference, lack of feeling
8. _____ consciousness	H. good and bad feelings at the same time toward one thing
9. _____ déjà vu	I. state of violent excitement accompanied by tremors
10. _____ delirium tremens	J. subconsciously suggesting to oneself a change in behavior

Set 2

Column A	Column B
1. _____ delusion	A. ability to understand another's feelings
2. _____ dependence	B. irresistible craving for a drink
3. _____ dipsomania	C. self-centered person
4. _____ disorientation	D. condition in which a person has excessive energy
5. _____ dyslexia	E. false idea portrayed or perceived as true
6. _____ egocentricity	F. difficulty in reading
7. _____ empathy	G. state of needing something for psychic support
8. _____ extroversion	H. wandering of the mind
9. _____ fixation	I. inability to realize time, place, or identity
10. _____ hallucination	J. person whose feelings are turned outward
11. _____ hyperactivity	K. mental development has stopped at a particular point

Set 3

Column A	Column B
1. ____ insomnia	A. irresistible urge to steal
2. ____ introversion	B. uncontrollable sexual desire in women
3. ____ kleptomania	C. inability to sleep
4. ____ malingering	D. self-love
5. ____ narcissism	E. feelings turned inward
6. ____ negativism	F. pretending to have poor health
7. ____ nymphomania	G. general term meaning turning away from normal
8. ____ perversion	H. irresistible urge to start fires
9. ____ pyromania	I. sleep-walking
10. ____ psychosomatic	J. tendency to resist commands by doing the opposite or doing nothing
11. ____ somnambulism	K. illness of the body that is influenced by the mind

9. The following terms are related to defense mechanisms. Use the list to complete the statements.

compensation	fantasize
conversion	idealization
denial	identification
displacement	

1. The act of changing a mental problem into physical illness is called ________.
2. The process by which a person identifies the qualities of another person as his or her own qualities is called ________________.
3. Refusal to believe that something stressful exists is called ______________.
4. The mental activity of transferring an emotion from one object to another is called ________________.
5. The effort to counterbalance a fault by stressing a quality is referred to as ________________.
6. When people have extravagant daydreams, they are said to ______________.
7. The mechanism by which a person overestimates the qualities of another person is referred to as ________________.

10. In the following sentences, terms are related to defense mechanisms.

1. The mental act of pushing an idea back into the subconscious is called:
   A. repression.
   B. regression.
   C. both of the above.
2. Diverting energy from an immediate goal to a higher goal is called:
   A. suppression.
   B. sublimation.
   C. both of the above.
3. The subconscious process of turning toward oneself the feelings one has for another person is called:
   A. introjection.
   B. projection.
   C. both of the above.
4. Determining that one's own unacceptable behavior is acceptable is called:
   A. identification.
   B. rationalization.
   C. both of the above.
5. The mental activity of introducing one's own faults or qualities into one's understanding of another person is called:
   A. projection.
   B. substitution.
   C. both of the above.
6. Stopping an impulse, feeling, or painful thought is referred to as:
   A. conversion.
   B. suppression.
   C. both of the above.
7. Going backward to an earlier level of development is called:
   A. regression.
   B. sublimation.
   C. both of the above.
8. The act of making up for an area of deficiency by concentration on another goal is called:
   A. idealization.
   B. substitution.
   C. both of the above.

11. The following sets of terms are related to the diagnosis and treatment of mental disorders. Use the list of therapies to complete the statements.

Set 1

crisis-intervention therapy	milieu therapy
conjoint therapy	psychotherapy
family therapy	reality-oriented therapy
group therapy	shock therapy

1. The form of treatment in which a person's environment is changed is called ________________.
2. The term that means the treatment of mental disorders is ________________.
3. The treatment aimed at familiarizing a person with the real world is called ________________.
4. Therapy aimed at both individuals involved in a problem is called ________________.
5. Helping a person come through a major emergency is called ________________.
6. The form of treatment involving members of a person's family is called ________________.
7. Inducing a state of shock by electrical current or chemicals is referred to as ________________.
8. The form of treatment dealing with several persons with problems at the same time is called ________________.

Set 2

hypnosis	psychosurgery
psychoanalysis	transactional analysis
psychodrama	

1. The treatment of mental disorders by such techniques as frontal lobotomy is referred to as ________________.
2. The inducement of a sleeplike state during which a person is susceptible to suggestion is called ________________.
3. ________________ is a form of group therapy in which persons act out roles of suggested characters.
4. During ________________ an attempt is made to understand the interplay between individuals.
5. The systematic review of the thought processes of an individual is called ________________.

PRETEST/ POSTTEST **ANSWERS** FOR CHAPTER **22**

1.	**1.** D	**2.** F	**3.** C	**4.** E	**5.** A	**6.** B	
2.	**1.** A	**2.** B	**3.** A	**4.** C	**5.** A	**6.** C	**7.** B
3.	**1.** B	**2.** A	**3.** E	**4.** C	**5.** D		

4. **1.** B **2.** E **3.** H **4.** C **5.** A **6.** G **7.** F **8.** D

5.
1. paranoid
2. hysterical
3. explosive
4. schizoid
5. passive-aggressive
6. cyclothymic
7. antisocial
8. inadequate
9. obsessive-compulsive
10. asthenic

6.
1. sadism
2. incest
3. voyeurism
4. transvestism
5. exhibitionism
6. masochism
7. transsexualism
8. fetishism
9. pedophilia
10. homosexuality

7. **1.** G **2.** D **3.** A **4.** F **5.** B **6.** E **7.** C

8. **Set 1**
1. C **2.** H **3.** E **4.** A **5.** G **6.** B **7.** J **8.** F **9.** D **10.** I

Set 2
1. E **2.** G **3.** B **4.** I **5.** F **6.** C **7.** A **8.** J **9.** K **10.** H **11.** D

Set 3
1. C **2.** E **3.** A **4.** F **5.** D **6.** J **7.** B **8.** G **9.** H **10.** K **11.** I

9.
1. conversion
2. identification
3. denial
4. displacement
5. compensation
6. fantasize
7. idealization

10. **1.** A **2.** B **3.** A **4.** B **5.** A **6.** B **7.** A **8.** B

11. **Set 1**
1. milieu therapy
2. psychotherapy
3. reality-oriented therapy
4. conjoint therapy
5. crisis-intervention therapy
6. family therapy
7. shock therapy
8. group therapy

Set 2
1. psychosurgery
2. hypnosis
3. psychodrama
4. transactional analysis
5. psychoanalysis

GLOSSARY OF MEDICAL SPECIALTIES

allergist: physician who specializes in the diagnosis and treatment of allergies.

anesthesiologist: a physician who specializes in the administration of anesthetics. An *anesthetic* is a drug that takes away (*an*) feeling (*esthetic*).

cardiologist: physician who specializes in the diagnosis and treatment of heart (*cardio*) disease.

cardiovascular surgeon: physician who specializes in operations on the heart (*cardio*) and blood vessels (*vascular*).

chiropodist: person who uses his or her hands (*chiro*) to treat foot (*pod*) ailments.

chiropractor: person who attempts to restore normal function of the body by using (*pract*) his or her hands (*chiro*) to manipulate the structures of the body, especially the spine.

coroner: person, sometimes a physician, whose chief function is to investigate any death that is not clearly attributable to natural causes.

dentist: person who has received a degree and is licensed to practice dentistry. Dentistry involves the diagnosis and treatment of diseases of the teeth and related structures. All branches of dentistry collectively are referred to as *odontology*.

dermatologist: physician who specializes in the diagnosis and treatment of diseases of the skin (*derma*).

endocrinologist: physician who diagnoses and treats diseases of the endocrine system.

endodontist: dentist who specializes in the diagnosis and treatment of diseases of the inside (*endo*) of the tooth (*dont*) including the root canal.

epidemiologist: person who studies (*olog*) diseases that spread from person to person (*epidemi*), or who examines patterns of diseases to find possible causes.

gastroenterologist: physician who specializes in the diagnosis and treatment of diseases of the stomach (*gastro*) and intestinal (*entero*) tract.

general surgeon: physician who operates on organs in the abdominal cavity and many other types of surgery.

geneticist: physician who deals with genetics, or the science of heredity.

gerontologist: person who specializes in the care of the elderly (*geronto*) or in the science of *geriatrics.*

gynecologist: physician who diagnoses and treats diseases of the reproductive systems of nonpregnant females.

hematologist: physician who diagnoses and treats diseases of the blood (*hema*).

histologist: physician who specializes in the microscopic study of tissues.

immunologist: physician who deals with immunity.

internist: physician who specializes in the diagnosis and treatment of conditions of the adult that are treated by nonsurgical means.

nephrologist: physician who diagnoses and treats diseases of the kidney (*nephro*).

neurologist: physician who specializes in the diagnosis and treatment of diseases of nerves and the nervous system.

neurosurgeon: physician who operates on nervous tissue including the brain.

obstetrician: physician who is involved in the care of women in pregnancy, before, during, and after delivery.

oculist: physician who is skilled in the examination and treatment of the eye.

oncologist: physician who diagnoses and treats tumor (*onc*) conditions.

ophthalmologist: physician who diagnoses and treats conditions of the eye (*ophthalm*).

optician: person who makes or sells glasses to improve vision (*opt*) using directions given by an oculist or ophthalmologist.

optometrist: person who measures (*metr*) the focusing power of the eye (*opto*).

oral surgeon: physician who operates on structures of the mouth (*oral*).

orthodontist: doctor of dentistry who specializes in the treatment aimed at straightening (*ortho*) teeth and correcting malocclusions of the jaw.

orthopedic surgeon: physician who operates on the skeletal system.

osteopath: person who practices osteopathy. *Osteopathy* is a treatment based on manipulation of the bones (*osteo*) and skeleton to treat disease (*pathy*).

otorhinolaryngologist: physician who specializes in the diagnosis and treatment of disease of the ear (*oto*), nose (*rhino*), and throat (*larynx*). Sometimes called an *ENT specialist.*

pathologist: person who studies the cause, nature, and course of diseases (*patho*), particularly in the laboratory.

pediatrician: physician who specializes in the diagnosis and treatment of diseases of children (*ped*).

physiatrist: physician who specializes in physical medicine or the diagnosis and treatment of conditions with the aid of physical (*phys*) agents such as heat, cold, and mechanical devices. Primarily deals with diseases that affect the physical movement of the body.

physician: person (*ian*) who is legally qualified to practice medicine (*physic*).

physiologist: person who specializes in the science dealing with the functions of living organisms or their parts.

plastic surgeon: person who operates to treat or restore malformed, injured, or lost parts of the body.

preventive medicine: branch of medicine that deals with the prevention of diseases.

proctologist: physician who specializes in the diagnosis and treatment of conditions of the rectum and anus (*procto*).

psychiatrist: physician who specializes in the diagnosis and treatment of mental (*psych*) diseases.

psychologist: a nonphysician specialist in the science of the mind (*psycho*).

radiologist: physician who uses radioactive (*radio*) substances for examination and treatment and interprets x-ray pictures taken for medical purposes.

rheumatologist: physician who specializes in the diagnosis and treatment of rheumatism, especially diseases of the structures of the joints.

specialist: physician who limits a medical practice to a particular (*special*) branch of medicine, usually having received advanced training and certification to practice by a group of reviewers known as a specialty board.

thoracic surgeon: physician who performs operations on structures in the chest (*thorac*).

urologist: physician who specializes in the diagnosis and treatment of diseases of the urinary (*uri*) system in the male and female and the reproductive system of the male.

GLOSSARY OF PREFIXES AND SUFFIXES

PREFIXES

a-, an-	without, absent
ab-	away from
acro-	extremity, tip
ad-	to, toward
alba-	white
allo-	another, different
ambi-	both
ambly-	dull
amphi-	both, double
ana-	up, back again
andro-	male
angi(o)-	vessel, duct
anis(o)-	unequal
ankyl(o)-	crooked, bent, stiff, fused
ante-, antero-	before
anti-	against
apo-	separation or deviation from
atel-	imperfect
auto-	self
bacter-	bacteria
bi-	two
bi(o)-	life
brachy-	short
brady-	slow
brevis-	short, slow
cac(o)-	bad, ill
cata-	down, through
centi-	100
chloro-	green
chromo-	color
circum-	around
cirrh-	yellow
clin(o)-	sloping toward or away from
co-, com-, con-	with, together
contra-	opposite, against
cry(o)-	cold
crypt(o)-	hidden
cyano-	blue
de-	away, not, down
deca-	10
demi-	one-half
dextr(o)-	right
di-, dis-	twice, doubly
dia-	through, between, completely
dis-	separation
dorso-, dorsi-	back
dys-	difficult, abnormal
e-	out
ecto-	outside, misplaced
endo-	within
epi-	on, upon, over
erythro-	red
eso-	within
eu-	good, normal
eury-	broad, wide
ex-	away from, out completely
extra-	outside of, in addition to, beyond
fore-	before, in front of

gen-	beginning, origin
glyco-, gluco-	sugar, sweet
gyn-, gyneco-	female
haplo-	single, simple
hemi-	half
hetero-	other, different
holo-	whole, all
homeo-	unchanged
homo-	same
hydra-, hydro-	water
hyper-	above, excessive, beyond
hypo-	below, under
idio-	peculiar to the individual, distinct
in-, im-	in, inside, without, not
infra-	below
inter-	between
intra-	within a part
ir-	against, into, toward
iso-	equal, same
juxta-	near
kata-	down, through
lepto-	small, slender, soft
leuko-	white
levo-	left
lute-	yellow
macro-	large
mal-	bad
medi-	middle
mega-	large
melano-	black
meso-	middle
meta-	beyond, over, between, change, next to
micro-	small
milli-	1000
mio-	less, smaller
mono-	one
multi-	many
neo-	new, strange
nigro-	black
noct(i)-	night
non-	not
normo-	normal
null(i)-	none
nyct(o)-	night
ob-	against
olig(o)-	little, small
opisth-	backward
ortho-	straight, erect, normal, correct
oxy-	sharp, acute
pachy-	thick
paleo-	old
pan-	all
para-	beside, beyond
path(o)-	disease, suffering
per-	excessive, through, by means of
peri-	around
phage(o)-	eat, consume
platy-	broad, wide
pleo-	more, many
plic(o)-	fold
plur(i)-	many, more
poikilo-	varied
poly-	many
post-	after
pre-	before
prim-	first
pro-	for, in front of, before
proso-	forward, anterior
prot(o)-	first
pseudo-	false
quadr(i)-	four

re-	back, again
retro-	behind, backward
rube-	red
schisto-, schizo-	split, divided
sclero-	hard
semi-	half
sinistr(o)-	left
steno-	contracted, narrow
stereo-	solid, three-dimensional, firmly established
sub-	beneath
super-	above, excessive, beyond
supra-	above, over
sym-, syn-	together, union
tachy-	fast
tele-	distant, far
telo-	end
terat(o)-	malformed, monster
ter(t)-	third
tetra-	four
therap-	treatment
thermo-	heat, warm
toxic-	poison
trachy-	rough
trans-	across, through, over, beyond
tri-	three
ultra-	above, excessive, beyond
uni-	one
xantho	yellow
xero-	dry

SUFFIXES

-a	*(pl) -ae*
-ac	pertaining to
-acy	that which is, pertaining to
-ad	toward, in the direction of
-agogue	leading, inducing
-agra	severe pain, seizure
-al	pertaining to
-algia	pain
-an	pertaining to, belonging to
-ance	quality or act of
-ar	pertaining to
-ary	related to, pertaining to
-ase	enzyme (chemistry)
-ate	that which is acted upon, salt made from acid (chemistry)
-atresia	abnormal closure
-cele	swelling, tumor, bulging hernia
-centesis	puncture of a cavity
-chezia, -chesia	discharge of a foreign substance
-cide	killer
-cis	cut
-clasis, -clasia	breaking up
-cleisis	closure
-cle, -cule, -culum, -culus	small
-cyst	sac or bladder
-desis	binding, fusion
-dom	state of being
-dynia	pain
-en	*(pl) -ina*
-ectasia, -ectasis	dilation or expansion of
-ectomy	excision, cutting out
-ema	swelling, distention
-ene	unsaturated compound (chemistry)
-et	facet

-ex	*(pl) -ices*
-facient	making or causing to become
-form	structure, shape
-fugal	driving or traveling away from
-ful	full of, characterized by
-gen	production of
-gram, -graphy	act or method of recording diagnostic information
-hood	state, quality of, condition
-ia, -iasis	a diseased condition
-ic	pertaining to
-ician	one charged with or skilled in care of
-id	condition
-ide	binary compound (chemistry)
-ies	*(pl) -ietes*
-ile	pertaining to, having the qualities of
-in, -ine	halogen, alkaloid, or nitrogen base (chemistry)
-ion	act of, state of, result of
-ious	capable of, causing
-is	*(pl) -es, -ides*
-ism	condition, act of, process
-ist	one charged with or skilled in
-itis	inflammation
-ity	quality of, state of
-ium	small
-ive	that which performs or tends toward
-less	without, not capable of
-lysis	setting free, dissolution
-ma	*(pl) -mata*
-malacia	softening
-meter	measure
-ness	quality of, state of
-nx	*(pl) -nges*
-oid	like
-ol	oil (chemistry)
-ole	small
-ology	science of
-olum	small
-olus	small
-oma	tumor
-on	*(pl) -a*
-or	that which, one who
-ory	process of, pertaining to, function of
-ose	having the qualities of, full of carbohydrate (chemistry)
-osis	a diseased condition
-ostomy	creation of a mouth or opening
-otomy	cut into
-ous	pertaining to
-pathy	suffering, disease
-penia	deficiency, lack
-pexy	fixation
-philia	love of
-phobia	fear of
-phylaxis	protection

-plasty	to mold or shape
-poiesis	production, formation of
-ptosis	dropping or downward displacement
-rrhage, -rrhagia	bursting forth
-rrhaphy	closure of by suturing, repair
-rrhea	flow, discharge
-rrhexis	rupture
-s	*(pl) -tes*
-scope, -scopy	looking at, examining
-sect	cut
-ship	state of, quality of
-some	tendency, like
-stasis	at a standstill
-staxis	hemorrhage
-sthenia	strength
-tion	act of, result of, process of
-tome	instrument for cutting
-tonia	stretching, tension
-tripsy	a rubbing, crushing
-trophic	related to nutrition, growth, development
-tropic	turning toward or changing
-u	*(pl) -ua*
-um	*(pl) -a*
-ure	act or result of action
-us	*(pl) -i, -era, -ora*
-vert	turn
-x	*(pl) -ces, -cis*
-y	having the nature or quality of
-yl	radical substance (chemistry)

GLOSSARY OF COMMON ABBREVIATIONS

aa	of each
A/B	acid-base ratio
ABD	abdomen
ac	ante cibum (before meals)
ACTH	adrenocorticotropic hormone
ad lib	as desired
Adm	admission
ADR	adverse drug reaction
Amb	ambulatory
AR	apical rate
ARD	acute respiratory distress
ASD	atrial septal defect
as tol	as tolerated
AV	atrioventricular arteriovenous
bid	bis in die (twice a day)
BP	blood pressure
BR	bed rest
BRP	bathroom privileges
BS	blood sugar
BUN	blood urea nitrogen
C	centigrade (°C)
CA	cancer cardiac arrest
Cath	catheter
CBC	complete blood count
cc	cubic centimeter
CCU	coronary care unit
cg	centigram
CHD	congenital heart disease coronary heart disease congestive heart disease
cm	centimeter
CNS	central nervous system
CPR	cardiopulmonary resuscitation
CSF	cerebrospinal fluid
CVA	cerebrovascular accident costovertebral angle
CVP	central venous pressure
D & C	dilatation and curettage
dim	diminutive
DM	diabetes mellitus
D & S	dilatation and suction
D5W	dextrose 5% in water
Dx	diagnosis
ECG	electrocardiogram
Ecoli	*Escherichia coli*
ED	emergency department
EEG	electroencephalogram
EKG	electrocardiogram
EMG	electromyogram
ENT	ear, nose, and throat
ER	emergency room
fx	fracture
g	gram
GI	gastrointestinal
GU	genitourinary
Hct	hematocrit
Hgb	hemoglobin
HO	house officer
HOB	head of the bed
hs	hour of sleep
Hx	history
hypo	hypodermically

I & O intake and output
ICU intensive care unit
IDDM insulin-dependent diabetes mellitus
IM intramuscular
IPPB intermittent positive-pressure breathing

mEq milliequivalent
MI myocardial infarction
ml milliliter
mm millimeter
Mn midnight

n.b. nota bene (note well)
Ng or ng nasogastric
NIDDM non-insulin-dependent diabetes mellitus
NPO null per os (nothing by mouth)

OD right eye (oculus dexter)
O_2 oxygen
OOB out of bed
OR operating room
os mouth
OS left eye (oculus sinister)
OU both eyes (oculus uterique)
oz ounces

P pulse
pc post cibum (after food; after meals)
PDR *Physicians' Desk Reference*
PEEP positive end-expiratory pressure
PERRLA pupils equal, round, and reactive to light and accommodation
PKU phenylketonuria
po per os (by mouth)
prn pro re nata (as needed; as desired)
qam every morning
qd quaque die (every day)
qh quaque hora (every hour)
q 2 h every 2 hours
qid quater in die (4 times a day)
qod quisque alius dies (every other day)
qs quantum sufficiat (a sufficient quantity)

R respiration
RBC red blood cell, red blood count
RDS respiratory distress syndrome
Rx recipe (take/prescription)

SOAP subjective, objective, assessment, plan
sc sub cutis (subcutaneously)
SOS si opus sit (if necessary)
SR sedimentation rate
stat statim (immediately)
sub l sublingual (under the tongue)

T temperature
T & A tonsillectomy and adenoidectomy
TIA transient ischemic attack
tid ter in die (3 times a day)

ung ointment
URI upper respiratory infection
UTI urinary tract infection

vol % volume percent
VS vital signs (T, P, R, and BP)

WBC white blood cell, white blood count

GLOSSARY OF TERMS RELATED TO AIDS

Terms related to the naming of the disease:

Acquired Immune Deficiency Syndrome (AIDS): acquired defect in the immune system that reduces a person's resistance to certain infections and cancers.

classic AIDS: person infected with the AIDS virus also has an opportunistic infection and actively shows symptoms of the disease.

opportunistic infection: infection by a bacterium, protozoan, or fungus that occurs when the immune system is deficient. The infecting agent is given the opportunity to cause disease because the normal defenses of the body are not able to ward off the disease.

Aids Related Complex (ARC): person infected with the AIDS virus and has symptoms less severe than those of classic AIDS. These symptoms are not related to an opportunistic infection, but are symptoms of many other diseases.

asymptomatic seropositivity: person's blood serum (*sero*) tests positive for the AIDS virus but the person has no symptoms (*asymptomatic*) of the disease.

AIDS dementia complex: subacute encephalitis associated with AIDS in which the person demonstrates memory loss, difficulty in concentrating, social withdrawal, and lethargy. This complex is associated with the sometimes erratic behavior of persons with AIDS.

Terms related to naming of the virus:

human immunodeficiency virus (HIV): the common name for the AIDS virus.

human T-cell lymphotrophic virus, type III (HTLV-III): another name for the AIDS virus.

lymphadenopathy associated virus (LAV): descriptive term related to the AIDS virus because one of the symptoms caused by the AIDS virus is lymphadenopathy.

Examples of "opportunistic" conditions:

cryptococcosis: fungal disease that can be spread to the meninges covering the brain and spinal cord and to the kidney and skin.

cytomegalovirus (CMV): virus that is related to the herpes group and can cause generalized symptoms in the general population but can lead to more severe illness in persons with the AIDS virus.

diffuse, undifferentiated non–Hodgkin lymphoma (DUNHL): lymphoma in which there is lymph enlargement and an enlarged spleen.

Kaposi's sarcoma (KS): cancer of the walls of blood vessels in the skin and in internal organs.

Pneumocystis Carinii Pneumonia (PCP): lung infection caused by a protozoan. The protozoan causes severe and often fatal pneumonia in immune-suppressed persons.

Terms related to transmission of the AIDS virus:

transmission categories: designation of persons with similar behaviors into groups (categories) in which the similar behavior results in spreading (transmission) of the virus from one person to another.

risk groups: categories of persons who are at risk for transmission of the AIDS virus.

heterosexual: person who engages in intercourse exclusively with a person of the opposite sex. This behavior is not considered a risk, unless one of the partners has previously engaged in other behaviors that would put him or her at risk.

blood transfusion: persons who receive blood transfusions are considered to be at risk. The blood currently being used for transfusions is tested for the AIDS virus. Persons who have had transfusions in the past are still considered to be at risk, because it is not known how long the AIDS virus can live in the body without showing symptoms.

homosexual: person who engages in intercourse exclusively with a person of the same sex. The term "gay" is sometimes used to refer to males. A lesbian is a female who practices homosexuality.

receptive anal intercourse: sexual practice in which the penis, or other object, is inserted into the anus of a receptive partner. Because of the thin wall of the anal area, there is danger that the wall will be injured, thus allowing the AIDS virus to enter the bloodstream. Persons who engage in this type of sex are considered an at-risk group.

bisexual: person who engages in intercourse with both sexes.

bidirectional heterosexual transfer: spread of the AIDS virus from opposite sexes. The spread can be in both (*bi*) directions, that is, from male to female, or female to male.

vertical transmission: spread of the AIDS virus from one generation to the next. Vertical refers to the line on a chart from mother to child. This is also known as transplacental transfer.

transplacental transfer: the virus goes through (*trans*) the placenta and is spread (*transfer*) from the mother to the baby.

casual contact: term used to denote any behavior involving contact with another person that does not result in the transfer of blood, semen, or vaginal secretions. Examples are kissing, hugging, or using the same dishes or bathroom facilities. Persons who only have casual contact with others are not an at-risk group.

intravenous drug abuse (IVDA): risk behavior in which a needle is inserted into a vein (*intravenous*) and the blood from the veins is withdrawn into a syringe, mixed with an illegal drug and then pushed back into the vein. This is considered a risk behavior if the syringe and needle may be contaminated by a person with the AIDS virus. This is caused by the practice of needle sharing, which increases the risk.

safe sex: practice of using precautions during any sexual encounter including vaginal, oral, or anal sex. The precaution consists of using a condom to trap the semen and prevent blood or vaginal fluid from spreading from one person to another.

abstinence: practice of avoiding any sexual contact with another person. Contact is limited to casual types of behavior. Abstinence is the *only* practice that ensures complete safety from the AIDS virus.

monogamous: practice of having one (*mono*) marriage partner (*gamous*). In AIDS discussions the word is used to describe the practice of limiting sexual contacts, either heterosexual or homosexual, to one person.

GLOSSARY OF TERMS RELATED TO TRANSPLANTATION

Terms related to transplantations:

transplantation: act of taking an organ or tissue from one place and placing it in another.

graft: common synonym for transplant.

heterotopic: graft in which the organ or tissue is transplanted into a different (*hetero*) place (*topic*) than the normal location.

orthotopic: grafts that are surrounded by the same kind of tissue, or located in the normal (*ortho*) place (*topic*) for that particular tissue or organ.

privileged sites: selection of a location (*site*) for an organ or tissue that protects it from rejection.

segmental grafts: graft in which only a part (*segment*) of an organ is transplanted or grafted. This term usually refers to endocrine gland grafts.

whole organ grafts: grafting or transplanting of whole organs such as the kidney or heart.

multiple organ procurement: effort to retrieve as many organs as possible from a single donor.

Terms denoting types of transplant:

allo-: combining form that means a condition differing from the normal, or referring to another or other.

allotransplantation: transplantation of tissue from one individual into the body of another individual of the same species, but of a different genotype from the donor.

allograft: same as allotransplantation.

allogenic: transplant between a donor and recipient with different genetic characteristics.

autotransplantation: organ transplanted (*transplantation*) from one part of a person's own (*auto*) body to another.

autogenous: another term for transplantation within the individual's own body.

autologous: related to oneself. Similar to autogenous.

cadaver: person who has died, but there has been preservation of either the whole body or specific organs to be used for transplant. Also known as cadaveric transplant.

donor: person furnishing, or giving (donor) the organ or tissue for transplantation.

heterotransplantation: the transplant of tissue or organs from one species to another (hetero). This is an old term that is not frequently used.

host: person who receives transplanted tissue or organs.

recipient: person who receives transplanted tissue or organs. Similar to host.

genotype: term that refers to the type of genetic tissue either the donor or recipient has.

islet autographs: islet cells of the pancreas are harvested and reimplanted into the person's own (*auto*) body.

iso-: a prefix that may refer to an immunity to antigens of tissues of genetically dissimilar individuals of the same species. Isoimmune is an example.

isogeneic: term that means to have the same (*iso*) genetic (*geneic*) structure.

living donor transplantation: living person donates an organ for transplantation to another person. This usually refers to donation of a kidney.

living related transplantation: living person who is donating the tissue or organ is a relative of the recipient.

living unrelated transplantation: living person who is donating the tissue or organ is not a blood relative of the recipient.

syngeneic: term denoting tissues that have identical genotypes such as in identical twins.

xenograft: a graft in which tissue from a different (*xeno*) species is used. An example is porcine (*pig*) skin grafts used in the treatment of burns.

xenotransplantation: another name for allograft.

Terms related to organ selection:

histocompatibility: used to determine tissue (*histo*) match (*compatibility*) between a donor organ and a recipient. The system consists of HLA-A-B and HLA stands for human leukocyte antigen.

immunosuppression: treatment to intentionally reduce (*suppress*) an immune response when foreign tissue, such as transplanted tissue or organ, is placed into a host body.

matching: process of selecting a recipient in whom to transplant a specific organ or tissue. This is done to increase the chance of acceptance of the organ by the recipient's body.

rejection: an immune reaction against transplanted tissue that results in the loss of the tissue.

tissue specific antigen: matching of the donor organ with the host tissue to increase the chance of success.

tissue typing: a process used in the selection of the host for the donor organ. This is also done to increase the chance of acceptance of the organ by the recipient's body.

GLOSSARY OF SYMBOLS

↑	increase, elevated
↓	decrease
∢	angle
>	more than, greater than
<	less (resembles the letter *L* for *l*ess)
°	degree
ʒ	dram (approximately 1 teaspoon)
℥	ounce (30 millimeters (ml), approximately 3 tablespoons)
=	equal
+	positive
−	negative
♀	female
♂	male
c̄	with
s̄	without

BIBLIOGRAPHY

Austrin MG and Austrin HR: Young's learning medical terminology, ed 6, St Louis, 1987, The CV Mosby Co.

Bates B: A guide to physical examination, Philadelphia, 1987, JB Lippincott Co.

Cerili GJ: Organ transplantation and replacement, Philadelphia, 1988, JB Lippincott Co.

Dorland's illustrated medical dictionary, ed 26, Philadelphia, 1985, WB Saunders Co.

Glanze WD: Mosby's medical and nursing dictionary, ed 3, St Louis, 1989, The CV Mosby Co.

Gruendemann BJ and Meeker MH: Alexander's care of the patient in surgery, ed 8, St Louis, 1987, The CV Mosby Co.

Jablonski S: Dictionary of medical acronyms and abbreviations, St Louis, 1987, The CV Mosby Co.

Koop E: Surgeon General's report on AIDS, US Department of Health and Human Services, U.S. Public Health Service, Washington, DC, 1988.

LaFleur MW: Exploring medical language, ed 2, St Louis, 1989, The CV Mosby Co.

Mandell G, Douglas RG, and Bennett J: Principles and practice of infectious diseases, New York, 1985, John Wiley & Sons Inc.

Reeder, S and Leonide M: Maternity nursing, ed 16, Philadelphia, 1987, JB Lippincott Co.

Sabiston D: Textbook of surgery, ed 13, Philadelphia, 1986, WB Saunders Co.

Way L, editor: Current surgical diagnosis and treatment, ed 8, Norwalk, Conn, 1988, Appleton & Lange.

West J: Best and Taylor's physiological basis of medical practice, Baltimore, 1985, Williams & Wilkins.

Wyngaarden J and Smith L, editors: Cecil's textbook of medicine, Philadelphia, 1985, WB Saunders Co.

INDEX

G

H

S